Sports Medicine *and* Rehabilitation

A Sport-Specific Approach

Second Edition

Sports Medicine *and* Rehabilitation

A Sport-Specific Approach

Ralph M. Buschbacher, MD

Professor and Chair
Department of Physical Medicine and Rehabilitation
Indiana University School of Medicine
Indianapolis, Indiana

Nathan D. Prahlow, MD

Assistant Professor of Clinical Physical Medicine and Rehabilitation
Department of Physical Medicine and Rehabilitation
Indiana University School of Medicine
Indianapolis, Indiana

Shashank J. Dave, DO

Assistant Professor of Clinical Physical Medicine and Rehabilitation
Department of Physical Medicine and Rehabilitation
Indiana University School of Medicine
Indianapolis, Indiana

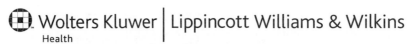

Wolters Kluwer | Lippincott Williams & Wilkins
Health
Philadelphia • Baltimore • New York • London
Buenos Aires • Hong Kong • Sydney • Tokyo

Acquisitions Editor: Robert Hurley
Senior Managing Editor: David Murphy, Jr.
Project Manager: Alicia Jackson
Manufacturing Coordinator: Kathleen Brown
Director of Marketing: Sharon Zinner
Designer: Stephen Druding
Cover Designer: Bess Kiethas
Production Service: International Typesetting and Composition

© 2009 by LIPPINCOTT WILLIAMS & WILKINS, a WOLTERS KLUWER business
530 Walnut Street
Philadelphia, PA 19106 USA
LWW.com

Printed in the USA

Library of Congress Cataloging-in-Publication Data

Sports medicine and rehabilitation : a sport-specific approach /[edited by]
Ralph M. Buschbacher, Shashank Dave, Nathan D. Prahlow. — 2nd ed.
    p. ; cm.
  Includes bibliographical references and index.
  ISBN-13: 978-0-7817-7745-2
  ISBN-10: 0-7817-7745-3
  1. Sports injuries—Patients—Rehabilitation.   2. Sports physical therapy.
I. Buschbacher, Ralph M.   II. Dave, Shashank.   III. Prahlow, Nathan D.
  [DNLM: 1. Athletic Injuries—rehabilitation.   2. Exercise.   3. Sports
Medicine. QT 261 S764965 2009]
  RD97.S747 2009
  617.1'027—dc22

                                                                    2008018515

Care has been taken to confirm the accuracy of the information presented and to describe generally accepted practices. However, the authors, editors, and publisher are not responsible for errors or omissions or for any consequences from application of the information in this book and make no warranty, expressed or implied, with respect to the currency, completeness, or accuracy of the contents of the publication. Application of the information in a particular situation remains the professional responsibility of the practitioner.

The authors, editors, and publisher have exerted every effort to ensure that drug selection and dosage set forth in this text are in accordance with current recommendations and practice at the time of publication. However, in view of ongoing research, changes in government regulations, and the constant flow of information relating to drug therapy and drug reactions, the reader is urged to check the package insert for each drug for any change in indications and dosage and for added warnings and precautions. This is particularly important when the recommended agent is a new or infrequently employed drug.

Some drugs and medical devices presented in the publication have Food and Drug Administration (FDA) clearance for limited use in restricted research settings. It is the responsibility of the health care provider to ascertain the FDA status of each drug or device planned for use in their clinical practice.

To purchase additional copies of this book, call our customer service department at (800) 638-3030 or fax orders to (301) 223-2320. International customers should call (301) 223-2300.

Visit Lippincott Williams & Wilkins on the Internet: at LWW.com. Lippincott Williams & Wilkins customer service representatives are available from 8:30 am to 6 pm, EST.

10 9 8 7 6 5 4 3 2 1

Ralph M. Buschbacher, MD
To Lois, Michael, Peter, John, and Walter

Nathan D. Prahlow, MD
To Julie, Jonathan, Caleb, and Joshua

Shashank J. Dave, DO
This book is dedicated to my residents
and medical students, whose brightness
and curiosity reminds me every day
why I went into medicine

CONTRIBUTORS

Andrea L. Aagesen, DO
Resident Physician
Department of Physical Medicine and Rehabilitation
University of Michigan
Ann Arbor, Michigan

Peter W. Bailey, MD
Resident
Department of Physical Medicine and Rehabilitation
Mayo Clinic
Rochester, Minnesota

Dennis A. Bandemer, Jr., DO
Rehabilitation Physicians PC
Farmingtm Hills, Michigan

Andrea J. Boon, MD
Consultant
Department of Physical Medicine and Rehabilitation
Mayo Clinic
Rochester, Minnesota

Angela T. Carbone, MD
Assistant Professor of Clinical Physical Medicine
    and Rehabilitation
Department of Physical Medicine and Rehabilitation
Indiana University School of Medicine
Indianapolis, Indiana

Chris Carr, PhD, HSPP
Sport and Performance Psychologist
Coordinator, Sport and Performance
    Psychology Program
St. Vincent Sports Performance Center
Indianapolis, Indiana

Gary P. Chimes, MD, PhD
Assistant Professor
University of Arkansas for Medical Sciences
Little Rock, Arkansas

Sara Christensen Holz, MD, PhD
Assistant Professor
Department of Orthopaedics and Rehabilitation
University of Wisconsin
Madison, Wisconsin

Shashank J. Dave, DO
Assistant Professor of Clinical Physical Medicine
    and Rehabilitation
Department of Physical Medicine and Rehabilitation
Indiana University School of Medicine
Indianapolis, Indiana

Jeff Fields, MD
Sports Medicine Fellow
Department of Family Medicine
Indiana University School of Medicine
Indianapolis, Indiana

Meenakshi Garg, MD, MPH
Department of Family Medicine
Indiana University Center
    for Sports Medicine
Indianapolis, Indiana

Nabiha N. Gill, MD
Staff Physician
Richard L. Roudebush VA Medical Center
Indianapolis, IN
Assistant Professor
Department of Physical Medicine
    and Rehabilitation
Indiana University School of Medicine
Indianapolis, Indiana

Elizabeth A. Grossart, MD
Department of Orthopedics and Rehabilitation,
    Physical Medicine Service
Brooke Army Medical Center
Fort Sam Houston, Texas

Patti Hunker, MS, ATC, LAT, CCRC
Methodist Sports Medicine/The Orthopedic
    Specialists
Indianapolis, Indiana

Neeru Jayanthi, MD, USPTA
Assistant Professor
Departments of Family Medicine and Orthopaedic
    Surgery and Rehabilitation
Loyola University Medical Center
Maywood, Illinois

Grant Lloyd Jones, MD
Team Physician
Department of Athletics
Associate Professor
Department of Orthopaedic Surgery
The Ohio State University
    Medical Center
Columbus, Ohio

Michael Khazzam, MD
Department of Orthopaedic Surgery
University of Missouri—Columbia
Columbia, Missouri

Donald C. LeMay, DO
Team Physician
Department of Athletics
The Ohio State University
Division of Sports Medicine
OSU Sports Medicine Center
Ohio State University
Columbus, Ohio

Gerard A. Malanga, MD
Director, Pain Management, Overlook Hospital
Director Physical Medicine and Rehabilitation
Sports and Spine Fellowship, Atlantic Sports Health
Associate Professor, Physical Medicine and Rehabilitation
University of Medicine and Dentistry
    of New Jersey Medical School
Summit, New Jersey

Kevin M. Marberry, MD
Assistant Professor, Orthopaedic Surgery
Assistant Team Physician, University of Missouri
Department of Orthopaedic Surgery
University of Missouri—Columbia
Columbia, Missouri

Anthony Margherita, MD
West County Spine Sports Medicine
Saint Louis, Missouri

Todd C. Miller, MEd, ATC
Head Athletic Trainer
Department of Athletics
Instructor
School of Physical Education
Physical Activities Division
Ohio Wesleyan University
Delaware, Ohio

Johnny G. Owens, MS, PT
Department of Orthopedics and Rehabilitation,
    Physical Medicine Service
Brooke Army Medical Center
Fort Sam Houston, Texas

Jason Peter, DO
Director of Pain Medicine at St. John Macomb Hospital
Center for Physical Medicine and Rehabilitation
Warren, Michigan

Nathan D. Prahlow, MD
Assistant Professor of Clinical Physical Medicine
    and Rehabilitation
Department of Physical Medicine & Rehabilitation
Indiana University School of Medicine
Indianapolis, Indiana

Lance A. Rettig, MD
Volunteer Clinical Assistant Professor of Orthopaedic Surgery
Indiana University School of Medicine
Methodist Sports Medicine/The Orthopaedic Specialists
Indianapolis, Indiana

Mark Ritter, MD
Methodist Sports Medicine/The Orthopaedic
    Specialists
Indianapolis, Indiana

Jess D. Salinas, Jr., MD, FAAPMR
Medical Director
National Pain Institute
Lake Mary, Florida

Peter I. Sallay, MD
Methodist Sports Medicine/The Orthopedic
    Specialists
Indianapolis, Indiana

Dawn Schisler, BS, ATC
Graduate Assistant Athletic Trainer
University of Missouri—Columbia
Columbia, Missouri

Albert Gunjan Singh, MD
Resident Physician
Department of Physical Medicine
    and Rehabilitation
Indiana University School of Medicine
Indianapolis, Indiana

Matthew Smuck, MD
Assistant Professor
Interim Director
University of Michigan Spine Program
Ann Arbor, Michigan

Jay V. Subbarao, MD, MS
Clinical Professor
Department of Orthopaedic Surgery
    and Rehabilitation
Loyola University Medical Center
Maywood, Illinois

John L. Turner, MD, CAQSM
Assistant Professor of Clinical Family Medicine
Department of Family Medicine
Indiana University School of Medicine
Indianapolis, Indiana

Vicki L. Voils, PT
Methodist Occupational Health Center
Indianapolis, Indiana

Julia J. Walker, MS
Indiana University School of Medicine
Indianapolis, Indiana

Eric J. Watson, DO
Resident
Department of Physical Medicine
    and Rehabilitation
Mayo Clinic
Rochester, Minnesota

Sports Medicine is an exciting field. However, the usual approach to a sports medicine text-concentrating on anatomic regions, such as shoulder, elbow, hand, etc., can be a bit dry. Working with athletes who are passionate about their sports, is anything but dry. The purpose of this book is to acquaint or reacquaint the reader with a basic background of individual sports along with the diagnosis and treatment of the most common conditions encountered in those sports. It is our hope that this makes the chapters more interesting and readable. We also hope that it will allow the clinician to speak on the athletes' terms, regarding their sport and their special needs, requirements, and training modifications.

Athletes can be a demanding group. They are dedicated to their sport. They and their coaches often do not wish to change their techniques, cutback in their training schedule, or make any modifications. It is up to the clinician to be able to explain the need for various treatments and interventions, as well as to help the athletes make modifications that will still allow them to maximize their fitness and skill level.

We have assembled an outstanding group of authors for this book; many of them have extensive athletic backgrounds, which has helped them to approach the topic with the athletes' perspective. We hope that readers enjoy this book as much as we have enjoyed putting it together.

Ralph M. Buschbacher, MD
Nathan D. Prahlow, MD
Shahank J. Dave, DO

CONTENTS

Sports Medicine *and* Rehabilitation

A Sport-Specific Approach

Second Edition

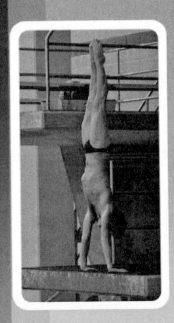

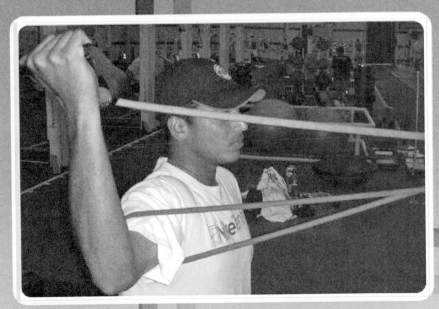

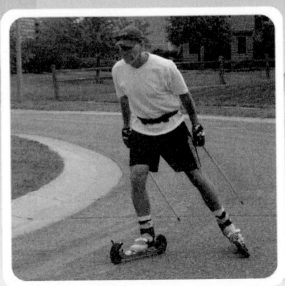

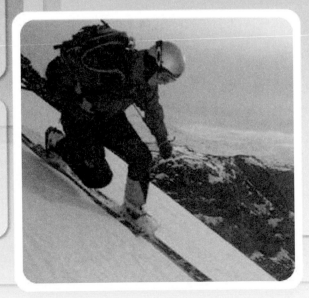

Preparticipation Physical Evaluation

T he preparticipation physical evaluation (PPE) is a well-known but poorly understood intervention with great psychological impact but often limited ability to accomplish its intended goals. Recent work has begun to codify and standardize the PPE to a greater extent, but there is still debate about the most appropriate content and application of athletic screening principles. In general, preparticipation screening is defined as the "systematic practice of medically evaluating large, general populations of athletes before participation in sports for the purpose of identifying (or raising suspicion of) abnormalities that could provoke disease progression or sudden death."[1] Despite general medical and lay support, the PPE is in transition both in its application and the evidence to support its use.

For many years athletes have undergone annual examination for clearance to compete in sports with three *primary goals:*

1. To identify life-threatening or disabling diseases and conditions.
2. To identify diseases or conditions that may put that athlete at increased risk for injury.
3. To ensure the participant, physician, and organization meet institutional, association, or governmental requirements.

Recently, the PPE has been recognized for its potential to improve the health of athletes by meeting other *secondary goals:*

1. To determine the general health of athletes.
2. To serve as an entry point for adolescents into the health care system.
3. To provide opportunity for discussion on health and lifestyle.[2]

New evidence and understanding about the real risk of athletic participation, combined with a refined understanding of how to truly identify those at risk, will hopefully lead to the most appropriate screening of our athletes. Ideally, the PPE should serve as a timely and effective method to minimize the dangers of sports while enhancing the overall health of the athletic population.

PREPARTICIPATION PHYSICAL EVALUATION PROCESS

The majority of PPEs are performed on competitive athletes. A competitive athlete is defined as "one who participates in an organized team or individual sport that requires systematic training and regular competition against others."[1] However, with a more active, aging population and recent focus on exercise as a lifestyle, there are growing numbers of participants who need evaluation but are not engaged in any formal competitive sport. Most PPEs are accomplished through one of two scenarios: (i) mass examination of athlete cohorts by physicians (often) associated with supervising organizations, or (ii) examination by the athlete's personal physician with provision of appropriate documentation to the necessary organization. There is debate over the needed qualifications for providers of the PPE, and guidelines often vary significantly by state. Since 1997, there has been a 64% increase in the states that allow nonphysicians to perform athletic screening. Eighteen states currently permit chiropractors or naturopathic practitioners to evaluate athletes.[1] The third PPE monograph[2] recommends a licensed medical doctor (MD) or doctor of osteopathy (DO) because this allows the provider to manage the broad range of problems potentially encountered during the PPE. Whichever practitioner performs the PPE, it is critical that all three primary objectives be met and needed follow-up testing or treatment be coordinated.

The various testing scenarios each have benefits and drawbacks. Often, mass PPE events or coordinated teams of examiners provide efficient and systematic screening to large numbers of athletes. Ideally, these events are organized to allow for involvement of specialists for particular evaluation components. Unfortunately, the impersonal approach can prevent athletes from disclosing delicate information, or may lead to disconnected evaluations unless communication is robust. When utilizing mass screening there must be a final review of all gathered information by a trained physician.

Younger athletes often have no contact with the health care system outside of an annual PPE, which places much importance on this interaction. Ideally, each person is seen by a personal physician who knows the athlete and can place new symptoms or findings into the context of existing problems. Established trust with a physician promotes honest conversations about delicate issues including drug and alcohol use, birth control, and sexual habits. When problems do arise, the primary physician is more likely to have the necessary medical records and may be in a position to communicate more effectively with parents or guardians. Ethical concerns over whose needs are being served first by the physician (institutional, organization, or team needs versus the individual athlete's needs) are minimized through the use of established physician relationships.

There are no universally accepted standards or practices for screening athletes at the high school or collegiate level. Clearance routinely consists of a medical history, family history, and physical examination, but the content of each component varies greatly. A review of state guidelines found that 81% of states have adequate questionnaires, up from 60% in 1997.[1] High schools rely heavily on individual physicians who complete clearance forms, as well as mass screenings delivered by volunteer practitioners with variable comfort and competence with the required evaluations. Most PPEs at this level occur just before the sport season and often do not leave time for further testing or management of identified problems before competition begins. Due to the large cohort of high school athletes (estimated at 5 to 6 million), logistic impediments are considerable.

The National Collegiate Athletic Association (NCAA) mandates preparticipation evaluation for all Division I, II, and III athletes before the first practice or competition. These athletes are routinely cleared through an organized examination led by a team physician (often formally associated with the institution) with the support of athletic trainers and on-campus health centers. Collegiate evaluations occur with more lead time and typically afford the opportunity to address any concerns. A review of collegiate evaluation forms found that 75% adequately address national recommendations.[3]

History and Physical Examination

Although there is some data on cardiac clearance, there is little evidence that particular components of the remainder of the PPE have the sensitivity or specificity to identify athletes at risk for significant injury or death. With those limitations in mind, the PPE in its entirety is still thought to be the best screening tool available, and its overall effectiveness depends upon systematic questioning and a focused physical examination. The third PPE monograph recommends a number of questions for the historical portion of the examination.[6] This PPE is designed to be applicable for many settings and competitive levels, while providing efficient and practical recommendations that are likely to identify athletes at risk.

Where possible, the history questions have been drawn from the Youth Risk Behavior Surveillance System, which has been validated in similar applications.[4] The minimalist will limit the scope of a PPE to a cardiovascular and musculoskeletal evaluation; however, the use of the PPE in a broader context of systematic health care for youth and young adults is becoming more widespread. Medical history-taking focuses on known health problems, medications and supplements, allergies, and surgical history. Review of personal history for heat illness, neurologic symptoms, cardiovascular symptoms, musculoskeletal symptoms, and symptoms of asthma is also included. Questions about menstrual patterns and nutrition are becoming more important, especially in those female athletes at risk for female athletic triad (impaired eating, dysmenorrhea, osteoporosis). Immunization history is critical in light of the more common contagious diseases seen in young populations such as meningococcus and hepatitis. Sexual history is important, but truthful answers are not anticipated on most written questionnaires or mass screening encounters.

The components of the physical exam may vary by application and athletic group being screened, but the third PPE monograph guidelines establish a standard that serves to direct most practitioners. Table 1-1

TABLE 1-1	Components of the Prepariticipation Physical Examination

Physical characteristics: Height, weight, % body fat
Vital signs: Heart rate, blood pressure (may include multiple readings)
General appearance
Eyes: Visual acuity, differences in pupil size
Ears: Hearing
Nose
Throat/oral cavity
Lungs
Cardiovascular system: Cardiac auscultation, radial and femoral pulses
Abdomen: Masses, tenderness, organomegaly
Genitalia (males only)
Skin: Rashes, lesions
Musculoskeletal system: Often low-yield, but can include range of motion, strength, stability, and symmetry of the neck, shoulder, arm, elbow, forearm, wrist, hand, fingers, back, hip, thigh, knee, leg, ankle, foot, and toes

Adapted from Prepariticipation Physical Evaluation Task Force. *Prepariticipation Physical Evaluation.* 3rd ed. Minneapolis: McGraw-Hill/The Physician and Sports Medicine; 2005.

lists the recommended examination. A comprehensive examination such as this does not have outcome data to support its use; nevertheless, there is generally wide acceptance of this more-than-minimal physical examination.

Height, weight, and calculation of body mass index (BMI) will help determine those in need of nutritional counseling or adaptation. Obesity is a growing concern among youth in the United States and a predictor of many chronic diseases that impact our population. Early identification allows for diet and exercise modification and incorporation of healthier habits. Obesity is a particularly ominous predictor of future health, as obese white males between the ages of 20 and 30 years live on average 13 fewer years, and obese black males lose around 20 years of life expectancy. Obese white females on average live 8 years less while obese black females lose 5 years of life expectancy.[5]

Blood pressure readings are crucial for identification of prehypertensive and hypertensive states. Both the short-term risks of participation and the long-term health outcomes are impacted by elevated blood pressure. Care should be taken to identify hypertension based on established norms in children and

adolescents; these values are now based on gender, age, and height.[6] HEENT (head, eyes, ears, nose, and throat) examination is for the general health of these areas, with particular attention paid to visual acuity and pupil reactivity and size, so that testing after any injury is comparable to a known baseline.

The cardiovascular examination includes auscultation for murmurs that may reflect underlying pathology that increases risk for sudden death or that may limit the exercise capacity of an athlete (Table 1-2). Detection of murmurs is most critical, and care should be taken to provide a quiet environment for auscultation. Often the clinician must distinguish between innocent flow murmurs and murmurs that require further testing.

The yield of any type of musculoskeletal examination is low in asymptomatic athletes with no history of injury. In fact, the history alone has been shown to detect 92% of significant musculoskeletal injuries.[7] Despite the poor evidence of disease detection, it is still standard to perform a thorough musculoskeletal examination on athletes before clearance for competition. Brief, repeat examination for returning players can suffice if an updated history suggests no interval injury.

The PPE: Practical Application

Taking the scientific evidence and combining it with traditional practices that are now informed by established guidelines, one is still left with room for significant disagreement on what constitutes the best PPE. Screening recommendations must take into account not only the scientific evidence to support each evaluation strategy, but the practical consideration of adopting expensive or resource-intensive methods. Many athletes and organizations cannot sustain more than is included in the current recommendations. Even with recent advances in the science and use of PPEs, a 2003 review of published articles on the PPE concluded that "the PPE for athletes does not satisfy the basic requirements for medical screening."[8]

A Closer Look: Can the PPE Reduce Cardiac Risk?

The sudden death of an athlete is one of the most devastating and publicized events in sports. Athletes are held in high regard and represent the healthiest and fittest of our population, and as such, the death of an athlete is not an expected event. However,

TABLE 1-2	American Heart Association Recommendations for Participation Cardiovascular Screening of Competitive Athletes

Medical history*

Personal history

1. Exertional chest pain/discomfort
2. Unexplained syncope/near-syncope[†]
3. Excessive exertional and unexplained dyspnea/fatigue, associated with exercise
4. Prior recognition of a heart murmur
5. Elevated systemic blood pressure

Family history

6. Premature death (sudden and unexpected, or otherwise) before age 50 years due to heart disease, in ≥1 relative
7. Disability from heart disease in a close relative < 50 years of age
8. Specific knowledge of certain cardiac conditions in family members: hypertrophic or dilated cardiomyopathy, long-QT syndrome or other ion channelopathies, Marfan syndrome, or clinically important arrhythmias

Physical examination

9. Heart murmur[‡]
10. Femoral pulses to exclude aortic coarctation
11. Physical stigmata of Marfan syndrome
12. Brachial artery blood pressure (sitting position)[§]

*Parental verification is recommended for high school and middle school athletes.
[†]Judged not to be neurocardiogenic (vasovagal); of particular concern when related to exertion.
[‡]Auscultation should be performed in both supine and standing positions (or with Valsalva maneuver), specifically to identify murmurs of dynamic left ventricular outflow tract obstruction.
[§]Preferably taken in both arms.[37]
From Maron BJ, Thompson PD, Ackerman MJ, et al. Recommendations and considerations related to preparticipation screening for cardiovascular abnormalities in competitive athletes: 2007 update. *Circulation.* 2007;115:1646.

underlying cardiac diseases are often silent and may be difficult to detect, yet the public often believes that such detection is always possible. Despite the judicious use of modern technology, there will always be sudden cardiac death among athletes, because certain predisposing conditions are not detectable. The role of the physician, therefore, is to minimize that risk while staying within the constraints of a health care system with limited resources.

Sudden death is rare and occurs between 1 in 100,000 to 1 in 300,000 high school athletes, with only 20% of lesions being detectable before death.[9,10] In competitors 35 years and younger in the United States, fatal arrhythmias resulting from underlying structural abnormalities account for 95% of all sudden deaths; 36% of deaths are also associated with hypertrophic cardiomyopathy, and 13% with anomalous coronary arteries.[11,12] Italian screening programs have found approximately 25% of athletic sudden death is attributable to arrhythmogenic right

ventricular cardiomyopathy.[13,14] Figure 1-1 reviews the common causes of sudden cardiac death. In athletes over the age of 40, undetected atherosclerotic disease is the leading cause of sudden death.[15,16]

Medical evaluations aim to detect these structural or functional abnormalities and make appropriate clinical decisions on clearance for competition. The most commonly used testing methods include a thorough history and physical examination, 12-lead electrocardiogram, and screening echocardiogram. Application of each method varies significantly by age of athlete, level of competition (recreational, school related, elite travel team, professional, etc.), organizational level (community youth sports, high school, NCAA divisions, professional, etc.), and the available resources. Many professional sports use a comprehensive testing program including cardiac stress testing, echocardiography, and a panel of blood tests to detect any possible abnormality. To apply that type of full testing would be cost-prohibitive in the

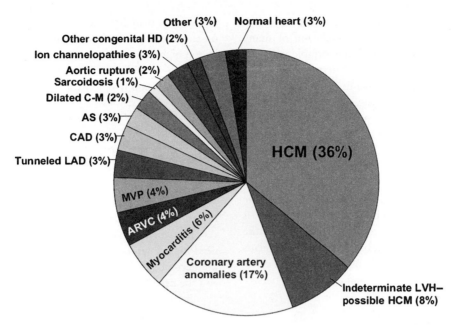

FIGURE 1-1 Cardiovascular causes of sudden death. (HCM indicates hypertrophic cardiomy-opathy; LVH, left ventricular hypertrophy; ARVC, arrhythmogenic right ventricular cardiomy-opathy; MVP, mitral valve prolapse; LAD, left anterior descending; CAD, coronary artery disease; AS, aortic stenosis; C-M, cardiomyopathy; and HD, heart disease.) (From Maron BJ, Thompson PD, Ackerman MJ, et al. Recommendations and considerations related to preparticipation screening for cardiovascular abnormalities in competitive athletes: 2007 update. *Circulation.* 2007;115:1645.)

general athletic population, and evidence is lacking that shows it superior to more standard approaches.

Electocardiogram

The 12-lead electrocardiogram (EKG) has been proposed for PPE screening by many groups and has been the subject of conflicting evidence. More favored by European and international groups, it has met resistance in the United States due to lack of clear outcome evidence as well as very poor cost-benefit ratios. In a study of more than 1,700 U.S. military recruits, abnormal EKGs were found in 34% of healthy soldiers, but only 7 of these findings changed the management plan and only 2 individuals had potentially dangerous cardiac disease.[17] In another study of more than 1,000 athletes, EKGs were compared to echocardiograms for identification of significant underlying cardiac disease. The sensitivity of EKGs was only 50% and positive predictive accuracy was only 7%.[18] By modeling conservative estimates of cost to provide EKG screening to competitive U.S. athletes at all

levels and utilizing the known incidence of detectable disease, one can calculate the cost to prevent a single sudden cardiac death. One study estimates a $3.4 million cost for each life saved, although others have less costly estimates.[1]

In contrast to these models, there is actual data outcome from the Italian screening program. In 1982, Italy began a nationwide screening program mandated by law that requires a 12-lead EKG as part of the PPE for all participants in competitive sports. The results of that program show the incidence of sudden cardiovascular death in athletes has substantially declined, while the incidence in the general population has remained steady. Moreover, the reduction was predominantly due to a lower incidence of death from detectable cardiovascular abnormalities and an increase in identification of athletes with cardiomyopathies.[19]

This mix of speculation and study data factors into the ongoing debate over the routine use of EKGs for PPE. Mandated EKG testing could result in false-positive tests that promote unnecessary additional testing and fear, or false-negative tests that miss disease. There is the potential for exclusion of many providers who would not feel comfortable with the increased responsibility of EKG interpretation. Cost and accessibility would continue to be major concerns, but even in the long-standing and robust Italian PPE structure there are estimates that up to 50% of eligible athletes do not undergo EKG testing as mandated by law.[20] Currently, 92% of North American professional athletic teams utilize EKG testing to routinely screen their athletes, and these percentages drop as one moves down the competitive structure toward high school, where EKG use is extremely rare.[21] Perhaps future research will end the debate in the United States, but until then physicians must weigh the real and psychological benefits against resource expenditure and practical barriers.

Echocardiogram

Many common causes of sudden cardiac death are anatomic and therefore theoretically detectable by echocardiography. Conditions such as hypertrophic cardiomyopathy, mitral valve prolapse, aortic stenosis, and Marfanoid aortic abnormalities can be detected in many cases; however, distinguishing them from normal adaptations seen in the athletic heart can be challenging. On the other hand, several high-risk cardiac conditions, such as anomalous coronary arteries and cardiac muscle ion channel dysfunction, cannot be detected even with sophisticated echocardiography. In one series of more than 5,000 athletes screened with echocardiography, no cases of hypertrophic cardiomyopathy or other life-threatening conditions were identified.[22] Costs are high and data supporting the use of screening echocardiography are limited, so even at elite levels only 13% of North American professional teams use echocardiography for preparticipation evaluation.[21] The echocardiogram should be reserved for workup of other suspicious findings from the history or physical examination.

Exercise Stress Testing

Stress testing of asymptomatic individuals older than 35 years has been considered as a screening measure, but supporting evidence is lacking. A cohort of more than 3,600 patients with risk factors for coronary artery disease was evaluated using exercise stress EKGs.[23] Of the 62 who subsequently had a cardiac

event, fewer than 20% had any detectable abnormality on stress testing. The false-negative rate is thought to be too high for exercise stress testing to be practical as a screening modality. Exercise stress testing is typically reserved for use in symptomatic athletes with risk factors for cardiac disease.

CURRENT PRACTICES—WHAT SHOULD CHANGE?

When comparing primary care sports medicine practitioners to cardiologists, there has been shown to be very little interobserver agreement as to which athletes need further cardiac testing.[24] This brings to question the accuracy of standard preparticipation evaluation and the need for enhanced testing strategies.

Because cardiac pathology is the most concerning athletic risk, it makes sense to focus the majority of effort on detection and further evaluation of these conditions to best determine safety and clearance issues. The 36th Bethesda Conference guidelines and the American Heart Association (AHA) recommendations offer the most concise and current recommendations for cardiac screening, diagnostic testing, and clearance guidelines.[1,25] Consensus is building in Europe to routinely apply 12-lead EKG testing as a component of the PPE. The AHA has stated that "on humanitarian medical grounds it supports any public health initiative to identify adverse cardiac abnormalities" but that it cannot ignore the "many epidemiological, social, economic, and other issues that impact screening." The International Olympic Committee and the European Society of Cardiology have both made recommendations for screening all athletes with 12-lead EKGs, but the 2007 AHA and third PPE monograph recommendations do not include EKGs as part of standard screening protocols.[26,27]

MEDICAL–LEGAL CONSIDERATIONS

No uniform laws exist in the United States that describe, direct, or mandate the legal duties of preparticipation screening. Unlike Italian law, which details the content of cardiovascular screening and holds physicians criminally negligent for improper clearance of at-risk athletes, U.S. lawmakers have left PPE in the hands of physicians.[1] Laws vary by state, but generally require physicians to practice established standards and use reasonable care in preparticipation evaluation.

The law recognizes that physicians are in the best position to make judgments about the proper screening and examination methods as well as the standards that must be met. Physicians who use published guidelines such as the third PPE monograph or the 2007 American Heart Association Guidelines will generally be protected from claims of malpractice.[1] Physicians who volunteer for mass PPE screenings need to consider their state's Good Samaritan laws, as those vary greatly by location and many malpractice policies do not cover care delivered in a pro bono setting.

An equally important legal consideration is the rights of athletes who have been found to have a high-risk condition and are not medically cleared for competition. In these situations, the physician must document complete disclosure of the risk to athletes (and parents, if the athlete is under the age of 18). Unfortunately, there are cases in which the athlete has refused to comply, and may even pressure the physician to give approval. Federal enactments such as the 1973 Rehabilitation Act and the 1990 Americans with Disabilities Act protect individuals, and the U.S. courts have at times upheld an athlete's right to participate even without medical clearance. Athletes and parents may wish to sign exculpatory waivers or risk-release documents that absolve both the physician and the sponsor from legal ramification should a significant injury or death result from participation. It is advised that legal representation for both the physician and the sponsoring institution be involved in these cases to ensure suitable outcomes for all. The validity of such waivers and the legal protection they offer varies from state to state.

A final legal consideration is the protection of privacy for the individual's medical and health information. The 1996 Health Insurance Portability and Accountability Act (HIPAA), as well as the 1974 Family Education Rights and Privacy Act (FERPA), serve as federal guidelines for the appropriate sharing of an athlete's medical information. Protected health information is that which "identifies an athlete relating to past, present, or future physical or mental health conditions" and is protected from disclosure without the individuals' expressed consent. The HIPAA standards allow for the release of medical information without an individual's permission for treatment, consultation, referral, or notification of family. The decision for clearance is protected under these guidelines and may be shared with appropriate staff or administrators.[2] However, the medical facts leading to the decision remain confidential and may not be shared.

CONCLUSION

The goals of prepartipation physical evaluation must be continually referenced to maintain proper perspective and to protect athletes from reasonably preventable harm. Recommendations for cardiac screening vary among experts, and the evidence offers no conclusive answer as to what must be included; evidence for other portions of the examination is extremely limited. Practical considerations in the entire process are paramount, as the number of individuals needing clearance each year in the United States alone is staggering. Public health concerns, along with reduction of risk in each individual, must be balanced against available resources and the acceptable levels of danger inherent in exercise and sport. Rigorous use of the published guidelines is currently the best method to achieve the stated goals of the PPE and to ensure the safest possible conditions for athletic competition. Future research is needed to further clarify the need for various examination component and screening methods.

REFERENCES

1. Maron BJ, Thompson PD, Ackerman MJ, et al. Recommendations and considerations related to prepartipation screening for cardiovascular abnormalities in competitive athletes: 2007 update. *Circulation.* 2007;115:1643–1655.
2. Prepartipation Physical Evaluation Task Force. *Prepartipation Physical Evaluation.* 3rd ed. Minneapolis: McGraw-Hill/The Physician and Sports Medicine; 2005.
3. Pfister GC, Puffer JC, Maron BJ. Prepartipation cardiovascular screening for U.S. collegiate student-athletes. *JAMA.* 2000;283:1597–1599.
4. Grunbaum JA, Kann L, Kinchen SA, et al. Youth risks behavior surveillance—United States, 2001. *MMWR.* 2002;51:1–62.
5. Fontaine KR, Redden DT, Wang C, et al. Years of life lost due to obesity. *JAMA.* 2003;289:187–193.
6. High Blood Pressure in Children. Available at: http://www.americanheart.org/presenter.jhtml?identifier=2130. Accessed December 2, 2007.
7. Gomez JE, Landry GL, Bernhardt DT. Critical evaluation of the 2-minute orthopedic screening examination. *Am J Dis Child.* 1993;147:1109–1113.
8. Carek PJ, Mainous A III. The prepartipation physical examination for athletics: a systematic review of current recommendations. *BMJ.* 2003;327:E170–E173.
9. Maron BJ, Shirani J, Poliac LC, et al. Sudden death in young competitive athletes: clinical, demographic, and pathologic profiles. *JAMA.* 1996;276:199–204.
10. Van Camp SP, Bloor CM, Mueller FO, et al. Nontraumatic sports deaths in high school and college athletes. *Med Sci Sports Exerc.* 1995;27:641–647.

11. Liberthson R. Sudden death from cardiac causes in children and young adults. *N Engl J Med*. 1996;334:1039–1044.

12. Maron BJ. Risk profiles and cardiovascular preparticipation screening of competitive athletes. *Cardiol Clin*. 1997;15:473–483.

13. Corrado D, Thiene G, Nava A, et al. Sudden death in young competitive athletes: clinic-pathologic correlations in 22 cases. *Am J Med*. 1990;9:588–596.

14. Corrado D, Basso C, Thiene G. Essay: sudden death in young athletes. *Lancet*. 2005;366:S47–S48.

15. Maron BJ, Epstein SE, Roberts WC. Causes of sudden death in competitive athletes. *J Am Coll Cardiol*. 1986;7: 204–214.

16. Roberts WO, Maron BJ. Evidence for decreasing occurrence of sudden cardiac death associated with the marathon. *J Am Coll Cardiol*. 2005;46:1373–1374.

17. Lesho E, Gey D, Forrester G, et al. The low impact of screening electrocardiograms in healthy individuals: a prospective study and review of the literature. *Mil Med*. 2003;168:15–18.

18. Pelliccia A, Maron BJ, Culasso F, et al. Clinical significance of abnormal electrocardiographic patterns in trained athletes. *Circulation*. 2000;102:278–284.

19. Corrado D, Basso C, Pavei A. Trends in sudden cardiovascular death in young competitive athletes after implementation of a preparticipation screening program. *JAMA*. 2006;296:1593–1601.

20. Pelliccia A, Maron BJ. Preparticipation cardiovascular evaluation of the competitive athlete: perspectives from the 30-year Italian experience. *Am J Cardiol*. 1995;75:827–829.

21. Harris KM, Sponsel A, Hutter AM Jr., et al. Brief communication: cardiovascular screening practices of major North American professional sports teams. *Ann Intern Med*. 2006;145:507–511.

22. Katcher MS, Maron BJ, Homoud MK. Risk profiling and screening strategies. In: Sudden cardiac death in the athlete. Estes NAM, Deeb NS, Wang PJ, eds. *Sudden Cardiac Death in the Athlete*. Armonk, NY: Futura Publishing; 1998.

23. Siscovick DS, Ekelund LG, Hyde JS, et al. Sensitivity of exercise electrocardiography for acute cardiac events during moderate and strenuous physical activity (the lipid research clinics coronary primary prevention trial). *Arch Intern Med*. 1991;151:325–330.

24. O'Connor FG, Johnson JD, Chapin M, et al. A pilot study of clinical agreement in cardiovascular preparticipation examinations: how good is the standard of care? *Clin J Sport Med*. 2005;15:177–179.

25. Maron BJ, Douglas PS, Graham TP, et al. Task force 1: preparticipation screening and diagnosis of cardiovascular disease in athletes. *J Am Coll Cardiol*. 2005;45:1322–1326.

26. Bille K, Brenner JI, Kappenberger L, et al. Sudden deaths in athletes: the basics of the Lausanne Recommendations of the International Olympic Committee. *Circulation*. 2005;112(suppl II):830.

27. Corrado D, Pelliccia A, Bjornstad HH, et al. Cardiovascular pre-participation screening of young competitive athletes for prevention of sudden death: proposal for a common European protocol: consensus statement of the Study Group of Sport Cardiology of the Working Group of Cardiac Rehabilitation and Exercise Physiology and the Working Group of Myocardial and Pericardial Diseases of the European Society of Cardiology. *Eur Heart J*. 2005;26:516–524.

Sport Psychology: Psychological Concepts and Interventions

T he field of sport and exercise psychology explores the relationship between psychological factors and optimal performance. Sport psychology is slowly becoming an integral aspect to the holistic care of the sports medicine patient. The physician who specializes in sports medicine should have some knowledge regarding the various facets of sport and performance psychology, as many of these skills are relevant to the care and management of an athletic and active population.

"Performance psychology" is used in this chapter to represent the various environments under which mental skills enhancement can be useful. "Sport psychology" represents the use of mental skills training within the sport and exercise domain. It has been found that many of the techniques used with elite athletes have had comparable success with elite musicians, actors, and dancers. Therefore, the skills that are addressed in this chapter, although related to the sports environment, may also be helpful for various forms of performance.

Topics addressed in this chapter include a brief review of the history and current issues of sport psychology, a summary of "mental skills" training techniques, and a discussion of specific performance concerns related to the injured athlete. If a sports medicine professional is to establish a holistic philosophy of care, the understanding of underlying psychological processes, along with a model of care, is necessary.

HISTORY AND CURRENT ISSUES

Sport psychology dates back to the turn of the 20th century.[1] It is a relatively young discipline, yet it has a history unappreciated by most clinicians. The origins of sport psychology are patchy at best, with roots in both applied and academic sport psychology, which are primarily housed in departments of physical education/kinesiology. Rarely is sport psychology recognized as a specialty within psychology departments.

Since the U. S. Olympic Committee (USOC) hired its first full-time sport psychologist in 1985, the applied realm of sport psychology has continued to grow tremendously (the USOC now has five full-time licensed psychologists representing their Sport Psychology Department within the Division of Sport Science, with their latest hire in July 2007). Articles within the area of sport psychology then began being published. Division 47 (Exercise and Sport Psychology) in the American Psychological Association (APA) has also been established, recognizing the uniqueness offered to the field of psychology in sports. Other advancements in the field include the establishment of the Association for the Advancement of Applied Sport Psychology (AAASP) in 1986 and the beginning of the *Journal of Sport Psychology* in 1979. In 1991, as a way to further advance this burgeoning field, AAASP established criteria designating a "certified consultant" in the field of sport psychology as a way to improve the clarity and understanding of a sport psychologist.[2] More recently, the APA Division 47 has established a proficiency document for members to help guide the unique training standards (e.g., education, training, supervision) that a psychologist would be wise to undertake in order to practice in the field of applied sport and performance psychology.

The applied realm of sport psychology has been growing rapidly in use and popularity since the 1990s. This use, however, has not been limited to elite athletes, such as those represented at the Olympic Games. Applied sport psychology is also finding utilization at the collegiate, high school, and youth levels.

MENTAL SKILLS IN SPORTS

This section will cover some of the basic psychological skills that are used with mental training and performance enhancement. This overview highlights some of the specific psychological skills that enhance confidence, composure, and focus with individuals who use these skills.

Many coaches and athletes attempt to put in more physical practice to correct mistakes made during competition. The mistakes, however, many times are due to mental breakdowns as opposed to physical or technical ones. In these cases, the athletes actually need to practice *mental*, not physical, skills. Similarly, sports medicine physicians working with athletes may not realize how mental skills can be used in their work.

Even though coaches, athletes, and sports medicine physicians agree that more than 80% of the mistakes made in sports are mental, they often still do not attempt to learn or teach mental skills that will assist athletes on the field or during rehabilitation.[3] Sports medicine and other physicians' lack of knowledge about mental skills may prevent them from being used in their work with athletes (as patients). Even though physicians may tell their athletes to "just relax" as they go through rehabilitation of an injury, they do not provide them with the knowledge of how to do so. Mental skills in sports are often viewed as part of an individual's personality and something that cannot be taught. Many physicians feel that injured athletes either have or do not have the mental toughness to progress through rehabilitation. Mental skills, however, *can* be learned.

Goal Setting

Goal setting is one of the primary mental skills used by athletes. Csikszentmihalyi discusses goal setting as one of the necessary components of achieving a "flow" experience.[4] He describes "flow" as an experience in which a person achieves peak performance. Other terms used for this "flow" experience are "in the zone," "autopilot," and "playing unconscious."

It is not typically a problem to get athletes to identify goals. They do, however, need instruction on setting *reasonable* goals and developing a program that works to achieve them.

It has been demonstrated in empirical research that goal setting can enhance recovery from injury.[5] Several goal-setting principles have been identified that provide a strong base to building a solid goal-setting program.

Set Specific Goals

Research illustrates that setting *specific* goals produces higher levels of performance than planning no goals at all or goals that are too broad.[6] Yet many times physicians tell patients to "do their best" regarding their recovery. Although these goals are admirable, they are not specific and do not help athletes move toward optimal performance. Goal-setting needs to be *measurable* and stated in *behavioral* terms. Instead of an athlete setting his or her goal to "get better," physicians can help these injured athletes set a more appropriate goal like "increasing leg press weight by 5% over the next 2 weeks."

Set Realistic but Challenging Goals

The research indicates that goals should be challenging and difficult, yet attainable.[7] Goals that are too easy do not present a challenge, and therefore can lead to less than maximal effort. Goals that are too difficult many times lead to failure, which can result in frustration. This frustration may lead to lower morale and motivation. In between these two extremes are challenging and realistic goals.

Set Both Long- and Short-Term Goals

Many times injured athletes discuss a long-term goal of returning to play after a serious injury. This goal is necessary and provides the final destination for the athletes. It is important, however, for physicians to help them focus on short-term goals as a means to attain long-term goals. For example, a physician can make certain that an injured athlete sets daily and weekly goals in the rehabilitation process. One way to employ this principle is to picture a staircase with the end or long-term goal at the top of the staircase, the present level of performance at the base of the stairs, and the short-term goals as the steps in between.

Set Performance Goals

It is important for sports medicine physicians to assist patients in setting goals related to performance process rather than outcomes, such as returning to play. Murphy discusses "action goals" versus "result goals" being extremely important and often missed by physicians.[8] With action-focused goals, athletes concentrate their energies on the actions of a task as opposed to the outcome. Action goals give focus to the task at hand, are under the athlete's control, and produce confidence and concentration. Result-focused goals, however, are not productive and often lead to slower recovery. These types of goals give focus to irrelevant factors, things outside the control of the athlete, and tend to produce anxiety and tension.

Write Down Goals

Sport psychologists have recommended that goals be written down and placed where they can be easily seen on a daily basis.[8,9] Athletes may choose to write them on index cards and place them in their locker, locker room, or bedroom. Many times physicians and athletes spend much time with goal-setting strategies only to see them end up never actually being utilized.

Develop Goal-Achievement Strategies

This aspect of goal setting is often neglected as goals are set without appropriate strategies to achieve them. An analogy to this faulty process is taking a trip from Indianapolis to San Jose without having a map. It will take one much longer to reach the final destination without a map.

Provide Goal Support

Research in the sport psychology literature has demonstrated the vital importance significant others play in helping athletes achieve goals.[10] In fact, it has been shown that exercise adherence is strongly affected by spousal support.[11] Sports medicine physicians need to enlist the support and help of parents, faculty, friends, and others to help athletes focus on the actions required to achieve success (i.e., returning to play).

Evaluate Goal Achievement

Evaluating progress toward goals is one of the most important aspects of goal setting, yet it is frequently overlooked. Injured athletes may spend considerable time in setting goals and devising programs, but it will be for naught if they do not regularly monitor their progress in achieving these goals. To draw an analogy from philosophy, just as an unexamined life is not worth living, unexamined goal setting is not worth doing.

Interventional Skills

Arousal Control

Have you ever watched the NCAA basketball finals and wondered how a player can make a free throw or last second shot with thousands of people screaming and millions of people watching on television? If you are like most, we wonder in amazement at how athletes are able to remain calm during such times of high pressure and anxiety. The fact is, however, that these athletes *are* actually nervous—they do have "butterflies" in their stomachs. The skill, however, that they have developed is to use this anxiety as a way to perform their very best, to make the butterflies "fly in formation," so to speak. Similarly, when athletes become injured, they typically experience affective, somatic, and cognitive anxiety.

The theories of arousal regulation are many, but too extensive for the present chapter. For a review and more explicit detail of these theories, see Van Raalte and Brewer.[12]

Breathing

Perhaps the most simple, yet most important, technique for regulating anxiety is breathing.[13] It is common for athletes to take short, quick breaths when confronted with a stressful event or situation, such as rehabilitating an injury. This action may result in muscles becoming tense and fatigued, both of which will prevent optimal performance in recovery. Taking slow, deep breaths allows athletes to improve oxygen intake and reduce their heart rate; both will assist them in recovery.

Muscle Relaxation

One of the most potentially damaging aspects of anxiety for athletes is muscle tension.[14] If an athlete's muscles are tense, he or she will not be able to perform the kinesthetic tasks required by the sport or rehabilitation process in a free-flowing and smooth manner. Therefore, for athletes to perform their best, they must learn to relax their muscles. If their muscles are not relaxed, the athlete's movements will be rigid, short, and tight.

Concentration and Focus Skills

Knowing *what* to focus on, and *when* to focus on it is essential to optimal athletic performance. Highly talented athletes often fail to achieve their best performance not due to a lack of ability, but rather to an inability to focus on the "cues" that are necessary for optimal performance. For example, a baseball pitcher may be able to throw an excellent 85-mph slider in his warm-up, but if he is unable to throw it in a game situation, he is not likely to have optimal performance.

Imagery

What is the mystery in imagery that has helped elite athletes, such as Jack Nicklaus, Tiger Woods, and Greg Louganis, compete so well? There is no mystery at all. Imagery is a human capacity that many people do not know about and/or have chosen not to use.

Imagery is a process by which sensory experiences stored in memory are internally recalled and performed in the absence of external stimuli.[8] Furthermore, imagery is more than visualization, more than just the sense of vision. To maximize its potential, imagery must be a multisensory event, involving as many of the senses as possible, including the senses of sound, touch, and movement.

Imagery has many uses for athletes, including regulating arousal level and rehabilitation from injury.[5,15] Imagery is useful for coping with pain and injury by speeding recovery as well as keeping athletic skills from deteriorating.

Concentration

Concentration is the ability to focus all of one's attention on the task at hand. For physicians and their athletes, concentration is being able to direct all attention to the recovery process. When athletes experience anxiety, however, maintaining attention on the task at hand becomes more difficult. Concentration also becomes more narrow and internally directed toward worry, self-doubt, and other task-irrelevant thoughts.[16]

Part of the definition of concentration involves paying attention to relevant environmental cues. This ability to give one's full attention to only the relevant parts of a task is sometimes very difficult to do. Think about a football player recovering from a serious knee injury. Which cues are relevant and which are irrelevant? Relevant cues include the rehabilitation process—keeping appointments with the physical therapist, good goal setting, and following the physician's recommendations regarding treatment. Irrelevant cues, however, might include the thoughts of friends or the next opponent on the schedule. These cues have absolutely nothing to do with rehabilitation. The physical actions required to rehabilitate the knee do not change, regardless of the next opponent.

Physicians can be extremely beneficial in helping athletes maintain the concentration levels on the task at hand (i.e., rehabilitating an injury). First, physicians can remind their patient that just as they are skilled in maintaining focus in high-pressure situations

(e.g., an athlete shooting free throws to win a game), they can do this same thing in the recovery process.

Second, patients can use cue words to help bring their full attention to the tasks in rehabilitation. For example, a tennis player recovering from an elbow injury might use the term "stay loose" as she lifts weights to strengthen the elbow, or the word "breathe" to remind herself that deep breathing will help relaxation during times of intense pain.

Furthermore, much research has demonstrated that routines can focus concentration and be extremely helpful to mental preparation.[17,18] The mind can easily wander during rehabilitation. Injured athletes might worry about losing their position or the reactions of coaches and teammates. These are the times at which routines are ideal.

In summary, to develop an effective mental skills plan, an athlete/patient may incorporate the use of many specific and defined behavioral skills in a structured manner. This type of detailed skill development requires more than a simplistic ("they aren't tough enough") approach. Rather, it is a systematic plan of skills that are individualized to account for the patient's age, skill level, sport-specific demands, and individual abilities.[19]

PSYCHOLOGICAL FACTORS WITH ATHLETIC INJURY

An inevitable aspect of sports participation is the risk of athletic injury. Injuries ranging from lacerations to ligament sprains to fractured bones are an undeniable aspect of the sports world. For the sports medicine professional, this is common sense. Yet to fully treat the injured athlete, what is done for his or her psychological (compared to physical) recovery? For example, to inform a patient that he is to have an anterior cruciate ligament reconstruction that will require surgery followed by extensive rehabilitation before his return to play is one aspect of care. What if the injury occurs 2 weeks before a championship contest? At this point, a significant emotional, mental, and behavioral dynamic will occur that should be treated.

The purpose of this brief section is to review some of the expected emotional, behavioral, and cognitive responses of the injured athlete. Heil has written a comprehensive text that addressed many of the psychological dynamics of the injured athlete.[20] For purposes of this section, the following stages of response to athletic injury will be highlighted.

Point of Injury/Immediate Postinjury

The most immediate emotional response at the point of injury is shock; the degree of shock may range from minor to significant, depending upon the severity of the injury. For example, an open fracture that is observed by the injured athlete may stimulate more of a shock response than a minor laceration. However, individual personality differences may impact the shock response. Additionally, the first denial response occurs, typically in an "I can't believe this happened" response. It is important to note that denial itself is an adaptive response that allows an individual to manage extreme emotional responses to situational stress.

Treatment Decision and Implementation

This stage is filled with uncertainty for the athlete; lack of knowledge of medical treatments and potential rehabilitation may create excess anxiety. This reactive anxiety to the injury and treatment decision may become anticipatory anxiety as surgery dates come closer. These anxiety responses may be mild, moderate, or severe in regard to the disruption of daily functioning for the athlete. A psychological referral for even mild anxiety may facilitate more effective coping and better response skills given the therapeutic relationship.

An additional factor to consider is the athlete's decision-making skills, as some athletes may not have a significant support system (e.g., parents) available at the time of making a decision about treatment. If surgery is required, and the athlete has no previous surgical experience, there may be an adaptive anxiety to manage the realities of anesthesia, pain, and physical restrictions. If the athlete is a collegiate student-athlete and far from home, there will be additional stressors due to the distance from the primary support network. It is often at this stage that a referral to a sport psychologist may best assist the athlete in recovery. The athlete may be more open to support during this time of decision making, and a psychologist can assist not only in the decision-making process but also with emotional support.

Early and Late Rehabilitation

Whether the intervention is surgical or nonsurgical, there may be a series of emotional, behavioral, and cognitive responses that follow the implementation of treatment. Primarily, there may be affective responses that appear atypical to the athlete's baseline behaviors. These emotional responses may be in the form of depression (acute), anger, confusion, and/or frustration. Again, individual differences will vary based on the athlete's personality style, adaptive coping skills, and social support network.

If there are delays in scheduled recovery times or disruptions in the healing process (e.g., infection), anger or withdrawal may become the affective response. Although anger is a difficult emotion to manage, a nonbehavioral display of anger is an adaptive response.

Return to Play

This stage of injury rehabilitation often presents with the dynamics of fear and relief. These emotional responses may conflict with one another during what appears to be a desirable period for the athlete: returning to competition. Fear of reinjury and fear of not being able to compete and perform optimally are typical affective responses for the athlete. When discussed and identified as normal adaptations to the emotional demands of competition and recovery, many athletes move through this stage well. When the athlete ruminates or obsesses about his or her full recovery status, the feelings of fear may create inhibition in rehabilitation, or perhaps even questions doubting his or her abilities.

SUMMARY

This chapter has briefly highlighted the area of sport psychology as it relates to performance psychology skills (mental training), including a historical overview and current topics overview. The use of mental training skills may be of interest to the practicing sports medicine professional in the treatment of patients. It is important that the sports medicine professional recognizes what sport or performance psychology represents within the paradigm of psychological interventions. Referring to an individual based on his or her training (licensed psychologist versus mental training consultant) is essential for the appropriate management of psychological issues related to performance. The issues related to the psychological rehabilitation of the injured athlete are of importance to the medical staff; the overview of affective responses will assist in understanding the normal and adaptive responses of the injured athlete.

REFERENCES

1. Wiggins DK. The history of sport psychology in North America. In: Silva JM, Weinberg RS, eds. *Psychological Foundations of Sport*. Champaign, IL: Human Kinetics; 1984:9–22.
2. Murphy SM. Introduction to sport psychology interventions. In: Murphy SM, ed. *Sport Psychology Interventions*. Champaign, IL: Human Kinetics Publishers; 1995:1–15.
3. Carr C, Kays T. Survey of Ohio State Athletics; Unpublished document, 1997.
4. Csikszentmihalyi M. *Flow: The Psychology of Optimal Experience*. New York: Harper & Row; 1990.
5. Weinberg RS, Gould D. *Foundations of Sport and Exercise Psychology*. Champaign, IL: Human Kinetics; 1995.
6. Weinberg RS, Weigand D. Goal setting in sport and exercise: a reaction to Locke. *J Sport Exercise Psychol*. 1993;15:88–95.
7. Locke EA, Latham GP. *A Theory of Goal Setting and Task Performance*. Englewood Cliffs, NJ: Prentice-Hall; 1990.
8. Murphy S. *The Achievement Zone*. New York: Putnam's; 1996.
9. Botterill C. Goal setting for athletes with examples from hockey. In: Martin GL, Hrycaik D, eds. *Behavior Modification and Coaching: Principles, Procedures, and Research*. Springfield, IL: Thomas; 1983:67–85.
10. Hardy CV, Richman JM, Rosenfeld LB. The role of social support in the life stress/injury relationship. *Sport Psychologist* 1993;5:128–139.
11. Dishman RK. *Exercise Adherence: Its Impact on Public Health*. Champaign, IL: Human Kinetics; 1988.
12. Van Raalte J, Brewer B. *Exploring Sport and Exercise Psychology*. Washington, DC: American Psychological Association; 1996.
13. Williams JM, Harris DV. Relaxation and energizing techniques for regulation of arousal. In: Williams JM, ed. *Applied Sport Psychology: Personal Growth to Peak Performance*. New York: McGraw-Hill; 2006:285–305.
14. Landers DM, Arent SM. Arousal-performance relationships. In: Williams JM, ed. *Applied Sport Psychology: Personal Growth to Peak Performance*. New York: McGraw-Hill; 2006:206–284.
15. Caudill D, Weinberg R, Jackson A. Psyching-up and track athletes: a preliminary investigation. *J Sport Psychol*. 1983;5:231–235.
16. Nideffer RM, Sagal MS. Concentration and attentional control training. In: Williams JM, ed. *Applied Sport Psychology: Personal Growth to Peak Performance*. New York: McGraw-Hill; 2006:382–403.
17. Cohn PJ, Rotella RJ, Lloyd JW. Effects of a cognitive behavioral intervention on the preshot routine and performance in golf. *Sport Psychologist*. 1990;4:33–47.
18. Moore WE. Covert–overt service routines: the effects of a service routine training program on elite tennis players. Unpublished doctoral dissertation, University of Virginia, 1986.
19. Orlick T. *Psyching for Sport: Mental Training for Athletes*. Champaign, IL: Leisure Press; 1986.
20. Heil J. *Psychology of Sport Injury*. Champaign, IL: Human Kinetics; 1993.

Tissue Injury and Healing

Musculoskeletal injuries are an inevitable result of sports participation. According to the 1992 National Institutes of Health (NIH) report, there are 3 million injuries annually in the United States directly related to organized sports.[1] However, the actual number of injuries is much greater, because many are not documented due to the lack of standardized reporting requirements and participation in unorganized sports. Currently, a reportable injury must meet all of the following criteria: occurs during a scheduled practice or game, requires medical attention, and results in restriction or exclusion of participation for one or more days.[2–4]

Football accounts for 81% of all reported injuries annually. Football also has the highest incidence of catastrophic injuries, with gymnastics and ice hockey close behind. However, when looking at the injury rate per 1,000 athlete exposures as reported by Rice and the National Collegiate Athletic Association (NCAA),[5] female track and field athletes have the highest injury rate, followed by male wrestlers, female soccer players, male football players, and female gymnasts.

Tissue injuries from sports can be classified as macrotraumatic or microtraumatic. Macrotraumatic injuries are usually due to a strong force—such as a fall, accident, collision, or laceration—and are more common in contact sports such as football and rugby. These injuries can be primary (due to direct tissue damage) or secondary (due to transmission of forces or release of inflammatory mediators and other cytokines). Microtraumatic injuries are chronic injuries that result from overuse of a structure such as a muscle, joint, ligament, or tendon. If the ability of the tissue to repair is exceeded by continued injury to the structure, the healing process becomes pathologic and a chronic reinjury occurs. This type of injury is more common in sports involving repetitive motion, such as swimming, cycling, and rowing.

OVERVIEW OF THE HEALING PROCESS

After an injury, the body attempts to limit tissue damage. *Inflammation* is a protective response designed to contain the injury, destroy damaged tissues and unwanted microorganisms, and dilute harmful mediators released as a result of the injury. It is the first step in the healing process, and involves migration and activation of cells, vascular responses, and systemic reactions. Inflammation activates the cascade of events necessary to heal tissues. The second phase of healing, *proliferation,* begins early in the inflammatory phase, usually after 3 to 5 days. Fibroblasts accumulate and the fibrin clot that was formed early is replaced with collagen. This initial collagen has little strength because it is randomly organized. The third phase of healing, *tissue remodeling,* involves replacing the random collagen with longitudinally arranged fibers (Fig. 3-1). This begins 1 to 2 weeks after the injury and may take months to years to complete. This process results in increased tissue strength. If the causative agent is not removed during the healing process, fibrosis can occur.[6]

SPECIFIC TISSUE INJURY

Tendon and Ligament Injury

Repair of ligaments requires migration of fibroblasts into necrotic and damaged tissue. Cell proliferation and matrix formation must occur for repair to be complete. Initially, a loose fibrous matrix composed of water, glycosaminoglycans, and type III collagen is produced by inflammatory cells. Vascular proliferation then occurs, and collagen and glycosaminoglycans fill the tissue deficit. During the next several weeks, the composition of the healing tissue is

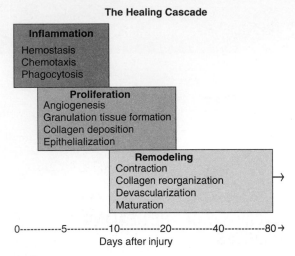

The Healing Cascade

Inflammation
Hemostasis
Chemotaxis
Phagocytosis

Proliferation
Angiogenesis
Granulation tissue formation
Collagen deposition
Epithelialization

Remodeling
Contraction
Collagen reorganization
Devascularization
Maturation

0------------5------------10------------20------------40------------80 →
Days after injury

FIGURE 3-1 Timing of the three primary stages of healing and key events in each stage.

changed. The amount of type I collagen increases, while decreases in type II collagen, glycosaminoglycan, and water content are observed. The type I collagen fibers then begin to hypertrophy and group together in bundles, increasing the tensile strength of the tissue. Alignment of the collagen is aided by tension in the tissues, so movement and gentle stress on the injured ligament is needed for proper tissue repair.

Remodeling, the next step in the process, improves the structure of the tissue. The volume of the repair tissue reduces during this stage. Upon completion of remodeling, the repaired tissue does not achieve the tensile strength of uninjured tissue, but the deficit is usually not sufficient to disturb the normal function of the ligament or joint.

The size of the tissue deficit, the type and location of the injured ligament, and the amount of loading on the repair tissues all affect the healing process. Healing can be maximized by stabilizing the injured structure and minimizing edema initially. Controlled loading of the ligament, with appropriate physical therapy during repair and remodeling, can also improve healing (Fig. 3-2).[7]

Tendon injury and repair is sometimes different from ligament repair. Tendon contains more collagen, mainly type I, and fewer glycosaminoglycans and fibrocytes. If the tissue deficit is small, resting tenocytes transform into tenoblasts and produce a new extracellular matrix. Tendon sheaths begin to proliferate after 3 to 4 days. Reorganization then occurs as it does in ligament repair, and the same factors that promote ligament healing promote tendon healing.[7]

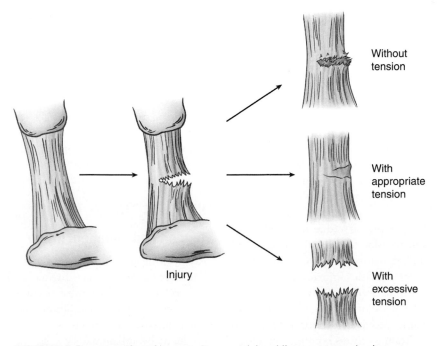

Without
tension

With
appropriate
tension

With
excessive
tension

Injury

FIGURE 3-2 Demonstration of how tension on an injured ligament or tendon impacts healing. (Courtsey Chi-Tsai Tang, MD.)

Muscle Injury

Muscle injury can result from lacerations, contusions, cramps, or compartment syndrome. No matter the type of injury, repair begins with the activation of a satellite muscle cell. This cell remains quiescent until growth factors and cytokines are released, causing the cell to differentiate into myotubules and muscle fibers. Tensile strength of the muscle is then enhanced by collagen synthesis.

If a muscle is lacerated, muscle cannot form across the deficit. Instead, a dense scar forms, and the continuity of the muscle is disrupted. Any portion of the muscle disrupted from the motor point is denervated. Thus, if the muscle is completely transected, a significant loss of strength is anticipated. If the laceration is partial, the ability of the muscle to generate force will be diminished, but to a lesser extent. For all muscle injuries, repair is affected by the type of muscle involved, type of injury, and metabolic condition of the muscle.

Myositis ossificans is another type of muscle injury that occurs from ossification of the muscle at the site of injury. This occurs most often following a muscle contusion. Reinjury shortly after the initial injury increases the risk of its development. It takes months for the ossification or calcification process to mature. Maturation is identified by loss of radioactive uptake on a triple-phase bone scan. If the ossification causes functional limitations, it can be removed surgically, but only after maturation. Surgery prior to maturation can result in accelerated bone formation and should be avoided. The body may resorb the ossification, but this process is slow and not guaranteed.

Compartment syndrome can also cause muscle damage and presents with either chronic recurring symptoms or from an acute injury. Excess fluid from hemorrhage or a rise in intracellular or extracellular fluid results in increased intracompartmental pressures when the compartmental volume is exceeded. This results in restricted blood flow and muscle ischemia. When this occurs from an acute injury, early detection and treatment with a fasciotomy is required to prevent irreversible tissue damage. Symptoms from chronic exertional compartment syndrome occur in association with specific physical activities and are relieved by rest. The diagnosis is made by pressure testing before and after symptomatic exercise. Treatments include activity modification or fasciotomy.[8]

Bone Injury

Normal bone is classified as cortical (compact) or cancellous (trabecular). Based on density, cortical bone makes up 80% of the bone in the body. Cancellous bone is less dense and more elastic. It undergoes more remodeling and endures more stress than cortical bone. Supporting tissues play a role in recovery from a bone injury. The periosteum assists with callus formation when a fracture occurs, and marrow provides progenitor cells for bone formation and remodeling.

Osteoporosis is a common disorder of the bone defined by low bone mass and altered bone architecture resulting in bone fragility and increased fracture risk. The overall risk of developing osteoporosis is three times higher in females than in males, and risk increases with age. Once a fracture has occurred, the associated morbidity and mortality is high.[9] There is growing research suggesting that exercise and adequate vitamin D and calcium intake can prevent osteoporosis, especially when started in youth. In adults, exercise can increase bone density in the spine by 1% to 2%.[10] The exact type and duration of exercise needed to achieve these results has not been determined. However, studies have indicated that resistance exercise promotes whole-body bone mineral density whereas endurance exercise promotes only lower-body bone mineral density.[11] Exercise also reduces the risk of falls, which also reduces fracture risk.[10,12,13] The mechanism of increased bone density associated with exercise is thought to be stimulation of bone formation from stress on the bone, and from hormonal changes.[11]

Bone can be damaged from ischemia, infection, direct injury from macrotrauma, or repeated microtrauma. Osteonecrosis is death of the bone and has been associated with ischemia, steroid or alcohol use, radiation, and sickle-cell disease. Inflammation follows the necrosis of bone and marrow. Mesenchymal tissues and capillaries invade the necrotic tissue. Osteoblasts begin to produce new bone matrix. Remodeling occurs through resorption of the necrotic bone and reorganization of new cells and matrix. A similar process, called osteochondrosis, can occur in children at traction apophyses.

Fractures are a common injury to the bone. As with muscles, ligaments, and tendons, inflammation is the initial phase in repair. Bleeding also occurs from the fracture site and provides hematologic cells and growth factors. Osteoprogenitor cells, mesenchymal cells, and fibroblasts migrate to the area of fracture.

The repair processes begins with formation of a soft callus made of fibrocartilage. A medullary callus bridges this initial callus.

Fracture healing is not always complete. Delayed union occurs when a fracture fails to heal as anticipated, but still shows evidence of biological activity and is still considered to be healing. A nonunion occurs when there is no evidence of clinical or radiologic healing after 6 to 9 months. A nonunion is classified as either atrophic or hypertrophic. Atrophic nonunions are avascular and lack the capacity to heal. They are usually treated with a bone graft. A hypertrophic nonunion has the capacity to heal, but lacks the membrane organization to do so. Stabilizing the bone via internal fixation with screws and plates is often required.

There are various modalities that can promote fracture healing. Ultrasound has been shown to promote fracture healing in clinical studies. Direct current applied to the fracture can also promote migration of inflammatory mediators and accelerate healing. Alternating current can promote collagen synthesis and calcification. Distraction can also stimulate bone formation and is used for hypertrophic nonunions, limb lengthening, and to correct deformities.

Nerve Injury

Nerve disorders occur from injury to the nerve axons, the insulating myelin sheath, or the supportive connective tissues that create the neural tube. When an axon is injured, it begins to swell, and the portion distal to the injury degenerates through a process called Wallerian degeneration. Macrophages migrate into the area and degrade the remaining axoplasm. The portion of the axon proximal to the injury will survive because it remains attached to the cell body. Axonal sprouts develop at the distal end of the surviving axon 1 week after the injury. The neural tube must be present for the sprouts to grow in the proper direction. Muscle that is cut off from its nerve supply will begin to atrophy and will not recover unless reinnervated. Because axon sprouts grow slowly, 1 to 3 mm/day, muscle recovery following axonal injury can be slow and will depend on the muscle's distance from the site of injury. If only a portion of the nerve supply to a muscle is disrupted, then intact nerves can form distal sprouts to innervate the orphaned muscle nearby. This usually occurs within a few weeks after nerve injury and provides a faster recovery of muscle strength.

If just myelin is injured it will recover as long as there are Schwann cells to produce new myelin. Until the myelin is repaired the nerve cannot transmit electrical signals down the axon. Recovery of nerve function can take weeks or months depending on the amount of myelin injured.

The remaining connective tissues that create the neural tube are more durable than the myelin and the nerve axons, so they are not typically injured in isolation. Injury to these connective tissues worsens the prognosis of a nerve injury, because the regeneration of axons depends on an available neural tube to direct proper growth of a new axon.

Nerve injuries are classified according to their severity by the Seddon or Sunderland criteria. The Seddon criteria are the more commonly used. They describe three types of injury: neurapraxia, axonotmesis, and neurotmesis. The Sunderland criteria describe five types of nerve injury, with type 1 corresponding to neurapraxia, type 5 corresponding to neurotmesis, and types 2, 3, and 4 representing different types of axonotmesis (Table 3-1).

Neurapraxia (Sunderland type 1) is usually caused by compression and involves injury to the myelin sheath only. If the lesion is large enough, it

TABLE 3-1	Details of Injured (+) and Noninjured (−) Nervous Tissues in the Five Types of Nerve Injury Based on the Sunderland Criteria and Corresponding Seddon Classification						
Sunderland	**Seddon**	**Myelin**	**Axon**	**Endoneurium**	**Perineurium**	**Epineurium**
Type 1	Neurapraxia	+	−	−	−	−
Type 2	Axonotmesis	±	+	−	−	−
Type 3	Axonotmesis	±	+	+	−	−
Type 4	Axonotmesis	±	+	+	+	−
Type 5	Neurotmesis	+	+	+	+	+

results in conduction block. Electrodiagnostic tests demonstrate normal conduction distal to the lesion, but blocked or slowed conduction across the lesion. Spontaneous activity, seen during needle electromyography (EMG) when a muscle is denervated by Wallerian degeneration of the axon, does not occur in neurapraxia. Decreased recruitment of motor units in the muscle may occur. Recovery takes weeks to months depending on the size of the injury.

Axonotmesis (Sunderland types 2, 3, and 4) is typically caused by a crush injury. This type of injury disrupts axons in addition to myelin. Schwann cells and portions of the neural tube remain intact. Initially, conduction studies resemble these of a neurapraxic injury. After 4 to 5 days, Wallerian degeneration occurs, and the axon distal to the lesion begins to degenerate. This results in an abnormal conduction distal to the lesion. Abnormal spontaneous activity is present during the EMG needle examination. Motor unit recruitment is absent if all axons are disrupted, or it may be present if some of the nerve's axons are undamaged. Because the neural tube is intact, the nerve is eventually able to repair with axonal regeneration.

Neurotmesis (Sunderland type 5) is a nerve transection injury. The axon, myelin, and entire neural tube are disrupted. Conduction studies distal to the injury will initially be normal because Wallerian degeneration has not yet occurred. Within a few weeks, the nerve conduction studies begin to show a lack of response. The EMG also demonstrates abnormal spontaneous activity along with lack of motor unit recruitment. Surgical intervention is sometimes used for complete nerve injuries in order to reconnect the connective tissues of the neural tube. Without surgery, no recovery is expected. With surgery, the degree of recovery depends on the success of axonal sprouting across the injured area and the distance of the injury to the affected muscles.

EFFECTS OF MEDICATIONS ON HEALING

Inflammation is an important part of the healing process. However, when prolonged, it can cause secondary tissue weakness, resulting in further injury and delays in repair and rehabilitation.[14,15] Nonsteroidal anti-inflammatory medications (NSAIDs) as well as corticosteroids are the most common medications used to reduce inflammation.

The mechanism of action of NSAIDs is to inhibit prostaglandin synthesis. Because prostaglandins are mediators of inflammation, inhibiting them reduces inflammation. The most common side effect of NSAIDs is gastrointestinal upset. More serious side effects include gastrointestinal bleeding and renal failure. These effects usually occur with prolonged use or with comorbid medical conditions. Some research suggests that NSAIDs have an inhibitory effect on bone synthesis. These studies have been conclusive in rats, with conflicting evidence about the effect in humans; therefore, avoiding NSAIDs in the early postoperative or posttraumatic phase is recommended.[16,17]

Corticosteroids are often used to treat acute or chronic injuries with associated inflammation. They work to suppress the initial events of inflammation by inhibiting capillary dilatation and migration of inflammatory cells, which limits tissue edema. However, corticosteroids can also cause tissue damage. Bone necrosis is the most significant complication reported with short-term, high-dose corticosteroid use. Subcutaneous fat necrosis and loss of skin pigmentation can also occur with injectable corticosteroids. Repeated corticosteroid injections can further weaken damaged tissue and can cause tendon rupture, especially in the rotator cuff and Achilles tendons. A study by Haraldsson et al. showed tensile strength of isolated collagen fascicles was diminished at 3 and 7 days after injection with corticosteroids.[18]

REHABILITATION

RICE (rest, ice, compression, and elevation) is a common algorithm used to treat acute musculoskeletal and sports injuries. Rest should be limited, and early mobilization is desirable whenever possible. Immobilization leads to contractures and muscle atrophy and can contribute to cardiovascular deconditioning and osteoporosis. These conditions are difficult to treat, and it is best to prevent them from occurring. Relative rest is encouraged when possible, and involves general conditioning exercises that do not aggravate the condition.

Immobilization is sometimes necessary, most often for fractures or tendon ruptures. This allows the injured segment to heal in the proper alignment and usually requires 2 to 6 weeks. An acutely inflamed joint or tendon, or a ligament sprain, should not be immobilized for more than a few days.

Ice is generally applied for 15 minutes every hour for the first few days after the injury, and can be used in conjunction with anti-inflammatory medication to control inflammation and pain. It is especially useful when treating tendonitis or bursitis.

Once inflammation and pain have subsided, range of motion should begin. Active range of motion is performed under one's own control, while passive range of motion occurs when another person or device produces the movement. Isometric exercises are used for strengthening when range of motion is restricted or needs to be avoided due to a fracture or acute inflammation of a joint. Otherwise, isotonic strengthening can begin within the painless arc of joint motion. Loss of proprioception occurs with injury to ligaments, tendons, or joints, and also with immobilization. Restoration of proprioception is an important part of rehabilitation in order to prevent further injury.

The final phase of rehabilitation is sports retraining. This is a critical step to reduce risk of further injury. Supervised activity-specific training is completed, followed by a slow and progressive return to full activity. This should be done gradually, with increases in duration and intensity of the activity occurring over many weeks. Cross-training is encouraged, especially with activities that do not produce any symptoms from the injury. With each increase in activity, signs of recurring pain or weakness should trigger a slowdown or a reversal to a tolerable level of activity. Unrestricted sports activity is not allowed until all of these steps have been completed and full-effort sports-specific activity is tolerated without symptoms.

REFERENCES

1. Conference on Sports Injuries in Youth. Bethesda, MD: National Institutes of Health; 1992. NIH Publication No. 93-3444.
2. Armsey TD, Hosey RG. Medical aspects of sports: epidemiology of injuries, preparticipation physical examination, and drugs in sports. *Clin Sports Med*. 2004;23:255–279.
3. Patel DR, Baker RJ. Musculoskeletal injuries in sports. *Prim Care*. 2006;33:545–579.
4. Patel DR, Greydanus DE, Luckstead EF. The college athlete. *Pediatr Clin North Am*. 2005;52:25–60.
5. Rice SG, Epidemiology and mechanisms of sports injuries. In: C.C. Teitz and B.C. Decker, Editors, Scientific Foundations of Sports Medicine, Philadelphia. WB Saunders, 1989.
6. Kumar V, Abbas AK, Faustu N. Tissue renewal and repair: regeneration, healing and fibrosis. In: Kumar V, Abbas AK, Faustu N, eds. *Pathologic Basis of Disease*. Philadelphia: Elsevier Saunders; 2005:81–118.
7. Best T, Kirkendall DE, Almekinders L, et al. Basic science and injury of muscle, tendon and ligaments. In: DeLee J, Drez D, Miller M, eds. *DeLee and Drez's Orthopaedic Sports Medicine: Principles and Practice*. 2nd ed. Philadelphia: Saunders; 2003:1–66.
8. Brennan FH, Kane SF. Diagnosis, treatment options, and rehabilitation of chronic lower leg exertional compartment syndrome. *Curr Sports Med*. 2003;2:247–250.
9. Takahashi K, Kawagoe J, Ohmichi M, et al. Hormone replacement therapy and osteoporosis. *Clin Calcium*. 2004;14:436–441.
10. Kelley GA, Kelley KS, Tran ZV. Exercise and lumbar spine bone mineral density in postmenopausal women: a meta-analysis of individual patient data. *J Gerontol A Biol Sci Med Sci*. 2006;57:559–604.
11. Benton MJ, White A. Osteoporosis: recommendations for resistance exercise and supplementation with calcium and vitamin D to promote bone health. *J Community Health Nurs*. 2006;23:201–211.
12. Cummings SR. A 55-year-old woman with osteopenia. *JAMA*. 2006;21:2601–2610.
13. Huntoon E, Sinaki M. The role of exercise in the prevention and treatment of compression fractures. *Mayo Clin Proc*. 2006;81:1400–1401.
14. Buckwalter J, Mow V. Basic science and injury of cartilage, meniscus and bone. In: DeLee J, Drez D, Miller M, eds. *DeLee and Drez's Orthopaedic Sports Medicine: Principles and Practice*. 2nd ed. Philadelphia: Saunders; 2003:67–120.
15. Buckwalter J, Woo S. Effects of medications in sports injuries at the tissue level. In: DeLee J, Drez D, Miller M, eds. *DeLee and Drez's Orthopaedic Sports Medicine: Principles and Practice*. 2nd ed. Philadelphia: Saunders; 2003;50–55.
16. Aspenberg P. Drugs and fracture repair. *Acta Orthop*. 2005;76:741–748.
17. Harder AT, An YH. The mechanisms of the inhibitory effects of nonsteroidal anti-inflammatory drugs on bone healing: a concise review. *J Clin Pharmacol*. 2003;48:807–815.
18. Haraldsson BT, Langber H, Aagaard P, et al. Corticosteroids reduce the tensile strength of isolated collagen fascicles. *Am J Sports Med*. 2006;34:1992–1997.

The Sports Medicine Approach to Musculoskeletal Medicine

M usculoskeletal medicine has become an increasingly prominent aspect of clinical practice. Many physicians seek to expand their practices in the areas of sports and musculoskeletal medicine. The purpose of this chapter is to provide the basis for the evaluation and treatment of individuals who sustain a wide range of musculoskeletal disorders and who seek assistance to address their musculoskeletal problems. The ways in which sports medicine approaches can be applied to the population of patients with a wide range of musculoskeletal problems will be explored. This chapter will use a "case-based" approach to illustrate the principles of musculoskeletal assessment. Four cases will provide examples that will illustrate how the various factors of the sports medicine assessment can be used for patient evaluation and treatment. Other chapters in this text will provide more specifically detailed approaches to the management of sports-specific injuries and their treatment.

PRINCIPLES AND PRACTICE OF SPORTS/MUSCULOSKELETAL MEDICINE

The basic premise of musculoskeletal evaluation and rehabilitation using sports medicine principles is that the rehabilitation process begins immediately following resolution of the acute-phase response to injury. Prolonged rest results in disuse atrophy, reduced cardiovascular endurance, and loss of activity or work-specific skills. The correction of muscle imbalance or specific biomechanic inefficiencies that will prevent reinjury and further time loss from a sport/activity is the goal of treatment. If one considers sport as the function, athletes are disabled if they are unable to participate. Similarly, the person with a musculoskeletal problem may be unable to participate in his or her life activities, whether or not they are associated with sports. Appropriate treatment and rehabilitation therefore minimizes or eliminates the potential for continued impairment by progressing the patient through the rehabilitation process with the end goal being return to activity.

The basis of the sports medicine approach to musculoskeletal evaluation rests on the fact that clinical excellence is necessary to achieve successful outcomes. Clinical excellence requires that the clinician gain the necessary skills to perform a well-structured and sufficiently detailed assessment. To perform an adequate sports medicine-oriented evaluation, knowledge should be acquired in the anatomy, biomechanics, and kinesiology of the musculoskeletal system and understanding gained in the mechanisms of acute and chronic overload injuries. As possible, the caregiver should attempt to understand common features of different movement patterns to allow appropriate assessment and understanding of the processes that induce overload. Therefore, an understanding of musculoskeletal anatomy and kinesiology, an ability to take a holistic approach to the evaluation and treatment of the individual, and an understanding of the integration of rehabilitation into the treatment continuum is required.

Standard static (range-of-motion, strength, neurovascular evaluation) and dynamic (evaluation of the musculoskeletal system in motion) assessment techniques are important to spine/musculoskeletal evaluation. Patients frequently have a relatively poor understanding of guidelines for return to their activities. Succinct guidelines based on sound rehabilitation principles for return to activity improve the patient's understanding of his or her problem and promote compliance with the program.

EVALUATING THE PATIENT—THE MYSTERY IS IN THE HISTORY

Sports-related injuries commonly occur when tissues or anatomic structures become overloaded, either acutely or chronically. These types of injuries are usually identifiable by the mechanism or type of injury or overload. Chronic musculoskeletal injuries or disorders are commonly less linked to a specific event and tend to be reported using more vague terminology relating to onset and degree. It is therefore imperative when obtaining the history from a musculoskeletal patient to establish patterns that correlate to the potential pathology. Exacerbating and remitting factors are important. Correlation to movement or activity patterns is useful to establish directional factors. These factors are illustrated by the cases described below.

Case Histories

Case 1: Auto Worker with Right Shoulder Pain

The patient is a 42-year-old man who reports vague-onset right shoulder pain over the past 6 months. He can describe no specific event or trauma that produced his symptoms. He describes symptoms that worsen with activity or movement. He is generally worse later in the day and more comfortable when he arises in the morning. He denies night pain and his shoulder does not awaken him from sleep. He feels that his symptoms have worsened somewhat since their onset. He had some initial benefit with the use of over-the-counter nonsteroidal agents, but notes less benefit currently. He works at an auto assembly plant where he rotates to different stations on the assembly line. He reports that he has the most problems with a painting station where he has to reach into the vehicle with a spray gun in his dominant right hand to paint areas that are not accessible to the robots on the assembly line. He plays softball recreationally but has had to discontinue this activity due to the pain it causes to his shoulder.

Case 2: Female Runner with Shin Pain

A 26-year-old experienced female runner is referred by a chiropractor with pain in both shins that she reports has worsened over the past 4 weeks. She has been training for a charity marathon event using her usual training routine for the past 2 months. She has seen her primary care physician, who felt that she was having shin splints. She has undergone active-release

therapy treatments with the chiropractor. She has been icing after her runs and notes some improvement with ice. She does not specifically describe one leg as worse than the other. She can relate no other changes to her routine. She notes that her pain has started coming on sooner and sooner on her runs. She does report a 10-pound weight gain over the past 2 years. She denies any night or rest pain. She has had a few episodes of pain in association with her regular daily activities such as climbing stairs. She changed shoes 6 months previously. She has been running on the same shoes for the past 6 months. She denies any sensory changes or sense of tightness or tenseness in the lower shin.

Case 3: Triathlete with Upper Extremity Weakness

A 29-year-old right-handed competitive triathlete comes to the office with vague complaints of weakness in the right shoulder. He is having increased difficulty with swimming, although he is able to do a freestyle stroke without a great deal of pain. He has a vague dull aching sensation that occurs when he is running. Resting his elbows on his aerobars does not affect his symptoms. He has been having problems with his strength-training program, with his right shoulder able to lift less weight in a variety of movements compared to his left. He is scheduled to compete in a half ironman race in 3 weeks.

Case 4: High School Athlete with a "Pulled Hamstring"

A 17-year-old 100-meter state champion runner presents with complaints of her third hamstring injury in as many months. She has had prior treatment with her primary care physician. She is a high-level athlete and has been approached by several colleges for possible scholarship opportunities. She reports that each time she has injured her hamstrings when coming out of the starting block during a race, after which she could not run. The treatment rendered for each of her prior two injuries consisted of rest, ice, and compression.

THE SPORTS MEDICINE EXAMINATION

Many parts of the examination are similar to those used in the general evaluation of any patient. Special emphasis for the static examination is placed on the details gleaned from the history of the events leading up to the acute or chronic injury, directed toward identifying the mechanism of injury and appropriate treatment. If indicated, the athlete's equipment or training/competitive environment may also require evaluation to determine if there are any external factors contributing to the injury. The examination consists of a static portion, similar to a standard musculoskeletal exam, and a dynamic portion, designed to evaluate the injured part in motion or to elicit injurious movement patterns.

The Static Examination

The static examination portion of the evaluation assesses strength, range of motion, posture, alignment, palpation, and neurovascular function. Understanding the specifics of the sport or activity that the patient may do is less important than a firm understanding of the anatomic and kinesiologic factors involved.

Muscle strength, balance, and symmetry are assessed clinically, and if necessary using a variety of testing modalities such as isokinetic dynamometry. Range of motion (ROM) is evaluated both in relative and absolute terms. Normal considerations of ROM are modified to incorporate the needed versus available range for a given activity and range restrictions or asymmetries that may be present. Although there is a broad spectrum of ROM compatible with injury-free activity, asymmetry is unusual in the absence of an acute or remote injury and should alert the clinician to potential mechanisms of injury.

Muscle Strength

Assessing muscle strength includes standard manual muscle testing (MMT) as well as tests to provide more detailed assessment of functional strength and symmetry. Most standard texts and medical school curricula provide information regarding techniques used to perform a general MMT examination. Static muscle testing provides general information regarding gross muscle function. Quantification of muscle strength using MMT, however, cannot be considered as the only measure from which strength loss can be identified, due to the fact that there can be significant strength loss without a change in muscle grade. Strength assessment is similarly evaluated in both absolute and relative terms. An athlete with strength imbalance of the vastus lateralis compared to the vastus medialis will manifest a higher propensity towards lateral patellar tracking.[1] Similarly, alteration of the

normal strength ratio between the quadriceps and hamstring muscles will result in a higher incidence of hamstring injuries in sprinters.[2,3]

Range of Motion

Substitution patterns used to compensate for lost range are also assessed by evaluating static positions. For example, a soccer player with inadequate hip flexor mobility attempting to kick a goal will compensate by increasing the amount of lumbar lordosis, predisposing to spondylolysis. Having the athlete extend the leg backwards will engage the pelvis early and demonstrate the lack of hip range.

Posture

Postural evaluation allows the examiner to evaluate the overall sagittal and coronal balance of the patient. A lack of postural control and balance will result in alterations of position that facilitate the injury process. It is often necessary to evaluate postural aspects that are far removed from the specific body part in question. For example, an athlete with poor trunk stability and a lumbar hyperlordosis may present with primary complaints involving the shoulder. A failure to identify the postural considerations for this patient will result in a less than optimal outcome.

Alignment

Various aspects of the examination require the determination of alterations in normal alignment and symmetry. For example, the alignment of the patella is important to diagnostically evaluate problems with the knee. Measurements for Q-angle, patella alta, or patellar rotation would be necessary in the evaluation of a person with knee pain. Similarly, pelvic height asymmetry serves as a marker for problems in the pelvis or at the lumbosacral junction.

Palpation

Palpation techniques allow the examiner to focus on the aspects of the athlete's injury that may result from specific bony, muscular, or soft-tissue–related pathology. Differentiating medial knee pain in the medial collateral ligament versus the pes anserinus, for example, guides other aspects of the examination.

Neurovascular Factors

A careful neurovascular examination will reveal potential neurologic contributions to the patient's problems. Thoracic outlet type pathology will often manifest with peripheral symptoms that can be traced to a central cause. Palpation and percussion will distinguish bony from ligamentous or musculotendinous pain generators.

Other Factors

A general physical examination will also provide clues to the nutritional status, hydration, and general health of the patient. Young women are particularly at risk due to the risks of eating disorders and athletic amenorrhea. The provider must be sensitive to the pressures and adaptive behaviors that can result in eating disorders. Psychological and secondary-gain issues frequently cloud the picture of sports injury and pain, especially in the adolescent athlete. When appropriate, the use of a counselor as part of the treatment process can be beneficial.

Dynamic Examination

"Kinetic chain" considerations are included in the dynamic examination phase of the assessment. In kinetic chain theory, when a limb or body segment is in contact with an immobile object (such as the floor), the chain of motion is described as "closed"; conversely, when there is no direct force against which the muscles work, the chain is "open."[3,4] Kinetic chain theory can be used to describe the methods through which movement occurs. Because parts of the body are links in the "chain," dysfunction at one level may affect adjacent or distal segments. For example, tight hip flexor muscles necessitate an increase in the lumbar lordosis when the person stands in order to maintain an upright position, thereby placing significant demands on the lumbar spine. Technique and form errors can be identified only if the patient is allowed to demonstrate the movement pattern in a minimally restrictive environment. Biomechanically inefficient and injurious movement patterns may only be found if the patient is observed walking, running, or lifting.

Injury acuity is manifested during this part of the examination, with movement patterns often helping to identify the cause of the patient's problems. An acute traumatic injury will preclude the patient from performing the desired movement and is associated with pain. Chronic overuse injuries allow the movement to be done, albeit with substitution and inefficient motion. Observation of the patient when fatigued will accentuate dynamic muscle weakness. Discouraged or depressed patients will exhibit body positions and facial expressions (if not overt emotions) that reveal their internal turmoil.

Included in the dynamic assessment is an evaluation of the patient's equipment, and if appropriate, the environment in which the activity takes place.

Case Examinations

Case 1: Auto Worker with Right Shoulder Pain

Static evaluation of this patient's scapular position with the arms at rest demonstrated that his right scapula was slightly depressed (Fig. 4-1A). With

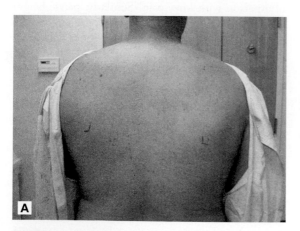 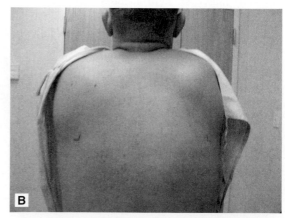

FIGURE 4-1 **A.** Static evaluation: With his arms at his sides, the right scapula is depressed compared to the left. **B.** Dynamic evaluation: With raising of the arms, the right scapula protects and elevates.

dynamic assessment, there was evidence of significant scapular protraction and elevation as compared to the unaffected side, indicative of a lack of scapular stability with resultant impingement (Fig. 4-1B). Weakness was noted in the scapular retractors, but there was no evidence of weakness in the serratus anterior. He had positive impingement findings that improved significantly when his scapula was manually corrected. His symptoms were virtually abolished with scapular taping.

Case 2: Female Runner with Shin Pain

On static examination, she demonstrated a valgus subtalar joint with the suggestion of internal rotation of the tibia. There was a mild lateral position to the patellae, but no significant knee valgus. There were no other postural deviations. Muscle strength was normal and neurovascular examination was unremarkable. There was point tenderness of the midshaft of the tibia on the right and at the distal tibia in the left. These areas demonstrated significant pain with vibration over the affected areas. With dynamic assessment, the patient demonstrated overpronation on gait evaluation. Her gait was apropulsive and worsened with increased gait speed from walking to running.

Case 3: Triathlete with Upper Extremity Weakness

Static examination demonstrated normal scapular position. Static posture was normal. Apprehension tests were positive. Impingement signs were positive. There was weakness noted in abduction and external rotation, graded as 4/5. All other muscles were normal with MMT. There were no sensory deficits. Dynamic examination showed altered swim-stroke mechanics with less elbow flexion prior to water entry using the affected limb. With further questioning, the patient related that he had discontinued using hand paddles during his swim workouts due to pain. His position on aerobars demonstrated no excessive forward flexion shoulder.

Case 4: High School Athlete with a "Pulled Hamstring"

Static examination demonstrated extremely well-developed quadriceps muscles bilaterally. There was mild swelling noted in the middle and proximal medial hamstrings. There was no discoloration or hematoma noted. Postural examination demonstrated no pelvic tilt or obliquity. There was tenderness noted in the medial hamstrings. Gross strength by manual muscle testing was normal in all muscles tested.

Range-of-motion assessment showed restricted hamstring, quadriceps, and hip flexor range. Neurovascular exam was unremarkable. Dynamic examination demonstrated weakness in both hamstrings with repeated eccentric loading in the prone position. There were no gross mechanical or technical faults noted with her sprinting position. Isokinetic dynamometry demonstrated a 5:1 strength imbalance between the quadriceps and hamstring muscles at 180 degrees per second (normal ratio is 3:2), suggesting a significant strength imbalance between the key muscles involved in her coming out of the block.

USING IMAGING MODALITIES TO SUPPLEMENT THE EXAMINATION

Increasingly, imaging modalities play an important role in evaluating the individual with a musculoskeletal injury. Bone scanning and Single photon emission computed tomography (SPECT) imaging can be used to assess the presence of stress fractures or spinal lesions.[5] Magnetic resonance imaging (MRI) scans allow imaging in areas otherwise not accessible to other imaging modalities.[6] The incorporation of arthrography can further enhance diagnostic accuracy. Ultrasound imaging is being used increasingly to evaluate disorders of tendons, bursae, and ligaments[7,8] at a lower cost than the other imaging modalities mentioned. Imaging modalities can provide an additional level of precision to the diagnostic assessment that is based on a sound history and clinical examination. Imaging cannot, however, serve as a replacement for a high-quality examination.

Case Imaging/Testing Results

Case 2: Female Runner with Shin Pain

Bone scan confirmed the presence of bilateral stress fractures in the tibiae (Fig. 4-2) in the location of the patient's tenderness on palpation and with vibration.[9,10]

Case 3: Triathlete with Upper Extremity Weakness

MRI demonstrated a tear in the glenoid labrum with a resultant cyst (Fig. 4-3) extending into the supra-scapular notch impinging on the suprascapular nerve.[11,12] Electromyographic (EMG) examination of the right shoulder girdle demonstrated significant denervation of the infraspinatus with all other muscles, including supraspinatus, demonstrating no abnormalities.

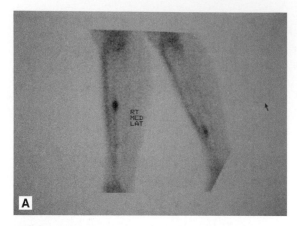
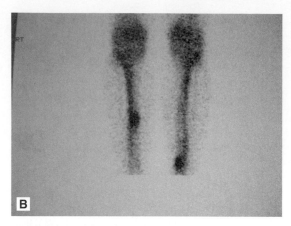

FIGURE 4-2 Bone scan confirms the presence of bilateral stress fractures in the tibiae, in the location of the patient's tenderness on palpation and with vibration. **A.** Lateral view. **B.** Anterior–posterior view.

TREATMENT PLANNING AND OUTCOMES

Treatment planning and implementation is based on the acuity of the condition and the abnormalities identified during the history and examination. In the acute situation, as shown in the fourth case, the application of RICE (rest, ice, compression, elevation) would be appropriate during the acute phase to reduce inflammation and hematoma formation, and to facilitate early healing. In subacute or more chronic

conditions, heat modalities such as superficial moist heat, ultrasound, and other modalities in combination with manual techniques may be of greater benefit to establish soft-tissue mobility and facilitate the healing process and the reestablishment of normal tissue characteristics.

Appropriate rehabilitation is a cornerstone of the sports medicine approach to the treatment of musculoskeletal disorders. Diagnosis-specific treatment results in improved outcomes and less downtime for the athlete. Rehabilitation progresses from the acute

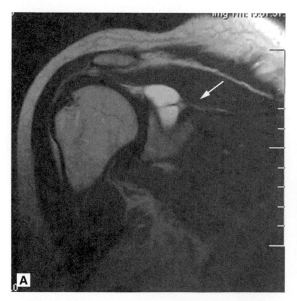
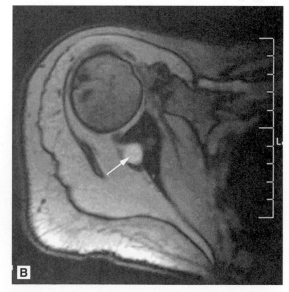

FIGURE 4-3 MRI demonstrated a tear in the glenoid labrum with a resultant cyst extending into the suprascapular notch impinging on the suprascapular nerve. **A.** Coronal T2 view demonstrating the cystic lesion. **B.** Axial T2 view of the lesion.

phase, where treatment is directed toward decreasing pain and inflammation and reestablishing range of motion, through functional progression with strength, balance, and function-specific activities.

In many cases, an athlete will be unable to return to all of their usual sports activity. Cross-training will often be utilized to return an athlete to sport sooner than would otherwise be possible. This is best illustrated by the second case, where the injured runner is progressed from water running, cycling, and elliptical training before returning to running. Cross-training allows the athlete to rest the injured area while still engaged in physical activity. This is sometimes called "relative rest," where the athlete continues with cardiovascular and training of the noninjured segments in the kinetic chain while resting the injured area.

The four cases used in this chapter have illustrated how accurate evaluation facilitates appropriate diagnosis and treatment. Each case is an example of the complexities associated with the evaluation and treatment of an individual with a sports or musculoskeletal disorder. The outcomes of these cases show how the sports medicine approach to musculoskeletal evaluation and treatment can result in an excellent outcome.

Case Outcomes

Case 1: Auto Worker with Right Shoulder Pain

The patient was evaluated diagnostically with scapular taping to stabilize the shoulder. He reported good results and was started on a scapular stabilization therapy program. He returned for reevaluation 3 weeks after initiation of treatment and reported an improvement in his pain complaints. By 6 weeks from the initiation of treatment, the patient reported that he was pain free and working at full capacity

Case 2: Female Runner with Shin Pain

The patient was instructed to ice the affected areas until her pain subsided. She discontinued running and initiated a nonweight-bearing, cross-training regimen with water running, swimming, and progression to elliptical training and bicycling. She was reexamined at 4 weeks and again at 8 weeks. She was nontender to palpation and demonstrated no vibratory tenderness. She returned to running in a gradual supervised manner. Based on the biomechanical alterations identified on the initial exam, she underwent diagnostic low-dye taping when she returned to running and noted a significant improvement in her

gait pattern and comfort level when running longer distances. She was prescribed foot orthotics and returned to all of her usual prefracture activities.

Case 3: Triathlete with Upper Extremity Weakness

Based on the MRI examination and the abnormalities identified on the EMG exam, the patient was recommended for surgical treatment with repair of the labrum and resection of the cyst. The patient was adamant about trying to race in an upcoming triathlon. To provide him with temporary benefit, the cyst was aspirated prior to the race, allowing him to participate. Two weeks following the triathlon he underwent surgical treatment, after which he initiated a therapy program to regain strength lost due to his neurologic deficit.

Case 4: High School Athlete with a "Pulled Hamstring"

The patient's acute hamstring injury was managed with ice, compression, and rest. Based on her isokinetic results and her dynamic assessment, she was initiated on a progressive strengthening program of her hamstring beginning with concentric activities progressing to eccentric loading. After 3 weeks, she began light running. After 4 weeks, she initiated sport-specific strengthening with special attention to her technique when coming out of the starting block. She was retested with isokinetic dynamometry and demonstrated a relative normalization of her quadriceps to hamstring ratio (3:1 ratio). She returned to racing and had an improvement of her sprint times. She was monitored for a 3-month period and had no recurrences.

REFERENCES

1. Nisell R. Mechanics of the knee: a study of joint and muscle load with clinical applications. *Acta Orthop Scand Suppl.* 1985;216:1–42.
2. Worrell TW, Perrin DH, Gansneder BM, et al. Comparisons of isokinetic strength and flexibility measures between hamstring injured and noninjured athletes. *J Orthop Sports Phys Ther.* 1991;13:118–125.
3. Crosier JL, Crielarrd JM. Causative factors in hamstring strains. *Med Sci Sports.* 2000;2:39–42.
4. Escamilla RF, Fleisig GS, Zheng N, et al. Biomechanics of the knee during closed kinetic chain and open kinetic chain exercises. *Med Sci Sports Exerc.* 1998;30:556–569.
5. Donohoe KJ. Selected topics in orthopedic nuclear medicine. *Orthop Clin North Am.* 1998;29:85–101.

6. Deutsch AL, Mink JH. Magnetic resonance imaging of musculoskeletal injuries. *Radiol Clin North Am.* 1989;27: 983–1002.

7. Kijowski R, De Smet AA. The role of ultrasound in the evaluation of sports medicine injuries of the upper extremity. *Clin Sports Med.* 2006;25:569–590.

8. Allen GM, Wilson DJ. Ultrasound in sports medicine—a critical evaluation. *Eur J Radiol.* 2007;62:79–85.

9. Young A, McAllister DR. Evaluation and treatment of tibial stress fractures. In: Kaeding CC, ed. *Clinics in Sports Medicine.* Elsevier, Philadelphia; 2006:117–128.

10. Scharf SC. The radionuclide bone scan in the evaluation of sports injuries. In: Freeman LM, ed. *Nuclear Medicine Annual.* Philadelphia: Lippincott-Raven; 1996:91–112.

11. Fritz RC, Helms CA, Steinbach LS, et al. Suprascapular nerve entrapment: evaluation with MR imaging. *Radiology.* 1992;182:437–441.

12. Cummins CA, Messer T, Nuber GW. Current concepts review: suprascapular nerve entrapment. *J Bone Joint Surg.* 2000;82:415–424.

Stretching and Injury Prevention

S tretching is an important component to any fitness or rehabilitation program. Its role in restoring and maintaining good joint range of motion, muscle strength, soft-tissue extensibility, balance, and coordination is supported by most clinicians. In our time of evidence-based medicine, however, there has been little good research supporting the "common sense" view that stretching has benefits. Some recent literature even reports that stretching prior to certain activities is not necessary, or may actually be detrimental. Media reports tend to jump to extremes, declaring that stretching is no longer recommended. Unfortunately, this could not be further from the truth. The actual truth about stretching is probably somewhere between the extremes reported in the media or advocated by fitness gurus. In the end, the public is left with a confusing message about stretching.

FUNCTIONAL ANATOMY

Approximately 40% of the human body by weight is made up of skeletal muscle.[1] Skeletal muscles are the muscles used to move our joints, support our bodies, transport us from one place to another, and move other objects. Each muscle is made up of many muscle cells, linked together through a variety of connective tissues. The individual muscle cells are thread-like, and may run the length of the entire muscle. Each muscle cell contains numerous subunits of myofibrils, which in turn contain the myofilaments actin and myosin. It is the movement of the actin myofilaments along the myosin myofilaments that uses energy and produces a muscle contraction (Fig. 5-1).[2]

Each individual muscle cell in a skeletal muscle is innervated by a motor nerve, often near the midpoint of the muscle. The nerve impulse spreads evenly away from the point of innervation, causing the muscle fiber to shorten along its length.[1] The strength of contraction depends upon the number of fibers activated. When a motor nerve sends a signal for a muscle fiber to contract, that individual fiber contracts with all of the force it is capable of producing at that moment. As greater strength is required, more muscle fibers are recruited, resulting in a stronger contraction. There are three types of muscle contractions: isometric—a static hold against equal resistance in which the muscle's length does not change; isotonic (or concentric)—an active, voluntary shortening of a muscle; and eccentric—an active, voluntary lengthening of a muscle.[2]

In order to modulate the forcefulness of a contraction, two specialized sensory organs exist in muscle tissue: the muscle spindle and the Golgi tendon organ. The muscle spindle is a group of 2 to 10 muscle fibers and is located in the muscle belly; it is primarily responsive to stretching and functions to sense length and rate of stretch in the muscle. The Golgi tendon organ is located in the musculotendinous junction; it is responsive to tendon tension and excessive stretching.[2] These receptors provide the central nervous system with information to control both movement and posture.[3]

CAUSES OF INJURY

Muscle injuries generally occur when the muscle tissue is working eccentrically within its normal range of motion or when it is exposed to a force that exceeds its strength. Common causes include excessive acceleration (or deceleration), poor body mechanics, or a combination of both.[4] Poor body mechanics contribute to problems when one group of muscles is strengthened excessively (such as from repetitive work tasks or sports

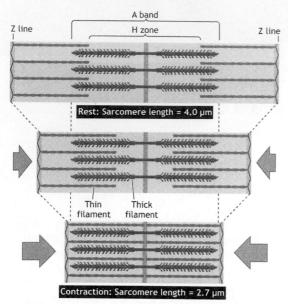

FIGURE 5-1 Muscle contraction. The basic unit of a muscle, the sarcomere, shortens as the actin (thin filaments) and myosin (thick filaments) move along each other. This shortening produces a muscle contraction. (From McArdle WD, Katch FI, Katch VL. *Exercise Physiology: Energy, Nutrition, and Human Performance.* 5th ed. Philadelphia: Lippincott Williams & Wilkins; 2001.)

motions), while the antagonistic muscles are held in a resting position for long periods of time. The resulting muscle imbalance can lead to poor posture, decreased range of motion, or even injury. The upper back/posterior shoulder girdle musculature, low back, thighs, and calves are commonly affected.

Muscle and tendon overuse also contributes to injury. Each sport has stereotypical movements that predispose the athlete to develop wear-and-tear injuries. It is beyond the scope of this chapter to describe the mechanisms for each of these injuries. The reader is referred to the chapter regarding the specific sport in question for further information.

RECOMMENDATIONS FOR STRETCHING

Stretching warrants consideration and implementation for the majority of the population at large. It is a simple way to restore and maintain good range of motion in our joints and extensibility in the muscles and connective tissues. Stretching protects our joints from excessive wear and tear by balancing the muscle

forces around the joints. Achieving and maintaining good postural alignment and negating the effects of prolonged positioning or excessive repetitive movements are also benefits. Stretching helps prepare the body for activity by increasing blood flow to the area and warming the muscles.[5] For all of these reasons, stretching—including warm-up and cool-down exercises—is generally accepted as promoting better performance and decreasing the number of injuries.[6]

The current literature supports stretching for several sports or activities, including football, tennis, soccer, volleyball, basketball, and gymnastics. The common features of these fast-moving sports include sudden changes in direction and jumping.[6] A stretching program should be a part of the general conditioning program and the precompetition warm-up periods of these sports.

Activities that produce less shock to the muscle, such as swimming, jogging, or cycling, seem to be helped less by stretching just prior to the activity. It appears that in these sports, muscles perform more efficiently when "tighter."[6] Stretching before an activity that requires strength (such as weight lifting) is not advantageous; stretching can cause a reduction of strength or force-generating power for nearly an hour poststretch. Even though stretching is not recommended just prior to these activities, a long-term general stretching program has been shown to be of benefit and is recommended. Also, stretching after exercise may be an alternative.

Stretching is easy to do. However, it needs to be performed with proper techniques; in some cases, instruction from a qualified professional may be of benefit. One should include a thorough evaluation of the musculoskeletal system prior to recommending a program.

Some basic rules to follow when stretching include:

1. Isolate a specific muscle.
2. Take the muscle to a comfortable pull without eliciting pain.
3. Hold the stretched position for 15 to 30 seconds statically (avoid ballistic or bouncing stretches).[7,8]
4. Perform the entire stretching routine on a regular basis. This may vary from once a day to periodically throughout the day.

A GENERAL STRETCHING PROGRAM

For each of the sports covered in this book, there are specific stretches that may be necessary, such as for the shoulder in baseball pitchers. It is beyond the

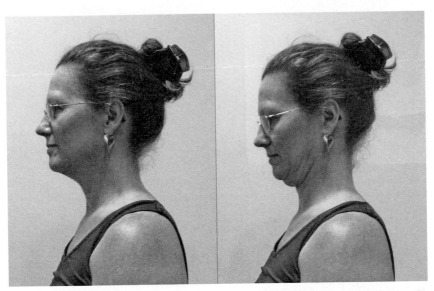

FIGURE 5-2 Suboccipital stretch. Sit upright, with good posture, and perform a small, downward nod, as shown on the right.

scope of this chapter to address all of these stretches. However, there are a number of areas that tend to be problematic for both athletes and the population in general that may be aided by proper stretching. The following stretches represent a good general stretching program that would be appropriate for the majority of subjects.

Suboccipital Region

An area of tightness that many people have is a forward-head posture. This often results from wearing multiple-vision glasses, where the user moves the head and neck to frame the desired field of view in the appropriate lens. This condition may also be associated with prolonged sitting or with working overhead. A stretch to counter this tightness is to sit in a good, erect position and perform a small downward nod (Fig. 5-2).

Upper Quarters

The shoulders, arms, anterior torso, and posterior torso tend to become rounded forward with prolonged reaching, such as with typing or driving. Large-breasted women may have a similar problem. In these situations, the biceps/chest stretch may be of benefit. It stretches multiple structures, including the proximal biceps, pectoralis major, and to some degree, the pectoralis minor. The execution of the stretch is shown in Figure 5-3.

Rib Cage

When the sternum is depressed, the thoracic spine is in a more kyphotic position. This posturing may be subsequent to a birth defect, a sternal injury, early breast

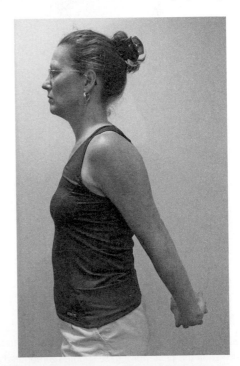

FIGURE 5-3 Biceps/chest stretch. This position stretches the proximal biceps and pectoralis muscles.

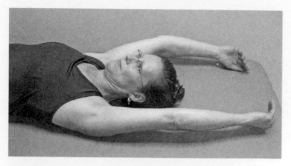

FIGURE 5-4 Latissimus dorsi stretch. This stretch is helpful for posterior shoulder and upper back pain.

stretch may be of benefit in this case as well. However, a muscle group often missed in a stretching program is the latissimus dorsi. Placing the arms overhead while laying supine stretches the latissimus dorsi effectively, as shown in Figure 5-4.

Lumbar Spine and Pelvis

Several dysfunctions common to the pelvis affect the curvature of the lumbar spine. An anteriorly tipped pelvis increases the lumbar lordosis; this could be the result of tightened hip flexors or lumbar paraspinal muscles. A posteriorly tipped pelvis leads to a flattened or reversed lordosis; this could be the result of tight abdominal muscles, gluteus maximus, or hamstring muscles. Good stretches to address these problems are hip flexor and superior quadriceps stretches. One must determine the areas with the greatest tightness to choose the proper stretches. For the iliopsoas and superior quadriceps, backward bending in a standing position is

development, or work in a bent-over position. Swimmers and runners may also exhibit this particular postural malalignment. This position can result in upper shoulder and back pain, periscapular pain, paraspinal pain, and can even adversely affect lung function. The biceps/chest

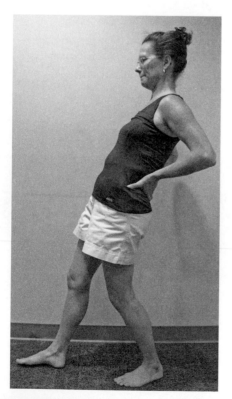

FIGURE 5-5 Iliopsoas and proximal quadriceps stretch. This stretches the posterior leg, so should be repeated for each side.

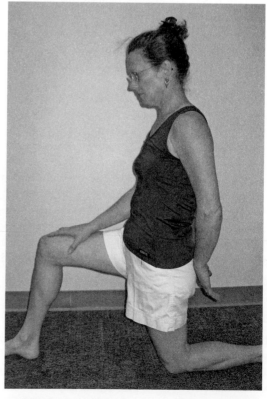

FIGURE 5-6 Distal quadriceps stretch. Bear weight on the knee and gently extend at the hip.

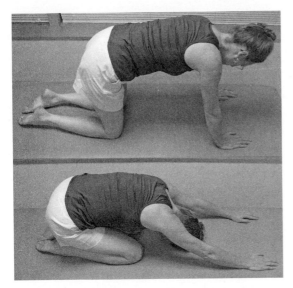

FIGURE 5-7 Quadruped stretch. The spine is kept in a neutral position in this stretch.

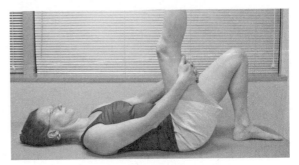

FIGURE 5-9 Hamstring stretch. Either the hands or a towel or belt may be used to hold the thigh in the position of stretch.

beneficial (Fig. 5-5). To stretch the more distal aspect of the quadriceps muscle, assume a half-kneel position and bear weight on the stretching-side knee (Fig. 5-6). The quadruped (all fours) position stretches multiple areas of the lower quarter by moving the buttocks backward towards the feet, keeping the spine in a neutral position (Fig. 5-7); this stretch may be beneficial for upper spine tightness as well. A good stretch for the

abdominal muscles is bending backward—while either sitting or standing—and maintaining a neutral position of the cervical spine (Fig. 5-8).

The hamstrings are muscles that can tighten up very easily, as is seen in vocations that require constant sitting, such as clerical workers and over-the-road truck drivers. Stretching while in the supine position allows the lumbar spine to remain in a neutral position. The leg to be stretched is held in 90 degrees of flexion at the hip with a towel or belt held around the thigh (the contralateral hip and knee are flexed), as shown in Figure 5-9. The stretch is then imposed by extending the raised knee to a comfortable pull. This stretch can be advanced to a standing position if the subject has good lumbar spine control.

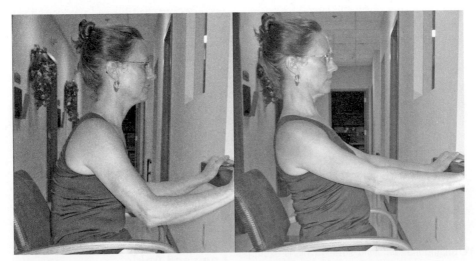

FIGURE 5-8 Abdominal stretch. This can be performed while sitting or standing. The cervical spine is held in a neutral position.

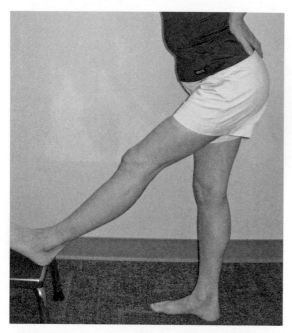

FIGURE 5-10 Standing hamstring stretch. The height of the stretch can be increased as tolerated. The hands may be placed on the back to keep the spine neutral.

The position of the stretched leg is dependent upon the person's flexibility, with the heel placed on a curb, step, or stool; the subject leans forward as demonstrated in Figure 5-10.

The iliotibial band is a massive tendon originating at the inferior iliac crest, where it envelops tensor fascia latae, and traversing down the lateral femur to insert on the lateral tibial plateau. The thick nature of the tissue makes it very difficult to stretch. When this

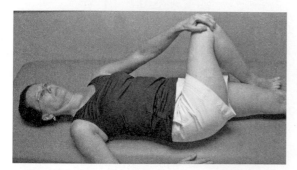

FIGURE 5-11 Supine iliotibial band stretch. This is useful when pelvic stability issues are present; the supine position stabilizes the pelvis.

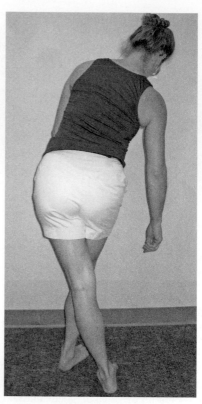

FIGURE 5-12 Standing iliotibial band stretch. In this example, to stretch the left side, cross the right leg over the left leg, then lean to the right.

structure tightens, it is usually the result of an overuse syndrome or prolonged positioning. The band becomes very painful and tender and can cause biomechanical problems either proximally or distally. With the proximal attachment on the inferior iliac crest, the sacroiliac joint can be affected by an iliotibial band syndrome. If pelvic instability issues are present, it is best to start stretching the iliotibial band in the supine position (Fig. 5-11). If pelvic symmetry and stability issues have been resolved or are not present, the iliotibial band may be stretched while standing. The stretch, shown in Figure 5-12, is performed by crossing the contralateral leg over the stretching-side leg, and then leaning away from the stretching side (for example, to stretch the left hip, cross the right leg over the left, then lean to the right).

Knee and Ankle

Tightness in the quadriceps may be associated with knee pain. When pain with squatting or stair climbing

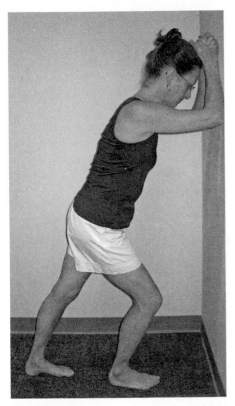

FIGURE 5-13 Gastroc-soleus stretch. The left calf is being stretched in the figure. To focus more on the soleus muscle, bend the knee of the stretching leg.

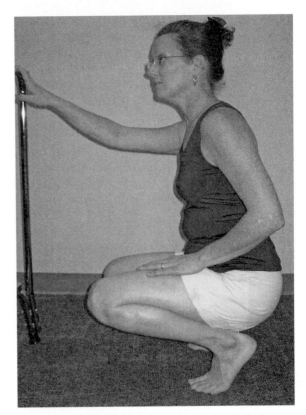

FIGURE 5-14 Foot stretch.

is present, quadriceps stretching (Figs. 5-5 and 5-6) may be of benefit. Tight hamstrings, in conjunction with the iliotibial band, may limit the excursion of the lower leg during walking and stair climbing; the stretches shown in Figures 5-9 to 5-12 may be helpful.

Gastrocnemius-soleus tightness might interfere with smooth stair descending. This tightness may be due to wearing heels or from being debilitated for an extended period; asymmetric tightness may be due to driving. Figure 5-13 illustrates a helpful stretch for this problem. Performing the same stretch with the knee bent will relax the gastrocnemius and allow the stretch to focus on the soleus. Finally, a foot stretch (Fig. 5-14) may be of benefit in these conditions, or in those with foot pain.

Forearms

Typing extensively places the arms in a single position for long periods of time. Other vocations or hobbies also involve a great deal of gripping, prolonged

positioning, and repetitive motions. To stretch the forearm flexor masses bilaterally, interlock the fingers and turn the hands palm-out from the body (Fig. 5-15). For Dupuytren's contractures, one may sit on the hands.

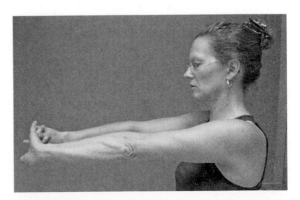

FIGURE 5-15 Forearm flexor stretch. Interlock the fingers and turn the hands palm-out.

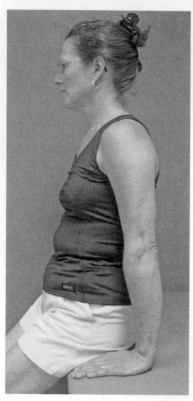

FIGURE 5-16 Epicondylitis stretch. Hyperextend the wrist for medial epicondylitis stretch; hyperflex the wrist for lateral epicondylitis stretch.

For medial epicondylitis symptoms, the shoulder is internally rotated (elbow turned outward) and the wrist is hyperextended; for symptoms of lateral epicondylitis, the wrist is hyperflexed (Fig. 5-16).

CONCLUSION

Regular stretching is good for us. It takes us out of prolonged positioning, it restores good muscle balance around joints, it gets our blood pumping to the tissues we are about to put into action, and it just makes us feel good.

For the majority of athletes, a regular stretching program can be of benefit. It must be kept in mind that in certain sports, such as weight lifting, stretching immediately before competition may be detrimental to performance.

REFERENCES

1. Guyton AC. *Human Physiology and Mechanisms of Disease.* 4th ed. Philadelphia: Saunders; 1987.
2. Jenkins DB. *Hollinshead's Functional Anatomy of the Limbs and Back.* 8th ed. Philadelphia: Saunders; 2002.
3. Barr ML, Kiernan JA. *The Human Nervous System: An Anatomical Viewpoint.* 5th ed. Philadelphia: Lippincott; 1988.
4. Baye D. Is it necessary to warm up for resistance training? Available at: http://www.baye.com/articles/warm_up.php. Accessed August 14, 2007.
5. Martin BJ, Robinson S, Wiegman DL, et al. Effect of warm-up on metabolic responses to strenuous exercise. *Med Sci Sports.* 1975;7:146–149.
6. Witvrouw E, Mahieu N, Roosen P. The role of stretching in tendon injuries. *Br J Sports Med.* 2007;41:224–226.
7. Lazarus K. To stretch or not to stretch. Available at: http://www.losalamosfitness.com/articles/To%20Stretch%20or%20not%20to%20Stretch.pdf. Accessed August 14, 2007.
8. Renne D. The importance of timing your flexibility training. Available at: http://www.fingerlakesrunningcompany.com/retail/common/community/article.asp?id=398. Accessed August 14, 2007.

Performance-Enhancing Sports Supplements

H undreds of nutritional supplements are marketed to improve athletic performance. It is estimated that dietary supplement sales in the United States exceed $20 billion annually.[1] These products are available in pharmacies, nutrition stores, gyms, and from numerous online retailers. In an attempt to gain a competitive advantage, many athletes not only use these products but also believe that the majority of their competitors are using such supplements.[2] At the 2000 Sydney Olympics, 78% of the athletes reported using supplements.[3] As the use of supplements continues to increase with athletes of all levels, it is also a growing and controversial area of sports medicine.

The federal government classifies a supplement as a product (other than tobacco) intended to supplement the diet, which contains one or more of the following: vitamins, minerals, herbs or other botanicals, amino acids, or any combination of these ingredients. By definition, supplements are substances that are not subject to Food and Drug Administration (FDA) regulation and therefore available without a prescription. The National Center of Complementary and Alternative Medicine (NCCAM) reports that studies of "herbal supplements have found differences between what's listed on the label and what's in the bottle. This means that one may be taking less— or more—of the supplement than what the label indicates." Because the federal government does not scrutinize supplements like it does prescription medications, there is more room for false claims and threats to safety.

So-called "doping" in sports involves the use of drugs that are banned by organizations that regulate competition, most famously, the International Olympic Committee. Examples include erythropoietin, steroids, and newer "gene doping." This subject is beyond the scope of this chapter, and the reader is

referred to http://www.wada-ama.org for more information.[4] This chapter will address those supplements most commonly claimed to be ergogenic aids. Due to the lack of regulation and scrutiny, there is often minimal data to support the numerous claims of performance benefit made by the manufacturers of many of these products. This list is not exhaustive, as new products are continually being introduced, but is meant to provide an overview of the most commonly used categories of products.

SYMPATHOMIMETICS

Sympathomimetics are substances that mimic the effects of the hormones epinephrine and the hormone/neurotransmitter norepinephrine. These drugs have not been consistently shown to be performance enhancing but are often used in attempts to increase mental alertness and energy. Pseudoephedrine (Sudafed), commonly used for the treatment of sinus congestion, is the archetypical and most commonly used supplement in this class. Bell showed that ingesting 0.8 to 1 mg/kg of pseudoephedrine 1.5 hours prior to activity improved cycling power output[5] and pace in a 10K run.[6] However, many other trials contradict theses findings, and have not shown such performance benefits.[7–10]

Pseudoephedrine is a chemical precursor in the illicit manufacture of methamphetamine and methcathinone, and many pharmaceutical firms have reformulated medications to use alternative decongestants. Federal policies also restrict sales of pseudoephedrine by limiting purchase quantities and requiring a minimum age with proper identification. There are several other commonly used sympathomimetics, including phenylephrine, pyclopentamine, and propylhexedrin, but there are few studies evaluating their ergogenic effects. The primary side effects of these substances are anxiety, agitation, headaches, elevated blood pressure, and cardiac arrhythmias.[7,8,10,11] The herbals ephedra and Ma Huang have similar structural properties and physiologic effects to pseudoephedrine. Sales of supplements containing these substances were banned by the FDA in April 2004 and should be avoided due to concern of adverse cardiovascular effects and even death.[12,13]

Ephedrine is a sympathomimetic and increases catecholamine levels in the brain and cardiovascular system. It was used initially to treat asthma and allergic rhinitis, but later found to promote weight loss, as common effects include bronchodilation, tachycardia, vasoconstriction, transient hypertension, nervousness, insomnia, appetite suppression, and headache.[12] Indeed, ephedrine was also shown to produce a two- to threefold increase in psychiatric and autonomic symptoms, including heart palpitations.[12]

CAFFEINE

Caffeine, as a member of the dimethylxanthine family, functions as an adenosine receptor antagonist with stimulant properties. Several studies, as reported by Graham, show caffeine to increase speed and/or power output in activities that last as little as 60 seconds or as long as 2 hours.[14] This effect has been associated with stimulation of the central nervous system and enhanced peripheral neuromuscular transmission and muscle contractility, although the exact mechanism is not completely understood. An increase in overall catecholamine levels has also been seen. There is less information about the effects of caffeine on strength, but it has been shown to favorably impact peak torque generated by the leg extensors and flexors.[15]

Numerous supplement companies have created products to capitalize on these properties and have used caffeine in combination with other supplements. One of the most promising supplement combinations was that of caffeine and ephedrine. Bell et al. found that supplementation with 5 mg/kg of caffeine along with 1 mg/kg of ephedrine could increase time to exhaustion due to exercise by 38% and improve anaerobic performance in untrained males.[16] Jacobs et al. studied the effect of 4 mg/kg of caffeine and 0.8 mg/kg of ephedrine on muscular endurance.[17] The study concluded that the combination of caffeine and ephedrine increased the number of repetitions and the total amount of weight lifted. It is important to note that in these studies, *caffeine supplementation alone was unable to produce any performance benefit,* and that *ephedrine use as a supplement is illegal* in the United States.

Adverse events seen with caffeine use are nausea, heart palpitations, headache, and muscle tension. Caffeine may behave as a mild diuretic, but no studies have shown a clear increased risk for dehydration.[18]

PROTEIN

Because skeletal muscle is composed primarily of protein, conventional wisdom holds that ingesting increased quantities of protein should increase the potential for building muscle. The U.S. Recommended Daily Allowance (RDA) for Dietary Reference Intakes for Energy, Carbohydrate, Fiber, Fat, Fatty Acids, Cholesterol, Protein, and Amino Acids (2002) recommends 46 g of protein daily for healthy males over the age of 18. This equates to about 0.65 g/kg for the average 70-kg male. This is even less than the 1989 RDA of 0.8 g/kg. Athletes, however, have traditionally been assumed to need significantly more protein than the average individual. Lemon et al. calculated the daily protein requirement of athletes to be 1.4 to 1.8 g/kg lean mass/day in order to maintain a positive nitrogen balance.[19,20] Despite the fact that these studies showed no difference in strength gains by maintaining a positive nitrogen balance, many athletes continue to use protein supplements based on this data.

An increased incidence of kidney stones and gout has been reported with high-protein diets and the cost of protein supplements can be prohibitive. Without evidence of performance benefit from supplementation, it may be wise to recommend a healthy, balanced diet as the only source of protein.

BRANCHED-CHAIN AMINO ACIDS

The branched-chain amino acids leucine, isoleucine, and valine—which are particularly high in concentration in skeletal muscle—are frequently promoted as ergogenic when supplemented in high quantities. However, no well-designed study has yet shown that branched-chain amino acid supplementation enhances performance.

L-CARNITINE

Carnitine is a quaternary amine whose physiologically active form is β-hydroxy-γ-trimethylammonium butyrate. This is found in meats and dairy products and is synthesized in the liver and kidneys from the essential amino acids, lysine and methionine. L-carnitine (the D-isomer is physiologically inactive) is thought to be ergogenic in two ways. First, by increasing free fatty acid transport across mitochondrial membranes, carnitine may increase fatty acid oxidation and utilization for energy, thus sparing muscle glycogen. Second, by buffering pyruvate, and thus reducing muscle lactate accumulation associated with fatigue, carnitine is proposed to prolong exercise tolerance. Despite these proposed mechanisms, Colombani et al. have shown that L-carnitine supplementation does not affect the metabolism or improve physical performance of endurance-trained athletes and does not alter their recovery.[21]

L-TRYPTOPHAN

L-tryptophan is an essential amino acid and has become popular as a supplement due to a theoretical mechanism by which it increases serotonin levels in the brain, thereby reducing the discomfort of prolonged muscular effort and delaying fatigue. One study in 1988 by Segura and Ventura[22] demonstrated a 49% increase in total exercise time to exhaustion when subjects ingested a total of 1.2 g of L-tryptophan (four 300-mg doses within 24 hours of exercise) versus placebo. Studies attempting to replicate these results, however, have shown no ergogenic effect of L-tryptophan.[23,24]

L-tryptophan supplementation has been linked to multiple cases of eosinophilia myalgia syndrome and 32 deaths.[25] Though these cases were probably due to contamination of an L-tryptophan produced by a single manufacturer, and not to the amino acid itself, they illustrate the concern of quality and purity of unregulated supplements.

HMB

β-hydroxy β-methylbutyric acid (HMB) is synthesized naturally from the amino acid leucine, which is found in high concentrations in muscles. During weight training and prolonged exercise, muscle damage leads to the breakdown of leucine and a resulting increase in HMB. It is proposed that high HMB levels decrease protein catabolism via a negative feedback mechanism, thereby creating a net anabolic effect.

Limited research seems to suggest that supplementation with HMB may increase muscle mass and strength. Nissen et al. have conducted randomized, double-blind, placebo-controlled studies[26,27] as well as a meta-analysis[28] to evaluate the ergogenic potential of HMB. In these studies, subjects receiving HMB supplements (1.5 or 3g/day) showed significant improvements in muscle mass, one-repetition maximum bench press, and percent body fat as well as significant decreases in muscle breakdown products (3-methylhistidine and creatine phosphokinase) when compared to placebo subjects. There are no currently reported side effects of HMB, but further studies are needed to adequately evaluate its safety.

CREATINE

Creatine (Cr) is produced endogenously by the liver from the amino acids L-arginine, glycine, and L-methionine or ingested from exogenous sources such as meat and fish (Fig. 6-1). Almost all the Cr in the body is located in skeletal muscle in either the free (Cr: ~40%) or phosphorylated (PCr: ~60%) form and represents an average Cr pool of about 120 to 140 g for an average 70-kg person. Taking creatine supplements is believed to increase the supply of phospohocreatine in muscles. It is hypothesized that Cr can act through a number of possible mechanisms as a potential ergogenic aid, but it appears to be most effective for activities that involve repeated short bouts of high-intensity physical activity.

Additionally, investigators have studied a number of different Cr loading programs; the most common program involves an initial loading phase of 20 g/day for 5 to 7 days, followed by a maintenance phase of 3 to 5 g/day for differing periods of time (1 week to 6 months). Absorption into muscles is thought to be enhanced when creatine is taken with a simple carbohydrate. Many manufacturers claim that their proprietary blend results in superior uptake into muscles, but there is a lack of published studies to validate these claims.

Numerous well-designed studies have demonstrated that creatine supplementation has an ergogenic

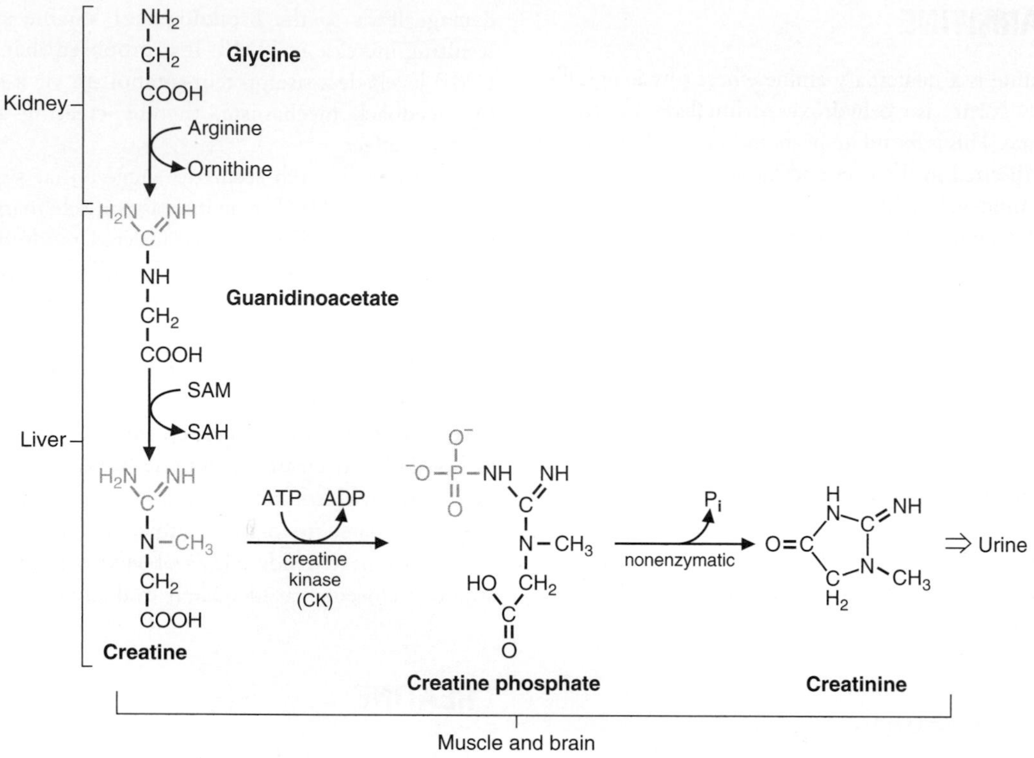

FIGURE 6-1 Creatine synthesis. Cr is produced endogenously by the liver from amino acids or ingested from exogenous sources such as meat and fish and excreted in the urine. (From Swanson TA, Kim SI, Glucksman MJ. *Biochemistry and Molecular Biology*. 4th ed. Baltimore: Lippincott Williams & Wilkins; 2007.)

potential. When measuring maximal force or strength, it generally appears that Cr does significantly impact force production regardless of sport, sex, or age.[29] Studies of endurance activities such as marathon running and swimming have not shown as strong benefits. Concomitant use of caffeine may block the effects of creatine.[30] There appears to be no strong scientific evidence to support any adverse effects, but it should be noted that there have been no studies to date that address the issue of long-term Cr usage.

NITRIC OXIDE

Biologically, nitric oxide (NO) has been shown to be important in a number of cellular communication processes and in the immune response. It is synthesized from the amino acid arginine (Fig. 6-2). NO has been the topic of many studies regarding its therapeutic benefit in cardiac patients, and supplementation with arginine has been shown to enhance exercise capacity in patients with stable angina.[31] More recent studies, focused on arginine supplementation in healthy individuals, have shown improved resistance to muscular fatigue as well as significantly lower blood lactate and ammonia levels after exercise.[32] Side effects of arginine, or NO, include dyspepsia and headaches.

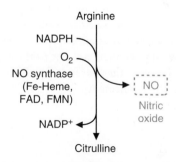

FIGURE 6-2 Nitric oxide synthesis from arginine. (From Swanson TA, Kim SI, Glucksman MJ. *Biochemistry and Molecular Biology*. 4th ed. Baltimore: Lippincott Williams & Wilkins; 2007.)

VITAMIN C

Very intense exercise, such as training for or running a marathon, can temporarily suppress immune function by slightly impairing the production of white blood cells. This may explain why 50% to 70% of athletes report upper respiratory infection symptoms in the second week after a marathon.[33] Taking vitamin C prior to intense exercise may help to prevent colds. Although not all studies agree, a subgroup of six studies of marathon runners, skiers, and soldiers exposed to significant cold and/or physical stress experienced, on average, a 50% reduction in common cold incidence with vitamin C supplementation.[34]

Vitamin C supplementation has not been shown to influence muscle recovery postexercise.[35] The dosage of vitamin C used in the studies ranges from 600 to 2,000 mg per day. For adults, the recommended tolerable upper intake level is 2,000 mg per day. Side effects include dyspepsia and an increased risk of kidney stones, and in very high doses of 5,000 mg per day there have been reports of male infertility. Chewable vitamin C supplements should be avoided, as their ascorbic acid can be caustic to teeth and erode enamel over time.

CHROMIUM PICOLINATE

Chromium is an essential trace mineral present in various foods, such as mushrooms, prunes, nuts, whole grain breads, and cereals. A normal American diet contains 50% to 60% of the RDA of chromium.[36] It has an extremely low gastrointestinal (GI) absorption rate, so supplement manufacturers have bound chromium with picolinate (CrPic) to increase the absorption and bioavailability.

Chromium supplementation became popular after it was found that exercise increases chromium loss, raising the concern that chromium deficiency may be common among athletes. Chromium seems to function as a cofactor that enhances the action of insulin, especially in carbohydrate, fat, and protein metabolism. Promoters of CrPic claim that it increases glycogen synthesis, improves glucose tolerance and lipid profiles, and increases amino acid incorporation in muscle.

Initial studies suggesting CrPic supplementation has an ergogenic effect have been shown to be flawed.[37] More recent studies by Clancy et al.[38] and Hallmark et al.[39] failed to demonstrate any significant improvement in percent body fat, lean body mass, or strength. Most studies of CrPic supplementation reveal no side effects except GI upset with dosages of 50 to 200 μg/day for less than 1 month. However, with CrPic ingestion at increased dosages and/or durations, there have been anecdotal reports of serious adverse effects including anemia, cognitive impairment, and interstitial nephritis.[37]

PYRUVATE (DIHYDROXYACETONE PYRUVATE, DHAP)

Pyruvate supplements have become popular with bodybuilders because it is believed that pyruvate can reduce body fat and enhance energy. Pyruvate supplies the body with pyruvic acid, which is a natural compound involved in energy metabolism (Fig. 6-3). Preliminary research suggested that pyruvate can help with weight loss and improve the capacity for endurance exercise.[40,41]

Pyruvate is not an essential nutrient, which means that the body can make all that it needs without supplementation. Morrison et al. have shown that oral pyruvate supplementation does not increase blood pyruvate content and does not enhance performance.[42] Side effects of pyruvate include stomach upset and diarrhea.

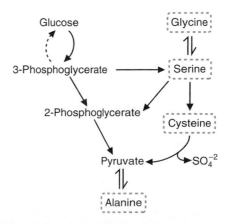

FIGURE 6-3 Pyruvate synthesis and its involvement in energy metabolism. (From Swanson TA, Kim SI, Glucksman MJ. *Biochemistry and Molecular Biology.* 4th ed. Baltimore: Lippincott Williams & Wilkins; 2007.)

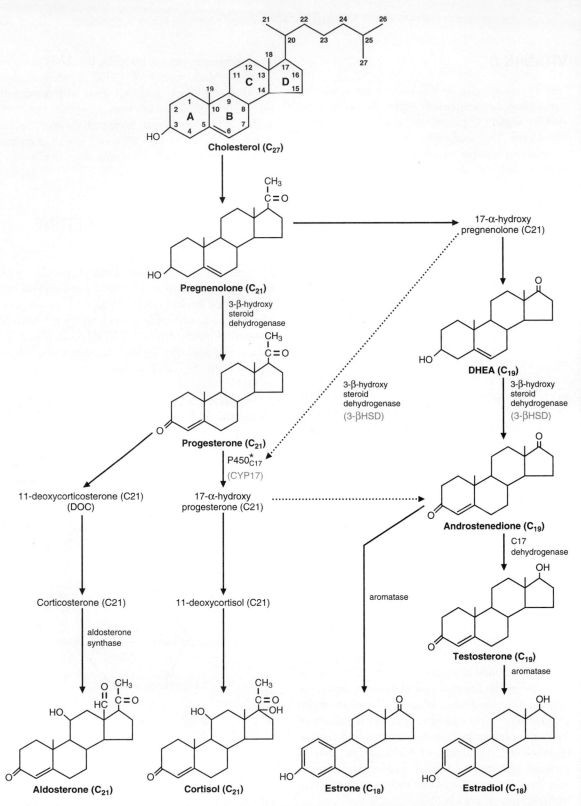

FIGURE 6-4 Androstenedione and dehydroepiandrosterone (DHEA) production. Note that cholesterol is involved in the production of both of these substances. (From Swanson TA, Kim SI, Glucksman MJ. *Biochemistry and Molecular Biology*. 4th ed. Baltimore: Lippincott Williams & Wilkins; 2007.)

RIBOSE

Ribose is used in the body as a precursor for making ATP molecules, as well as proteins, DNA, RNA, and other nucleotides. Some manufacturers claim that as a dietary supplement ingredient, ribose leads to increased ATP production and energy levels. Clinical trials have failed to substantiate these claims or show any improvement in performance with supplementation.[43,44] Some individuals taking high doses of ribose developed minor cases of diarrhea, while others had occasional mild and asymptomatic hypoglycemia.

GINSENG

A widely used alternative medicine worldwide, ginseng has been shown to have antioxidant and anti-inflammatory properties. Additionally, it has been claimed to improve mental alertness and athletic performance. Well-controlled studies to support these claims are not found in the literature.[45] Usual doses are 200 to 400 mg/day, but products may contain extract from one or several of many different plant species that contain ginsenosides. Side effects including nausea, headache, hypertension, and vaginal bleeding have been reported. Ginseng may also interact with warfarin, phenylzine, oral hypoglycemics, insulin, and caffeine, and should be used with caution.

ANDROSTENEDIONE

Androstenedione originates either from the conversion of dehydroepiandrosterone or from 17-hydroxyprogesterone, where it is further converted to either testosterone or estrone (Fig. 6-4). Despite studies showing that androstenedione supplementation does not produce significant changes in muscle mass or strength,[46,47] it was once a commonly used and quite popular supplement. However, in April 2004 the FDA banned the sale of androstenedione, citing that the drug poses significant health risks commonly associated with steroids.

DHEA

Dehydroepiandrosterone (DHEA), is a natural steroid prohormone produced from cholesterol in the adrenal glands, gonads, adipose tissue, brain, and skin. DHEA is the precursor of androstenedione, which can undergo further conversion to produce the androgen testosterone and the estrogens estrone and estradiol (Fig. 6-4). Several studies have confirmed the positive effects of DHEA administration in healthy elderly people, mostly aged > 70 years. Improvements in skin, bone density, and neuropsychological effects have been seen, including increased libido, sexual satisfaction, and patients' sense of well-being.[48] It is marketed as an agent that increases testosterone levels and lean body mass, despite a randomized placebo-controlled trial that found DHEA supplementation had no effect on lean body mass, strength, or testosterone levels.[47]

DHEA has been reported to have a multitude of side effects including hair loss and gynecomastia in men, virilization and menstral irregularities in women, as well as increased risk of ovarian, breast, and prostate cancer. However, a Cochrane database systematic review in 2006 showed there is no consistent evidence from the controlled trials that DHEA produces any of these adverse effects.[49]

CONCLUSION

Nutritional supplements can be marketed without FDA approval, which leads to many questions about product purity, safety, and efficacy. They come in many forms including herbals, sympathomimetics, hormone precursors, protein and amino acid derivatives, vitamin, minerals, and nutrients. Athletes who choose to ingest them need to understand the lack of evidence to support the performance-enhancing benefits for many supplements. Supplements are often marketed with unsubstantiated or exaggerated claims, and athletes may risk making decisions based on hearsay or incomplete information. Side effects are common for many supplements, and interaction with other medications is always a risk. Understanding the true impact and risk of any performance-enhancing substance is the key to safe use.

TABLE 6-1   Sympathomimetics/Stimulants

Supplement	Usual Dose	Advertised Benefits	Results of Scientific Studies	Side Effects
Ephedra/ephedrine/ Ma Huang	1 mg/kg	Increase energy and mental alertness	Increased endurance and strength; synergistic effects with caffeine	Illegal in United States due to adverse cardiovascular effects
Pseudoephedine	0.8–1 mg/kg		Some evidence for increased power output	Anxiety, agitation, headaches, minimal increase in blood pressure, cardiac arrhythmias
Caffeine	4–5 mg/kg	Increase energy and mental alertness	Some evidence for increased speed power and strength; possibly synergistic with ephedrine	Nausea, palpitations, headache, muscle tension
Ginseng	200–400 mg/day	Increased energy levels	No ergogenic effect	Nausea, headaches, hypertension, vaginal bleeding; interacts with several prescription medications

TABLE 6-2   Protein, Amino Acids, and Derivatives

Supplement	Usual Dose	Advertised Benefits	Results of Scientific Studies	Side Effects
Protein	1.4–1.8 g/kg	Muscle growth	No evidence for increased muscle size or strength with amounts greater than USRDA	Gout, kidney stones
Branched-chain amino acids	40–80 g/day	Muscle growth	No ergogenic effect	None reported
L-carnitine	2–4 g/day	Prolong exercise tolerance	Does not affect metabolism or improve performance	Palpitations, dyspepsia
L-tryptophan	1.2 g/day	Prolong exercise tolerance	One study showed benefit but has not been able to be replicated	Eosinophilia myalgia syndrome
HMB	1.5–3 g/day	Increase lean mass and strength	Increased lean mass and strength	None reported
Creatine	20 g/day for 5–7 days; then 3–5 g/day	Increase muscle mass and strength	Increased force production	None reported
Arginine (Nitric Oxide)	3–9 g/day	Increase muscle size, strength, endurance	Increased exercise capacity in patients with stable angina; some studies show increased endurance in healthy individuals	Dyspepsia, headaches

| TABLE 6-3 | **Vitamins, Minerals, and Nutrients** | | | |

Supplement	Usual Dose	Advertised Benefits	Results of Scientific Studies	Side Effects
Vitamin C	600–2,000 mg/day	Improved postexercise recovery	Decreased incidence of upper respiratory infection (URI) symptoms after significant physical stress	Dyspepsia, increased incidence of kidney stones
Chromium picolinate	50–200 µg/day	Increased lean mass and strength	No ergogenic effect	Aecdotal reports of anemia, cognitive impairment, interstitial nephritis
Pyruvate	7–25 g/day	Weight loss and increased endurance	No ergogenic effect	
Ribose	9–12 g/day	Increased energy levels	No ergogenic effect	Diarrhea, hypoglycemia

| TABLE 6-4 | **Hormone Precursors** | | | |

Supplement	Usual Dose	Advertised Benefits	Results of Scientific Studies	Side Effects
Androstenedione		Increase muscle mass, strength, testosterone levels	No increase in muscle mass or strength	Illegal in the U.S. due to side effects similar to anabolic steroids
DHEA		Increase muscle mass, strength, testosterone levels	Several beneficial effects in patients >70 yrs old; no effect on lean body mass, strength, or testosterone levels	Numerous reported, but *Cochrane Review* does not show consistent evidence to support any side effects

BANNED SUBSTANCES RESOURCES

National Collegiate Athletic Association.
http://www1.ncaa.org/membership/ed_outreach/health-safety/drug_testing/banned_drug_classes.pdf
World Anti-Doping Agency.
http://www.wada-ama.org/en/prohibitedlist.ch2
International Olympic Committee Medical Commission.
http://www.olympic.org/uk/organisation/commissions/medical/index_uk.asp
National Football League.
http://www.nflpa.org/pdfs/RulesAndRegs/ProhibitedSubstances. pdf

National Basketball Association.
http://hoopedia.nba.com/index.php/NBA/NBPA_Anti-Drug_Program_Prohibited_Substances

REFERENCES

1. Blendon RJ, DesRoches CM, Benson JM, et al. Americans' views on the use and regulation of dietary supplements. *Arch Intern Med.* 2001;161:805–810.
2. Juhn MS. Popular sports supplements and ergogenic aids. *Sports Med.* 2003;33:921–939.

3. Huang S, Johnson K, Pipe A. The use of dietary supplements and medications by Canadian athletes at the Atlanta and Sydney Olympic Games. *Clin J Sport Med.* 2006; 16:27–33.
4. World Anti-Doping Agency. http://www.wada-ama.org. Accessed October 21, 2007.
5. Bell DG. Effect of caffeine and ephedrine ingestion on anaerobic exercise performance. *Med Sci Sports Exerc.* 2001; 33:1399–1403.
6. Bell DG. Effect of ingesting caffeine and ephedrine on 10-km run performance. *Med Sci Sports Exerc.* 2002;34:344–349.
7. Gillies H. Pseudoephedrine is without ergogenic effects during prolonged exercise. *J Appl Physiol.* 1996;6:2611–2617.
8. Swain RA, Harsha DM, Baenziger J, et al. Do pseudoephedrine or phenylpropanolamine improve maximum oxygen uptake and time to exhaustion? *Clin J Sport Med.* 1997;7:168–173.
9. Chu KS. Doherty TJ, Parise G, et al. A moderate dose of pseudoephedrine does not alter muscle contraction strength or anaerobic power. *Clin J Sport Med.* 2002;12:387–390.
10. Hodges AN, Lynn BM, Bula JE, et al. Effects of pseudoephedrine on maximal cycling power and submaximal cycling efficiency. *Med Sci Sports Exerc.* 2003;35:1316–1319.
11. Coates ML, Rembold CM, Farr BM. Does pseudoephedrine increase blood pressure in patients with controlled hypertension? *J Fam Pract.* 1995;40:22–26.
12. Shekelle PG, Hardy ML, Morton SC, et al. Efficacy and safety of ephedra and ephedrine for weight loss and athletic performance. *JAMA.* 2003;289:1537–1545.
13. Haller C. Adverse cardiovascular and central nervous system events associated with dietary supplements containing ephedra alkaloids. *N Engl J Med.* 2000;343:1833–1838.
14. Graham TE. Caffeine and exercise: metabolism, endurance and performance. *Sports Med.* 2001;31:785–807.
15. Jacobson BH, Weber MD, Claypool L, et al. Effect of caffeine on maximal strength and power in elite male athletes. *Br J Sports Med.* 1992;26:276–280.
16. Bell D, Jacobs I, Zamecnik J. Effects of caffeine, ephedrine, and their combination on time to exhaustion during high-intensity exercise. *Eur J Appl Physiol.* 1998;77:427–433.
17. Jacobs I, Pasternak H, Bell D. Effects of ephedrine, caffeine, and their combination on muscular endurance. *Med Sci Sports Exerc.* 2003;35:987–994.
18. Juhn M. Popular sports supplements and ergogenic aids. *Sports Med.* 2003;33:921–939.
19. Lemon PW, Tarnopolsky MA, MacDougall JD, et al. Protein requirements, muscle mass/strength changes during intensive training in novice bodybuilders. *J Appl Physiol.* 1992;73:767–775.
20. Lemon PW. Effect of exercise on protein requirements. *J Sports Sci.* 1991;9:53–70.
21. Colombani P, Wenk C, Kunz I, et al. Effects of L-carnitine supplementation on physical performance and energy metabolism of endurance-trained athletes: a double-blind crossover field study. *Eur J Appl Physiol.* 1996;73:434–439.
22. Segura R, Ventura JL. Effect of L-tryptophan supplementation on exercise performance. *Int J Sports Med.* 1988;9: 301–305.
23. Stensrud T, Ingjer F, Holm H, et al. L-tryptophan supplementation does not improve running performance. *Int J Sports Med.* 1992;13:481–485.
24. Seltzer S, Stoch R, Marcus R, et al. Alterations of human pain thresholds by nutritional manipulation of L-tryptophan supplementation. *Pain.* 1982;13:385–393.
25. Teman AJ, Hainline B. Eosinophilia-myalgia syndrome. *Phys Sports Med.* 1991;19:81–86.
26. Nissen SL, Sharp R, Ray M, et al. The effect of the leucine metabolite beta-hydroxy beta-methylbutyrate on muscle metabolism during resistance-exercise training. *J Appl Physiol.* 1996;81:2095–2104.
27. Nissen SL, Panton J, Wilhelm R, et al. The effect of beta-hydroxy beta-methylbutyrate (HMB) supplementation on strength and body composition of trained and untrained males undergoing intense resistance training. *FASEB J.* 1996; 10:287.
28. Nissen SL, Sharp RL. Effect of dietary supplements on lean mass and strength gains with resistance exercise: a meta-analysis. *J Appl Physiol.* 2003;94:651–659.
29. Bemben, MG, Lamont HS. Creatine supplementation and exercise performance: recent findings. *Sports Med.* 2005;35: 107–125.
30. Vandenberghe K, Gillis N, Van Leemputte M. Caffeine counteracts the ergogenic action of muscle creatine loading. *J Appl Physiol.* 1995;80:452–457.
31. Ceremuzynski L, Chamiec T, Herbaczynsa-Cedro T. Effect of supplemental oral L-arginine on exercise capacity in patients with stable angina pectoris. *Am J Cardiol.* 1997;80:331–333.
32. Hauk J, Hosey R. Nitric Oxide therapy: fact or fiction? *Cur Sports Med Rep.* 2006;5:199–201.
33. Nieman D. Exercise, upper respiratory tract infection, and the immune system. *Med Sci Sports Exerc.* 1994;26:128–139.
34. Douglas RM, Hemilä H. Vitamin C for preventing and treating the common cold. *PLoS Med.* 2005;2:e168. Available at: http://medicine.plosjournals.org/perlserv/?request=getdocument&doi=10.1371/journal.pmed.0020168&ct=1. Accessed October 1, 2007.
35. Thompson D, Williams C, Garcia-Roves P, et al. Postexercise vitamin C supplementation and recovery from demanding exercise. *Eur J Appl Physiol.* 2003;89:393–400.
36. Clarkson PM. Do athletes require mineral supplements? *Sports Med Digest.* 1994;16:1–3.
37. Armsey TD Jr, Green GA. Nutrition supplements: science vs hype. *Phys Sports Med.* 1997;25:77–92.
38. Clancy SP, Clarkson PM, DeCheke ME, et al. Effects of chromium picolinate supplementation on body composition, strength, and urinary chromium loss in football players. *Int J Sport Nutr.* 1994;4:142–153.
39. Hallmark MA, Reynolds TH, DeSouza CA, et al. Effects of chromium and resistive training on muscle strength and body composition. *Med Sci Sports Exerc.* 1996;28:139–144.
40. Stanko RT, Robertson RJ, Spina RJ, et al. Enhancement of arm exercise endurance capacity with dihydroxyacetone and pyruvate. *J Appl Physiol.* 1990;68:119–124.
41. Kalman D, Colker CM, Wilets I, et al. The effects of pyruvate supplementation on body composition in overweight individuals. *Nutrition.* 1999;15:337–340.

42. Morrison MA, Spriet LL, Dyck DJ. Pyruvate ingestion for 7 days does not improve aerobic performance in well-trained individuals. *J Appl Physiol.* 2000;89:549–556.

43. Bertardi J, Zeigenfuss T. Effects of ribose supplementation on repeated sprint performance in men. *J Strength Cond Research.* 2003;17:47–52.

44. Op't EB, Van Leemputte, Brouns F, et al. No effects of oral ribose supplementation on repeated maximal exercise and *de novo* ATP resynthesis. *J Appl Physiol.* 2001;91:2275–2281.

45. Keifer D, Pantuso T. Panax ginseng. *Am Fam Physician.* 2003;68:1539–1542.

46. Nissen S, Sharp R. Effect of dietary supplements on lean mass and strength gains with resistance exercise: a meta-analysis. *J Appl Physiol.* 2003;94:651–659.

47. Wallace MB, Lim J, Cutler A, et al. Effects of dehy-droepiandrosterone vs androstenedione supplementation in men. *Med Sci Sports Exerc.* 1999;31:1788.

48. Genazzani AD, Lanzoni C, Genazzani A. Might DHEA be considered a beneficial replacement therapy in the elderly? *Drugs Aging.* 2007;24:173–185.

49. Grimley EJ, Malouf R, Huppert F, et al. Dehydroepian-drosterone (DHEA) supplementation for cognitive function in healthy elderly people. *Cochrane Database Syst Rev.* 2006;4:CD006221.

SECTION II

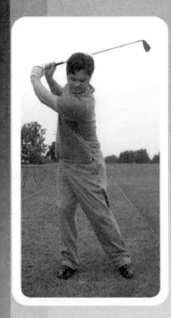

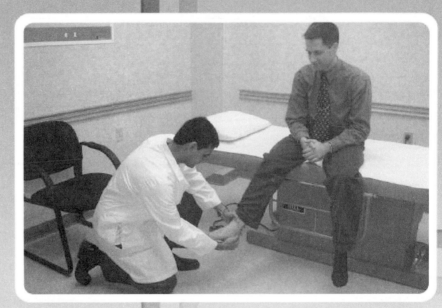

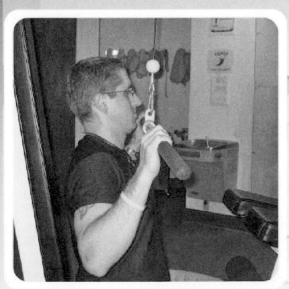

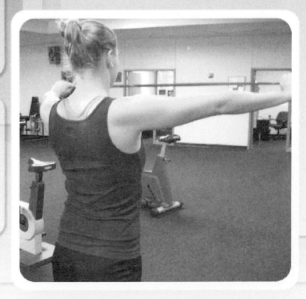

Baseball Injuries

It is estimated that half of all professional base-ball pitchers experience symptoms related to the elbow or shoulder joint at some point during their careers.[1] Forces generated during the throw create significant demands on the upper limb. Bennett, in 1959, was one of the first to report on injuries of the shoulder and elbow in pitchers.[2]

A significant amount of work has been devoted to the biomechanics of throwing. Understanding throwing motions is important in identifying the variable forces placed on the elbow and shoulder and the anatomic structures at risk. Appreciation of the mechanical stresses placed on the upper limb during a throw will help the clinician in diagnosing, treating, and rehabilitating these injuries.

Over 100,000 teams participate annually in Little League Baseball.[3] Many injuries are associated within the pediatric shoulder and elbow as a result of repetitive overhead throwing.[4,5] With the continued popularity of the sport and significant number of young throwers, investigators are now focusing on preventative measures.[3,4,6,7]

EPIDEMIOLOGY

In 2001, a survey of major league baseball injuries revealed that injury rates had slightly increased over the previous decade.[8] Chambless et al. reported on injuries in minor league baseball teams, suggesting that the injury rate is greater among the rookie-level teams compared with the higher-level minor league clubs.[9]

Among college players, the upper limb is the most common site of injury (58%), followed by the lower limb (27%), and the trunk/back (15%).[10] The most common injury is rotator cuff tendonitis. Strains and sprains were the most common etiology.[8–10] Contusions are a causative factor in 17% of the reported injuries.

Both collegiate and professional data suggest that pitchers and catchers are the most vulnerable to injury.[8,10]

Upper limb injuries cause the most time lost from play. Shoulder injuries most commonly occurred in pitchers (69%), followed by infielders (19%), and outfielders (12%).[10] At the collegiate level, the most common diagnoses at the elbow are ulnar collateral ligament sprains and forearm flexor strains.[10] Shoulder injuries are responsible for the greatest number of disability days at the professional level, followed by the elbow, knee, wrist/hand, and back.[8]

PITCHING BIOMECHANICS

Throwing is a complex coordination of trunk, upper limb, and lower limb motion. During the overhead throw, energy is transmitted from the trunk into the upper limb, generating significant loads across both the shoulder and elbow. The overhead throw can be broken down into five phases: wind-up, cocking, acceleration, deceleration, and follow-through (Fig. 7-1).[11] Abrupt changes in acceleration of the upper limb take place during the arm cocking and acceleration portions of the throw.[12] During the arm-cocking phase, the upper limb moves to a maximum external rotation of 140 to 180 degrees.[13] As the arm is positioned in abduction and external rotation, the angular velocity of the shoulder approaches 1,100 degrees/second.[14] The elbow range of motion required for pitching is a maximum of 120 degree of flexion in the early cocking or acceleration phase, and 19 to 38 degrees during the follow-through.[15]

The acceleration phase starts as the upper limb moves out of maximum external rotation. Associated with this is internal rotation of the glenohumeral joint and early extension of the elbow. During the acceleration phase, angular velocities of the shoulder

Stages of Pitching

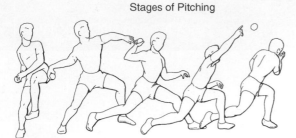

FIGURE 7-1 The five phases of the throwing motion include wind-up, stride and early cocking, late-arm cocking, acceleration, and deceleration and follow-through. (From DeLee JC, Drez D Jr., eds. *Orthopaedic Sports Medicine: Principles and Practice.* Philadelphia: Saunders; 1994:471, Fig. 15A-9. With permission.)

and elbow approach 7,000 degrees/second and 2,500 degrees/second, respectively.[12] Valgus stress loads across the medial elbow reach 64 Nm (Newton meter) during the throw.[15] Lateral compressive loads of the radiocapitellar joint approach 500 N (Newton) with overhead throwing.[15] Internal rotation torque about the shoulder approaches 67 Nm and anterior forces across the glenohumeral joint reach 310 N.[15]

SHOULDER ANATOMY AND INJURY

The scapulothoracic joint is a sliding, gliding joint between the scapular body and the posterior rib cage. Trapezius and levator musculature superiorly allows for elevation and abduction, and rhomboids control retraction toward the midline. The serratus anterior powers protraction of the scapula as well as aiding in abduction of the scapula. The scapula moves in a 1:2 ratio of scapulothoracic to glenohumeral abduction-adduction or flexion-extension. Scapulothoracic bursitis is chronic irritation of the bursa between the scapula and the chest wall. Usually treated conservatively, this bursitis causes painful snapping or crepitant movement. Refractory cases may require either arthroscopic or open surgical debridement.[16]

Scapular dyskinesis (sick scapula syndrome) describes alterations in normal scapular resting position or dynamic alterations in motion that lead to impingement symptoms.[17] The rehabilitation focus for scapular dyskinesis is regaining motor control and coordination of the periscapular musculature.

The glenohumeral joint is arranged to allow for maximal mobility. A small, shallow glenoid cavity combined with a large humeral head allows for much more motion than a similar-sized ball and socket, like the hip joint. Capsular soft-tissue restraints include the glenoid labrum and the glenohumeral ligaments. The labrum deepens the glenoid and aids in keeping the humeral head properly located. The glenohumeral ligaments also prevent humeral head subluxation throughout this joint's extensive range of motion by reinforcing the anterior capsule. The long head of the proximal biceps tendon inserts onto the superior labrum.

Dynamic stabilizers like the rotator cuff musculature help to keep the joint from dislocating or subluxating by centering the humeral head and depressing it into the glenoid. The subscapularis internally rotates the humeral head deeper into the glenoid while the infraspinatus and teres minor externally rotate the humeral head and act as check reins against anterior subluxation. The supraspinatus aids in abduction along with the deltoid.

Throwing velocity and power are largely generated by the legs, core trunk musculature, and the larger scapular muscles. The rotator cuff (R-C) functions to stabilize the humeral head, controlling rotation in the glenoid and provides only a small percentage of the force to move the arm anteriorly in a throwing motion. The R-C does, however, play a significant role in decelerating the arm during follow-through.[18]

Rotator cuff injuries range from irritation and tendonitis to the more serious partial-thickness articular or bursal-sided tears to full-thickness tears (Fig. 7-2). Much speculation and research has been directed toward explaining the exact mechanism for R-C injury. To date, no specific cause has been identified for R-C tears in throwers; rather, it is thought to be the result of multiple factors. These include intrinsic tendon-specific etiology, such as poor tissue mechanical properties, poor vascular supply, and poor healing capacity. Extrinsic factors include impingement of the R-C on the undersurface of the acromion, excessive anterior motion of the humeral head, alteration of the sequence of muscular contractions, and tightness of pectoralis minor.[19]

Internal impingement is a theory of particular interest, because it may explain some of the labral changes also seen in throwers. Specifically, an articular-sided posterior partial thickness R-C tear is identified along with posterior, superior labral tearing (Fig. 7-3). Proposed mechanisms are acquired anterior microinstability,

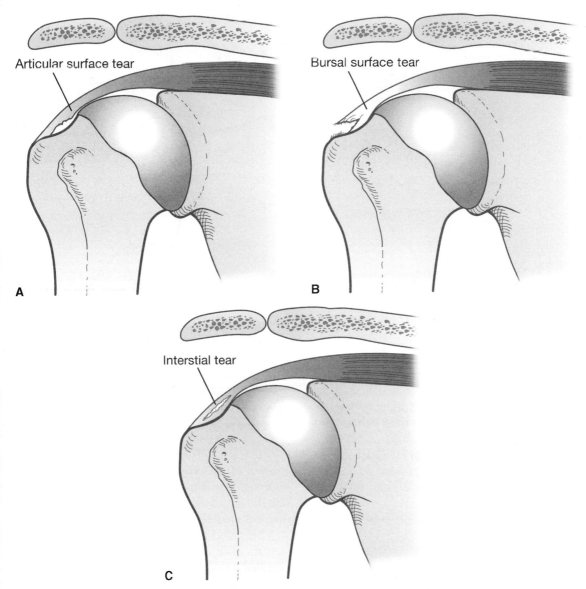

FIGURE 7-2 A. Articular surface tear. **B.** Bursal surface tear. **C.** Interstitial tear. (From Burkhart SS, Lo IKY, Brady PC. *Burkhart's View of the Shoulder: A Cowboy's Guide to Advanced Shoulder Arthroscopy.* Philadelphia: Lippincott Williams & Wilkins; 2006.)

which allows the humeral head to slide anteriorly impinging the posterior cuff on the glenoid/labrum; or an acquired, tight, contracted posterior capsule increasing the shear forces during the cocking phase of throwing.[20]

In the overhead athlete, rotator cuff "irritation" — defined as tendonitis, tendinosis, or partial-thickness tearing—is most commonly seen with repetitive microtrauma. The common complaints include pain,

decreased throwing velocity, tiredness, and lack of accuracy. Overhead athletes—most commonly pitchers—suffer this type of injury, and the initial approach is conservative. "Shutting down" the player by resting the shoulder, maintaining range of motion, and controlling the pain are the main tenets of conservative therapy.

Labral tears in throwers can be seen as isolated injuries, but are often associated with other pathology ranging from R-C tears to anterior or posterior

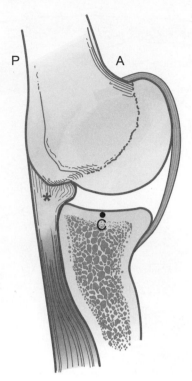

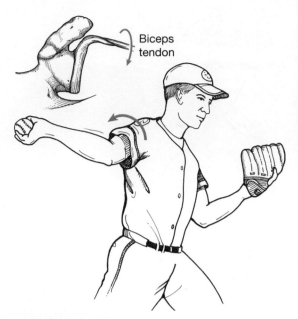

FIGURE 7-4 The peel-back mechanism of injury in the overhead athlete for type II superior labrum anterior and posterior (SLAP) lesions. (From Burkhart SS, Lo IKY, Brady PC. *Burkhart's View of the Shoulder: A Cowboy's Guide to Advanced Shoulder Arthroscopy.* Philadelphia: Lippincott Williams & Wilkins; 2006.)

FIGURE 7-3 In abduction and external rotation of the shoulder, the greater tuberosity abuts the posterosuperior glenoid, entrapping the rotator cuff between the two bones (*). (A, anterior; P, posterior; C, glenohumeral center of rotation.) (From Burkhart SS, Lo IKY, Brady PC. *Burkhart's View of the Shoulder: A Cowboy's Guide to Advanced Shoulder Arthroscopy.* Philadelphia: Lippincott Williams & Wilkins; 2006.)

instability. Glenohumeral dislocations often avulse the capsulolabral complex off the glenoid in the direction of the dislocation. Continued instability is often seen, especially in the younger athlete, and surgical repair of the labrum back to the glenoid is often required.

SLAP (superior labral anterior posterior) tears occur in the biceps (long head) anchor at the superior glenoid. These are often seen in throwers as well as in players who have fallen on an outstretched arm. SLAP tears are thought to be the result of excessive compression of the labral tissue or a "peel back" phenomenon (Fig. 7-4). Depending on the type of SLAP tear, surgical repair may be required (Fig. 7-5).[21]

The acromioclavicular joint (AC) joins the lateral end of the clavicle to the medial border of the acromion of the scapula. The AC joint allows for superior–inferior and anterior–posterior motion and

rotation of the clavicle. The trapezoid and conoid make up the coracoclavicular (CC) ligaments. These stabilize the clavicle, and are often injured with falls onto the shoulder.

Acromioclavicular separations are commonly seen after falls on the point of the shoulder, and are classified into types 1 to 6. Types 1 and 2 represent strains of the AC joint capsule and incomplete tearing of the trapezoid and conoid ligaments. Type 3 involves complete disruption of the AC joint capsule and the CC ligaments. Types 4 and 6 are also complete disruptions, with the clavicle displaced posteriorly and inferiorly, respectively. Type 5 is an exaggerated type 3 injury, with extensive tenting and damage of the soft tissues by the clavicle. Surgical reconstruction is routine for types 4 to 6 and for types 2 and 3 that remain unstable and painful. Persistent deformity is common for AC separations treated conservatively.[22]

The sternoclavicular joint (SC) is composed of the medial end of the clavicle adjoined to the manubrium by strong capsular ligaments. This joint also allows for rotation, superior–inferior, and anterior–posterior

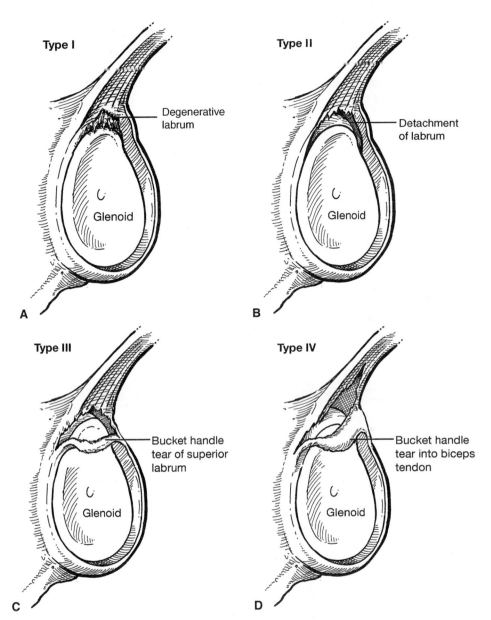

FIGURE 7-5 A. Type I superior labrum anterior and posterior (SLAP) lesion. **B.** Type II SLAP lesion. **C.** Type III SLAP lesion. **D.** Type IV SLAP lesion. (From Burkhart SS, Lo IKY, Brady PC. *Burkhart's View of the Shoulder: A Cowboy's Guide to Advanced Shoulder Arthroscopy.* Philadelphia: Lippincott Williams & Wilkins; 2006.)

motion. Sternoclavicular dislocations are relatively uncommon, but may occur after collisions or falls onto the point of the shoulder. Anterior dislocations are most commonly seen, but posterior dislocations with impingement of the great vessels in the neck can occur. Complaints include pain and deformity, but also can include dysphagia and venous congestion. Computed tomography (CT) scan best demonstrates SC dislocation and the orientation of the medial clavicle. Reductions of posterior SC dislocations should be done with the assistance of a vascular or cardiothoracic surgeon in case of great vessel damage.

Nerve injuries are relatively uncommon in baseball but should be part of the differential for a painful

| TABLE 7-1 | Interval Throwing Progression Program (Phase I). Each phase is titled according to the distance (in feet) that the athlete is to throw. Throwing program should be performed every other day, unless otherwise specified by physician or rehabilitation specialist. Advance to next step when throwing the specified number of throws without pain. |

45-Foot Phase

| Step 1 | A) Warm-up throwing
B) 45 feet (25 throws)
C) Rest 15 minutes
D) Warm-up throwing
E) 45 feet (25 throws) |
| Step 2 | A) Warm-up throwing
B) 45 feet (25 throws)
C) Rest 10 minutes
D) Warm-up throwing
E) 45 feet (25 throws)
F) Rest 10 minutes
G) Warm-up throwing
H) 45 feet (25 throws) |

60-Foot Phase

| Step 3 | A) Warm-up throwing
B) 60 feet (25 throws)
C) Rest 15 minutes
D) Warm-up throwing
E) 60 feet (25 throws) |
| Step 4 | A) Warm-up throwing
B) 60 feet (25 throws)
C) Rest 10 minutes
D) Warm-up throwing
E) 60 feet (25 throws)
F) Rest 10 minutes
G) Warm-up throwing
H) 60 feet (25 throws) |

90-Foot Phase

| Step 5 | A) Warm-up throwing
B) 90 feet (25 throws)
C) Rest 15 minutes
D) Warm-up throwing
E) 90 feet (25 throws) |
| Step 6 | A) Warm-up throwing
B) 90 feet (25 throws)
C) Rest 10 minutes
D) Warm-up throwing
E) 90 feet (25 throws)
F) Rest 10 minutes
G) Warm-up throwing
H) 90 feet (25 throws) |

120-Foot Phase

| Step 7 | A) Warm-up throwing
B) 120 feet (25 throws)
C) Rest 15 minutes
D) Warm-up throwing
E) 120 feet (25 throws) |
| Step 8 | A) Warm-up throwing
B) 120 feet (25 throws)
C) Rest 10 minutes
D) Warm-up throwing
E) 120 feet (25 throws)
F) Rest 10 minutes
G) Warm-up throwing
H) 120 feet (25 throws) |

150-Foot Phase

| Step 9 | A) Warm-up throwing
B) 150 feet (25 throws)
C) Rest 15 minutes
D) Warm-up throwing
E) 150 feet (25 throws) |
| Step 10 | A) Warm-up throwing
B) 150 feet (25 throws)
C) Rest 10 minutes
D) Warm-up throwing
E) 150 feet (25 throws)
F) Rest 10 minutes
G) Warm-up throwing
H) 150 feet (25 throws) |

180-Foot Phase

| Step 11 | A) Warm-up throwing
B) 180 feet (25 throws)
C) Rest 15 minutes
D) Warm-up throwing
E) 180 feet (25 throws) |
| Step 12 | A) Warm-up throwing
B) 180 feet (25 throws)
C) Rest 10 minutes
D) Warm-up throwing
E) 180 feet (25 throws)
F) Rest 10 minutes
G) Warm-up throwing
H) 180 feet (25 throws) |

| Step 13 | A) Warm-up throwing
B) 180 feet (25 throws)
C) Rest 15 minutes
D) Warm-up throwing
E) 180 feet (25 throws) |
| Step 14 | Begin throwing off the mound or return to respective position |

From Burkhart SS, Lo IKY, Brady PC. *Burkhart's View of the Shoulder: A Cowboy's Guide to Advanced Shoulder Arthroscopy.* Philadelphia: Lippincott Williams & Wilkins; 2006.

throwing motion. Tension and repetitive nerve injury can be seen both at the elbow and the shoulder due to the extreme stresses experienced during throwing. Tingling, numbness, and pain distal to the site of compression are the usual presenting symptoms. Most commonly seen is ulnar neuropathy at the elbow, discussed later in the text. Suprascapular nerve injury at the spinoglenoid notch may also be seen, but is frequently asymptomatic.

Vascular injuries are relatively uncommon. Aneurysms, intimal hyperplasia, or stenosis can partially or completely occlude the vessel, causing ischemia of the distal limb. Floating clot, or emboli, may also cause vascular symptoms. Repetitive stretch, compression, and microtrauma to these vascular structures is thought to cause vascular injuries. Obtaining the correct diagnosis is critical. Radiating pain, abnormal pulses, palpable thrills, petechia, and asymmetric temperature are signs and symptoms of vascular abnormality. When vascular damage is suspected, evaluation with ultrasound, arterio/venography, or magnetic resonance arteriogram (MRA) is essential for recognition.[23,24]

Conservative Approach for "Dead Arm"

A "dead arm" is the description many throwers use to describe a tired, painful, or weak shoulder or elbow, and may be caused by any number of the aforementioned diagnoses. The conservative approach to "dead arm" in the high-level pitcher is a trial of rehabilitation. The common approach is to rest the arm for 2 weeks while continuing with range-of-motion stretching, electrical stimulation, iontophoresis, icing, and massage. Other modalities include oral nonsteroidal anti-inflammation drugs (NSAIDs); corticosteroid injections can be used as adjuncts to control pain and swelling.[25] Once the inflammation and pain have resolved, then the thrower is progressed through a 4-week "return to throw" program. This helps restore strength, endurance, and proper throwing mechanics (Tables 7-1 and 7-2). The program gradually increases in intensity and duration, with the goal of returning the thrower back to previous level of competition while allowing for the arm to recover between workouts. Appropriate stretching and strengthening

---

TABLE 7-2 **Interval Throwing Progression Program—from the Mound (Phase II). All throwing off the mound should be done in the presence of a pitching coach to stress proper throwing mechanics.**

Stage One: Fastball Only

Step 1	Interval throwing 15 throws off mound 50%
Step 2	Interval throwing 30 throws off mound 50%
Step 3	Interval throwing 45 throws off mound 50%
Step 4	Interval throwing 60 throws off mound 50%
Step 5	Interval throwing 30 throws off mound 50%
Step 6	30 throws off mound 75% 45 throws off mound 50%
Step 7	45 throws off mound 75% 15 throws off mound 50%
Step 8	60 throws off mound 75%

Stage Two: Fastball Only

Step 9	45 throws off mound 75% 15 throws in batting practice
Step 10	45 throws off mound 75% 30 throws in batting practice
Step 11	45 throws off mound 75% 45 throws in batting practice

Stage Three

Step 12	30 throws off mound 75% warm-up 15 throws off mound 50% breaking balls 45–60 throws in batting practice (fastball only)
Step 13	30 throws off mound 75% 30 breaking balls 75% 30 throws in batting practice
Step 14	30 throws off mound 75% 60–90 throws in batting practice 25% breaking balls
Step 15	Simulated game: progressing by 15 throws per workout

From Burkhart SS, Lo IKY, Brady PC. *Burkhart's View of the Shoulder: A Cowboy's Guide to Advanced Shoulder Arthroscopy.* Philadelphia: Lippincott Williams & Wilkins; 2006.

exercises are used in conjunction with the throwing program to maintain strength and flexibility while decreasing the risk for reinjury. The entire program usually encompasses 6 weeks. If the thrower falls off the program pace, conservative therapy is often abandoned for surgical therapy.

If surgical repair is necessary, repair of soft-tissue structures, such as a rotator cuff, usually requires 6 weeks for biologic healing and several more weeks for return of motion and strength. Often, a "return to throw" program is begun approximately 12 to 14 weeks postoperatively.

ELBOW ANATOMY AND INJURY

The significant forces generated across the elbow during the throw are thought to create attritional changes within the important stabilizers of the elbow. Both bone anatomy and the ulnar and lateral collateral ligaments are important components of elbow stability. The osseous structures of the elbow are important stabilizers for varus and valgus stresses <20 degrees and >120 degrees.[26] The collateral ligaments are the primary restraints in an arc motion of 20 to 120 degrees.[26,27] The greatest stresses across the elbow occur at midflexion during the overhead throw. Therefore, the bony structures of the elbow play a lesser stabilizing role during throwing. The anterior bundle of the ulnar collateral ligament (UCL) is the primary stabilizer to valgus stress.[27,28] The origin of the ligament is the medial epicondyle. It has two bundles, anterior and posterior, with the insertion of the anterior bundle of the ligament on the sublime tubercle (Fig. 7-6).[27,29] The posterior bundle inserts on the ulna proper and is sometimes noted as a capsular thickening.[29] The radial head serves as a secondary restraint with some stability provided by the flexor-pronator mass.[26]

Cadaveric studies have demonstrated the anterior band of the ulnar collateral ligament to be the strongest and stiffest, with an average failure load of 260 N.[29] Fleisig et al. demonstrated that the ultimate failure load during pitching approaches that of an intact UCL with valgus stress.[15] Repetitive valgus stress can result in microtrauma, inflammation, attenuation, and eventual rupture of the UCL. The valgus loads placed across the elbow can lead to progressive UCL insufficiency and a spectrum of injury, primarily along the medial and posterior structures of the elbow. Pathology within the lateral compartment may also occur as a result of the significant repetitive valgus stress (Fig. 7-7).

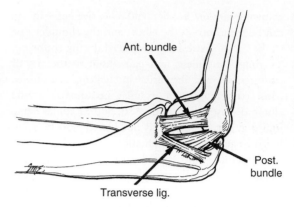

FIGURE 7-6 The ulnar collateral ligament originates at the medial epicondyle and inserts on the sublime tubercle. The medial elbow ligament complex consists of an anterior and posterior bundle. (From Morrey BF, Atlas SW. *Master Techniques in Orthopaedic Surgery: The Elbow.* 2nd ed. Philadelphia: Lippincott Williams & Wilkins; 2002.)

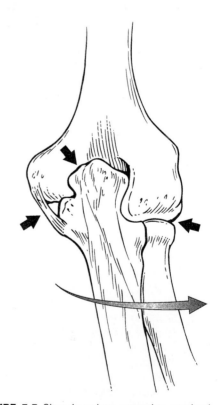

FIGURE 7-7 Sites in valgus extension overload: medial tension, lateral compression, and posterior impaction. (From Garrett WE, Speer KP, Kirkendall DT, eds. *Principles and Practice of Orthopaedic Sports Medicine.* Philadelphia: Lippincott Williams & Wilkins; 2000.)

Ulnar Collateral Ligament Insufficiency

History and physical examination are particularly helpful in the diagnosis of ulnar collateral ligament insufficiency. Throwers typically present with a history of medial elbow pain noted during the early phases of the throw. They often report a drop in their throwing velocity. Symptoms usually develop gradually, although occasionally, athletes may feel a "pop" or immediate soreness after one throw. Subsequently, the patient is unable to continue throwing. In chronic UCL injuries patients may be able to bat and perform most activities of daily living (ADLs) without pain. The athlete may note early fatigue or inability to achieve preinjury velocity.

On physical examination, soreness is reproducible over the UCL either at the sublime tubercle or at the medial epicondylar origin. Pain along the medial elbow with valgus stress test or the milking maneuver is suggestive of UCL insufficiency (Fig. 7-8).[30,31] The valgus stress test is performed with the arm externally rotated, while a valgus force is placed across the elbow positioned at 70 degrees of flexion. The medial joint is palpated for tenderness while performing the maneuver. The milking manuever is performed by positioning the forearm in full supination and 80 degrees of flexion. Valgus stress is produced by stabilizing the elbow and applying force by grabbing onto the thumb of the patient. With a constantly applied valgus force, the elbow is brought through an arc range of motion of 80 to 110 degrees, evaluating for medial elbow pain. It is important to assess for concomitant ulnar nerve pathology, for posteromedial joint line pain, and for soreness over the flexor pronator insertion.

Radiographs of the elbow may demonstrate posterior olecranon spurring, loose bodies, or a small avulsion injury to the medial epicondyle or sublime tubercle. Bilateral valgus stress films are obtained to assess for medial joint space opening. A positive test is noted if the injured elbow demonstrates a >2 mm medial joint space opening compared to the contralateral side.[31] Magnetic resonance imaging (MRI) of the elbow is a helpful tool to assess these injuries. Contrasted MRI studies of the elbow have been shown to be 97% sensitive in the detection of partial or complete tears of the UCL.[32] In addition to evaluation of the UCL, MRI is useful to assess for flexor-pronator pathology or intra-articular injuries.

An arthroscopic stress exam to assess for medial elbow instability may be positive in cases of the complete disruption of the UCL; however, the exam is

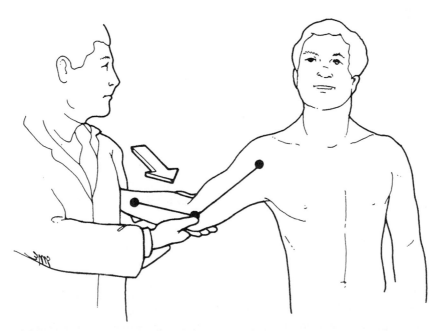

FIGURE 7-8 Valgus stress test produces pain and tenderness over the ulnar collateral ligament. (From Morrey BF, Atlas SW. *Master Techniques in Orthopaedic Surgery: The Elbow.* 2nd ed. Philadelphia: Lippincott Williams & Wilkins; 2002.)

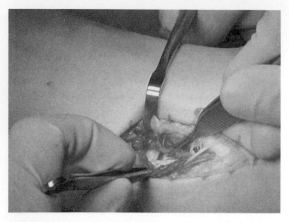

FIGURE 7-9 Intraoperative photograph of a muscle splitting approach to the ulnar collateral ligament. The ulnotrochlear joint opens 4 to 5 mm (forceps) with intraoperative valgus stress indicating an incompetent ligament.

sometimes equivocal or difficult to interpret.[33] Although all of the aforementioned diagnostic tests are helpful, the gold standard to confirm UCL insufficiency is to incise the ligament longitudinally and evaluate the degree of medial joint space opening while positioning the elbow at 70 degrees with valgus stress. Greater than 3 to 4 mm gapping of the ulnotrochlear joint with stress is indicative of UCL insufficiency (Fig. 7-9).

If UCL insufficiency is suspected, we recommend a period of nonoperative treatment. The patient is placed into a hinged brace with early range of motion. Terminal extension of the elbow may be limited during the early phases of rest. The goal of the first 4 to 6 weeks is full range of motion (ROM) and pain-free activity with ADLs. Once this has been achieved, flexor-pronator strengthening exercises are initiated. The patient is then taken through a return to a throwing program (Table 7-1). In the case of pitchers, a portion of the rehabilitation is dedicated to mound work (Table 7-2). Studies have demonstrated that approximately 40% of players with this injury are able to return to preinjury status after nonoperative treatment of these injuries. Throwers successfully undergoing nonoperative management typically return to their previous level of competition at approximately 6 months postinjury.[34] In general, we recommend at least 3 months of rehabilitation prior to surgical consideration. Athletes who are unable to return to their desired level of performance and who have persistent medial elbow pain with throwing may be candidates for surgery.

Valgus Extension Overload

With attenuation or insufficiency of the UCL, increased stress may take place at the level of the posteromedial compartment (Fig. 7-7). The posteromedial portion of the olecranon may impinge on the fossa, creating inflammation, chondral injury, or spur formation.[35] Valgus extension overload occurs as a result of posteromedial olecranon osteophyte impingement in the terminal phases of throwing. Patients note posteromedial elbow pain during deceleration and terminal extension while throwing. Occasionally, a drop in throwing velocity will be noted.

Examination may demonstrate soreness over the posteromedial joint line. The hallmark physical finding is a positive valgus extension overload test. The maneuver is completed by forcing the arm into full extension with a valgus load.[35] A positive result is the reproduction of posteromedial pain with the maneuver. If the diagnosis is unclear, a lidocaine injection within the posterior compartment of the elbow can be helpful. In some cases the cause of the olecranon spur may be secondary to ulnar collateral ligament insufficiency. During throwing, abnormal forces can be generated at the level of the posteromedial compartment in the presence of ulnar collateral ligamentous laxity.[35,36] Therefore, it is extremely important to examine the ulnar collateral ligament to evaluate for insufficiency in these patients.

Patients are evaluated with plain film radiographs including valgus stress views. Subtle findings such as mild posteromedial spurring may be difficult to appreciate on standard plain films. MRI and CT scan imaging studies of the elbow can be helpful to define changes within the posterior compartment or identify concomitant pathology.

The athletes are initially treated nonoperatively with rest, ice, and NSAIDs. Players may begin a return to throwing program once they are not tender to palpation and have a negative valgus extension overload test. If they fail to achieve meaningful pain relief with rest, or if symptoms recur with throwing, consideration is given to an intra-articular cortisone injection. An additional period of rest is recommended following injection. Once again, the patient is slowly returned to throwing.

During the rehabilitation phases we recommend a series of exercises designed to strengthen the flexor-pronator muscle group. If the patient has subtle UCL insufficiency, strengthening of the medial elbow flexor group may facilitate the player's return to throwing. Those athletes who fail rehabilitation may be candidates for arthroscopic posteromedial osteophyte debridement. Care is taken to avoid an overzealous resection of the spur.

Medial Epicondylitis/Strain

Both hitting and throwing place the flexor-pronator musculotendinous group at risk. The flexor-pronator muscles are thought to serve as dynamic stabilizers of the medial elbow.[37] The repetitive nature of both activities can create microtrauma at the level of the flexor-pronator insertion on the medial epicondyle. Subsequent inflammation with repeat injury may result in medial epicondylitis. Acute stress of the flexor-pronator mass may result in strain or injury at the level of tendinous insertion, including complete rupture.[38]

Baseball players who have injuries related to the flexor-pronator mass often complain of anteromedial elbow pain in the terminal phases of the throw or during follow-through of the batting swing. Pain may also be noted during activities that require lifting or twisting. Patients may also complain of concomitant numbness within the ring and small fingers indicating associated ulnar nerve irritation.

Athletes with medial epicondylitis or flexor-pronator strain may characteristically have pain along the anteromedial portion of the medial epicondyle. The milking maneuver and valgus extension overload test should not elicit pain in cases of an isolated injury to the flexor-pronator group. Increased discomfort is noted with resisted pronation and/or wrist flexion. This maneuver is performed with the elbow extended. Pain referred to the anteromedial elbow is suggestive of a flexor-pronator injury. Bilateral grip strength assessment may demonstrate decreased strength with the elbow in full extension compared to the contralateral side. Palpation of the ulnar nerve over the medial elbow and the elbow flexion test should be performed to assess for a possible neurogenic etiology.

Conservative treatment is the mainstay for these injuries. Athletes are treated with an initial period of rest, wrist cock-up splinting, and stretches. Ice and ultrasound application are additional modalities. Throwers are encouraged to withhold from throwing until pain at rest subsides and minimal tenderness is noted on examination. Once this is achieved, the athlete is gradually returned to throwing, usually over 1 to 3 weeks. The length of rest period determines the time required for pitchers to return to the mound.

In patients with medial epicondylitis who fail to improve with initial nonoperative management or who are unable to return to preinjury status, consideration is given to a cortisone injection within the flexor-pronator insertion. Operative debridement and repair of the flexor-pronator origin may be required in patients with recalcitrant symptoms. The athlete is started on a return-to-throwing program once full, pain-free ROM and symmetric strength are demonstrated.

Olecranon Stress Fracture

In adults, stress fractures most commonly occur in the olecranon. Discomfort can be noted along the posterolateral border of the olecranon with throwing, usually during the acceleration phase.[39] Point tenderness over the site may be appreciated on physical exam. Plain film radiographs may be negative and require CT scan imaging for confirmation.

These injuries are initially managed on a conservative basis, with rest and protected range of motion. Once the athlete demonstrates pain-free ADLs and has no tenderness with palpation, the patient is initiated on a progressive return-to-throwing program. One study reported on successful nonoperative treatment of these injuries at the professional level.[39] If the patient is unable to progress through the program, surgical stabilization with a cannulated screw is considered.

Radiocapitellar Injury/Loose Bodies

As previously noted, high compressive loads of the lateral joint are achieved with valgus loads. Lateral joint injuries are more common in the adolescent overhead thrower. Occasionally, chondral injury of the capitellum or radial head may be noted in the adult thrower. Loose bodies may be generated from the lateral, posterior, or anterior compartments. Athletes with loose bodies of the elbow may complain of mechanical symptoms such as locking or catching. Examination can demonstrate effusion, joint line tenderness, and decreased range of motion. Plain film radiographs, CT scan, or MRI may demonstrate pathology. If loose bodies are present, elbow arthroscopy is indicated for removal.

Ulnar Neuritis

Irritation of the ulnar nerve can occur in the overhead thrower. Valgus loads may play a role in the development of ulnar neuritis in a subset of throwers.

Approximately 40% of patients with ulnar collateral ligament insufficiency have ulnar nerve symptoms.[40] Most commonly the patients present with numbness and tingling within the ulnar two digits. The athlete usually has symptoms only during or after throwing. On occasion, paresthesias maybe noted with ADLs. The player may complain of medial elbow discomfort and decreased velocity.

Examination should document the status of the nerve with regard to sensory and motor function. Static two-point assessment of the ulnar two digits is completed. The dorsal sensory portion of the ulnar nerve branches 8 cm proximal to the wrist and provides cutaneous innervation to the dorsalulnar hand. Decreased sensation in the distribution of the dorsal sensory branch is suggestive of ulnar nerve irritability proximal to the Guyon canal. Paresthesias in the ring and small finger while performing the elbow flexion test are consistent with pathology of the ulnar nerve at the elbow. A Tinel test with palpation of the ulnar nerve over the cubital tunnel should be performed. The nerve should be assessed for subluxation or a snapping medial triceps. The presence of intrinsic weakness and atrophy indicate severe compromise of the ulnar nerve. Dynanometer bilateral grip strengths should be obtained. Comprehensive examination of the elbow is critical to assess for ulnar collateral ligament instability and posteromedial osteophytes as possible contributing causes for the ulnar nerve neuritis.

Our indications for obtaining electrodiagnostic studies include a failure of conservative treatment or a significant compromise of the ulnar nerve seen on exam. In the absence of abnormal sensory and/or motor abnormalities of the nerve, the athlete is treated nonoperatively. Initial treatment includes a period of ice, rest, NSAID administration, and application of an elbow pad. In patients with recalcitrant symptoms or nocturnal paresthesias, a night extension splint is recommended. Consideration may be given to assessment of throwing mechanics with possible modifications. If the thrower's complaints are mild and they are able to perform, then continued participation is permitted.

If the athlete's symptoms worsen or continue despite nonoperative modalities, then electromyographic/nerve conduction velocity (EMG/NCV) studies are obtained to assess the ulnar nerve. The study will serve as both a diagnostic and prognostic tool. The likelihood of the player responding to conservative treatment is decreased with abnormal needle EMG results or with a significant drop in nerve conduction velocity of the ulnar nerve across the elbow.

In patients who fail nonoperative management (minimum 3 to 6 months), operative treatment is considered. The recommended procedure is ulnar nerve transposition. Although good results have been achieved with submuscular and intramuscular techniques, we favor a subcutaneous transposition.[41] In cases where concomitant UCL insufficiency is also suspected, a reconstruction of the ligament is also performed. Postoperatively, patients are rehabilitated with early protected ROM. At 4 to 6 weeks, medial elbow strengthening exercises are introduced. Throwers are initiated on a return to a throwing program at 10 weeks. Pitchers are permitted to return to the mound at 4 months. Results have been favorable with 90% of patients returning to preinjury status.

Pronator Syndrome

In some cases, the throwers may experience symptoms related to pronator syndrome—compression of the median nerve in the proximal forearm. The nerve can be compressed at four anatomic locations as it passes from the brachium into the forearm: the ligament of struthers, the lacertus fibrosis, the pronator teres muscle, and the flexor digitorum superficialis arch. As the nerve enters the two heads of the pronator teres, muscle hypertrophy can cause compression. This is the most common anatomic location of pronator syndrome.[42]

Throwers may complain of generalized pain within the proximal forearm with activity. Paresthesias within the radial three digits are commonly noted and are more pronounced with repetitive activity. Unlike median nerve compression at the wrist, provocative maneuvers for carpal tunnel syndrome fail to reproduce the patient's symptoms. Physical exam findings suggestive of pronator syndrome include: reproduction of symptoms with resisted pronation and with resisted middle finger flexion. It may also be helpful to perform a marcaine block of the nerve within the proximal forearm and then have the athlete throw. If the injection relieves the symptoms with activity, then pronator syndrome should be considered. The diagnosis is largely clinical, with electrodiagnostic studies having low yield in identifying pronator syndrome.[42] Patients should be treated conservatively with NSAIDs, ice, rest, and intermittent splinting. Operative treatment may be considered for patients whose symptoms are refractory to conservative. The nerve is explored through an antero-medial incision with all potential sites of compression released.[43]

Radial Nerve Injury

The diagnosis of radial tunnel syndrome, although uncommon, may be considered in athletes who present with lateral elbow pain. In cases of recalcitrant lateral epicondylitis, compression of the radial nerve within the proximal forearm is a possible cause. Patients usually present with generalized posterolateral elbow discomfort. Unlike posterior interosseous nerve palsy, there are no motor deficits noted. Examination may demonstrate reproduction of pain with deep palpation over the radial tunnel, resisted middle finger extension, and resisted supination with the elbow extended. If rest, NSAIDs, and long-arm splinting fail to resolve symptoms over a 3- to 6-month period, then surgical exploration and release of the radial tunnel may be considered.

HAND AND WRIST INJURIES

Hand and wrist injuries in baseball are common.[10] Blunt injuries to the hand and wrist are often caused by a ball strike. Sprains and fractures are some of the more common injuries. Other reported injuries include dislocations, tendon rupture, laceration, and contusions.

Ligamentous injuries of the proximal interphalangeal (PIP) and metacarpal phalangeal (MP) joints are usually amenable to buddy taping and early mobilization. However, soft-tissue injuries of the thumb need to be carefully assessed for complete disruptions of the ulnar or radial collateral ligaments of the thumb MP joint. In most cases, differentiation between partial- and full-thickness ulnar collateral ligament tears can be made by physical examination. A full-thickness tear of the ulnar collateral ligament should be suspected in the absence of a firm end-point when applying a radial directed stress of the MP joint in full extension (Fig. 7-10). The contralateral thumb MP joint should always be evaluated for comparison. Greater than 30 degrees of laxity of the MP joint of the injured thumb compared to the contralateral side with radial stress is suggestive of a complete tear.[44]

A palpable lesion on the ulnar metacarpal head may be suggestive of a Stener lesion. This occurs as a result of distal avulsion of the ligament with retraction and interposition of the adductor aponeurosis. The

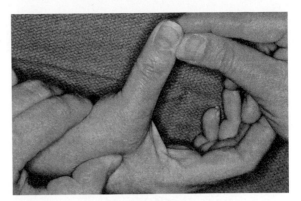

FIGURE 7-10 The ulnar collateral ligament of the thumb is assessed with a radially directed stress of the metacarpal phalangeal joint in full extension and 30 degrees of flexion. (From Strickland JW, Graham TJ. *Master Techniques in Orthopaedic Surgery: The Hand.* 2nd ed. Philadelphia: Lippincott Williams & Wilkins; 2004.)

ligament is held in a retracted position, and when left untreated, results in persistent laxity of the thumb MP joint.[45] Partial tears of the ligament often respond to 4 weeks of rigid immobilization. In the athlete, surgical repair should be considered in complete tears.

Baseball injuries to the hand and phalanges are usually low energy and may result in stable, minimally displaced fractures. Minimally displaced extra-articular fractures of the tubular bones of the hand can often be managed with early protected range of motion. However, the significant demands of the hand required for batting or catching make it difficult for the athlete participating in baseball to return to play earlier than 6 weeks following the injury. Intra-articular injuries of the hand, most notably of the PIP joint and thumb carpometacarpal joint (Bennet fracture), should be managed carefully and often require surgical stabilization.[46]

Hamate injuries are relatively uncommon in sports, accounting for approximately 3% of all carpal fractures.[47] The fracture can occur as a result of direct trauma while swinging a bat.[48] While gripping the bat, the handle is positioned overlying the ulnar palm. During a swing, the handle can impact the hook of the hamate, causing a fracture. Stark et al. reported that the fracture most commonly takes place at the end of a checked swing (stopping the bat in midswing); (Fig. 7-11).[48] The lead wrist (left wrist in a right-hand-dominant batter) is often involved because of its position nearest to the handle.[49]

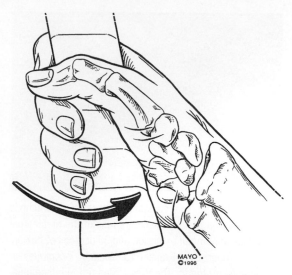

FIGURE 7-11 The butt end of the baseball bat strikes against the hook of the hamate as a potential mechanism of fracture. (From Berger RA, Weiss APC. *Hand Surgery.* Philadelphia: Lippincott Williams & Wilkins; 2003.)

Athletes may report discomfort along the hypothenar eminence that is exacerbated with gripping activities. With the close proximity of the hook of hamate to the ulnar nerve, occasional paresthesias may be noted. Pain is noted with palpation over the hamulus, which is located distal and radial to the pisiform. Diagnosis may not be readily confirmed on standard plain films. Carpal tunnel view or oblique views may demonstrate the fracture. If a hamulus fracture is suspected with no evidence of osseous injury on plain films, then CT scan is recommended.

If the fracture is diagnosed early and is not displaced, consideration could be given to nonoperative management. Even with prompt immobilization, union rates average 8 to 12 weeks.[50] Close follow-up is required because of the risk for displacement and nonunion. In cases of established nonunion and displacement of the hook, excision is recommended. Athletes are permitted to return to play once swelling and hypothenar pain has resolved.

Injuries to the ulnar side of the wrist in baseball may occur secondary to chronic loading with hitting, blunt trauma, or acute ulnar deviation and hyperdorsiflexion injury of the wrist while sliding into a base. Differential diagnosis for ulnar-sided wrist pain includes ulnar styloid fracture, triangular fibrocartilage complex tear (TFCC) tears, distal radioulnar joint (DRUJ) dysfunction, extensor carpi ulnaris tendonitis or instability, luntotriquetral (LT) tears, flexor carpi ulnaris tendonitis, and injury to the pisotriquetral joint. Careful physical examination of the ulnar wrist and plain films can help to localize the pathology. In some cases, MRI imaging may be required to assess for LT or TFCC injuries.

Fractures of the distal radial platform may occur while diving for a ball or as a result of a sudden hyperdorsiflexion load of the wrist such as sliding into a base. These injuries are usually low energy and may cause nondisplaced or minimally displaced fractures. Strict immobilization is required until radiographic union is achieved. Once the fracture is healed (6 to 8 weeks), the athlete is initiated on range-of-motion and strengthening, and is eventually transitioned into a functional progression program. Open reduction and internal fixation may be required in the case of significant displacement or intra-articular incongruity.

Neurovascular Injuries of the Hand and Wrist

Repetitive trauma to the ulnar portion of the hand can place the ulnar artery and nerve at risk. The ulnar neurovascular structures within the hand are well protected within the Guyon canal bordered by the hook of the hamate, pisiform, the volar carpal ligament, and the pisohamate ligament. The ulnar nerve and artery are felt to be at risk distal to the pisiform because of the lack of protective structures at this level. Repetitive loading in this area, such as catching a baseball, could result in secondary injury.[51]

Athletes with hypothenar hammer syndrome—internal injury to the ulnar artery as a result of blunt trauma—often complain of coolness of the digits and pain along the ulnar portion of the palm. Symptoms are often exacerbated by catching a ball or with repetitive gripping. In addition to neurologic assessment of the hand and wrist, the vascularity is carefully examined. Allen testing is performed to assess the patency of the ulnar artery. The entire upper limb is examined to rule out a more proximal etiology. In the case of suspected ulnar artery thrombosis, arterial Doppler exam, MRI arteriogram, and standard arteriogram may be indicated.[51]

Initial treatment includes rest, splinting, and the addition of padding to the ulnar portion of the hand.

Calcium-channel blockers and other sympatholytic medications may be helpful. In athletes with recalcitrant symptoms, surgery may be indicated with excision only of the thrombosed ulnar artery versus reconstruction with vein grafting.[52]

Catchers and pitchers may experience isolated digital ischemia. Several investigators have demonstrated the effect of padding on perfusion of the digits with repetitive loading.[53] The index finger of the catching hand is often involved.[54] The patient may report cyaniotic episodes, numbness, or pain within the involved digit.[55] Pitchers may develop vascular compromise within the digits as a result of lumbrical hypertrophy or compression by Cleland ligaments.[56] Examination should include vascular assessment of the involved upper limb with noninvasive Doppler exam. Treatment is similar to hypothenar hammer syndrome with additional padding as a primary treatment for catchers. In cases of refractory symptoms in pitchers, surgery may be indicated to decompress the neurovascular structures of the involved digit.

CONCLUSION

The evaluation and management of upper limb injuries can be quite difficult. The rehabilitation of these injuries can be even more difficult, as these athletes are often quite motivated to return to play. Careful evaluation at each step of the rehabilitation process is important, as is open communication between the athlete, the physician, and the therapist.

The extreme forces placed upon the throwing arm in baseball focus much of our attention on the injuries of the upper limb. One must be mindful that neck, mid and low back, and lower limb injuries also occur. Their evaluation and management is covered more fully in a number of other chapters in this book.

REFERENCES

1. Tullos HS, King JW. Throwing mechanism in sports. *Orthop Clin North Am.* 1973;4:709–721.
2. Bennett GE. Elbow and shoulder lesions of baseball players. *Am J Surg.* 1959;98:484–492.
3. Limpisvasti O, El Attrache NS, Jobe FW. Understanding shoulder and elbow injuries in baseball. *J Am Acad Orthop Surg.* 2007;15:139–147.
4. Sciascia A, Kibler WB. The pediatric overhead athlete: what is the real problem? *Clin J Sport Med.* 2006;16:471–477.
5. Chen FS, Diaz VA, Loebenberg M, et al. Shoulder and elbow injuries in the skeletally immature athlete. *J Am Acad Orthop Surg.* 2005;13:172–185.
6. Klingele KE, Kocher MS. Little league elbow: valgus overload injury in the pediatric athlete. *Sports Med.* 2002;32:1005–1015.
7. Lyman S, Fleisig GS, Andrews JR, et al. Effect of pitch type, pitch count, and pitching mechanics on risk of elbow and shoulder pain in youth baseball pitchers. *Am J Sports Med.* 2002;30:463–468.
8. Conte S, Requa RK, Garrick JG. Disability days in major league baseball. *Am J Sports Med.* 2001;29:830–831.
9. Chambless KM, Knudtson J, Eck JC, et al. Rate of injury in minor league baseball by level of play. *Am J Orthop.* 2000;29:869–872.
10. McFarland EG, Wasik M. Epidemiology of collegiate baseball injuries. *Clin J Sport Med.* 1998;8:10–13.
11. DiGiovine NM, Jobe FW, Pink M, et al. An electromyographic analysis of the upper extremity in pitching. *J Shoulder Elbow Surg.* 1992;1:15–25.
12. Pappas AM. Biomechanics of baseball pitching. *Am J Sports Med.* 1985;13:216–222.
13. Fleisig GS, Dillman CJ, Andrews JR. Biomechanics of the shoulder during throwing. In: Andrews JR, Wilk JE, eds. *The Athlete's Shoulder.* New York: Churchill Livingstone; 1994.
14. Fleisig GS, Dillman CJ, Andrews JR. Proper mechanics for baseball pitching. *Clin Sports Med.* 1989;1:151.
15. Fleisig GS, Andrews JR, Dillman CJ, et al. Kinetics of baseball pitching with implications about injury mechanisms. *Am J Sports Med.* 1995;23:233–239.
16. Lehtinen JT, Macy JC, Cassinelli E, et al. The painful scapulothoracic articulation: surgical management. *Clin Orthop Relat Res.* 2004;423:99–105.
17. Kibler B. Scapular involvement in impingement: signs and symptoms. *Instructional Course Lect.* 2006;55:35–43.
18. Tibone JE, Elrod B, Jobe FW, et al. Surgical treatment of tears of the rotator cuff in athletes. *J Bone Joint Surg Am.* 1986;68:887–891.
19. Conway J. Arthroscopic repair of partial-thickness rotator cuff tears and SLAP lesions in professional baseball players. *Orthop Clin North Am.* 2001;32:443–456.
20. Riand N, Boulahia A, Walch G. Posterosuperior impingement of the shoulder in the athlete. *Chir Orthop Reparatrice App Mot.* 2002;88:19–27.
21. Burkhart SS, Morgan CD, Kibler WB. The disabled throwing shoulder: spectrum of pathology. Part I: pathoanatomy and biomechanics. *Arthroscopy.* 2003;19:404–420.
22. Nuber G, Bowen MK. Acromioclavicular joint injuries and distal clavicle fractures. *J Am Acad Orthop Surg.* 1997;5:11–18.
23. DiFelice GS, Paletta GA Jr., Phillips BB, et al. Effort thrombosis in the elite throwing athlete. *Am J Sports Med.* 2002;30:708–712.
24. Arko FR, Harris EJ, Zarins CK, et al. Vascular complications in high-performance athletes. *J Vasc Surg.* 2001;33:935–942.
25. Bytomski JR, Black D. Conservative treatment of rotator cuff injuries. *J Surg Orthop Adv.* 2006;15:126–131.
26. Morrey BF, Tanaka S, An KN. Valgus stability of the elbow. A definition of primary and secondary constraints. *Clin Orthop Relat Res.* 1991;265:187–195.

27. Morrey BF, An KN. Articular and ligamentous contributions to the stability of the elbow joint. *Am J Sports Med.* 1983;11:315–319.

28. Callaway GH, Field LD, Deng XH, et al. Biomechanical evaluation of the medial collateral ligament of the elbow. *J Bone Joint Surg Am.* 1997;79:1223–1231.

29. Regan WD, Korinek SL, Morrey BF, et al. Biomechanical study of ligaments around the elbow joint. A definition of primary and secondary restraints. *Clin Orthop Relat Res.* 1991;271:170–179.

30. Morrey BF. Acute and chronic instability of the elbow. *J Am Acad Orthop Surg.* 1996;4:117–128.

31. Ball CM, Galatz LM, Yamaguchi K. Elbow instability: treatment strategies and emerging concepts. *Instr Course Lect.* 2002;51:53–61.

32. Timmerman LA, Schwartz ML, Andrews JR. Preoperative evaluation of the ulnar collateral ligament by magnetic resonance imaging and computed tomography arthrography. Evaluation in 25 baseball players with surgical confirmation. *Am J Sports Med.* 1994;22:26–31.

33. Rohrbrough JT, Altchek DW, Hyman J, et al. Medial collateral ligament reconstruction of the elbow using the docking technique. *Am J Sports Med.* 2002;30:541–548.

34. Rettig AC, Sherrill C, Snead DS, et al. Nonoperative treatment of ulnar collateral ligament injuries in throwing athletes. *Am J Sports Med.* 2001;29:15–17.

35. Wilson FD, Andrews JR, Blackburn TA, et al. Valgus extension overload in the pitching elbow. *Am J Sports Med.* 1983;11:82–88.

36. Ahmad CS, Park MC, El Attrache NS. Elbow medial ulnar collateral ligament insufficiency alters posteromedial olecranon contact. *Am J Sports Med.* 2004;32:1607–1612.

37. Park MC, Ahmad CS. Dynamic contributions of the flexor-pronator mass to elbow valgus instability. *J Bone Joint Surg Am.* 2004;86:2268–2274.

38. Barnes DW, Tullos HS. An analysis of 100 symptomatic baseball players. *Am J Sports Med.* 1978;6:62–67.

39. Schickendantz MS, Ho CP, Koh J. Stress injury of the proximal ulna in professional baseball players. *Am J Sports Med.* 2002;30:737–741.

40. Conway JE, Jobe FW, Glousman RE, et al. Medial instability of the elbow in throwing athletes: surgical treatment by ulnar collateral ligament repair or reconstruction. *J Bone Joint Surg.* 1992;74:67–83.

41. Rettig AC, Ebben JR. Anterior subcutaneous transfer of the ulnar nerve in the athlete. *Am J Sports Med.* 21: 836–839, 1993.

42. Johnson RK, Shrewberry MM. Median nerve entrapment syndrome in the proximal forearm. *J Hand.* 1979;4:48–51.

43. McCue FC, Alexander EJ, Baumgarten TE. Median nerve entrapment at the elbow in athletes. *Operative Techniques Sports Med.* 1996;4:21–27.

44. Heyman P, Gelberman RH, Duncan K, et al. Injuries of the ulnar collateral ligament of the thumb metacarpophalangeal joint. *Clin Orthop.* 1993;292:165–171.

45. Derkash RS, Matyas JR, Weaver JK, et al. Acute surgical repair of the skier's thumb. *Clin Orthop.* 1987;216:29–33.

46. Hastings H, Carroll C. Treatment of closed articular fractures of the metacarpophalangeal and proximal interphalangeal joints. *Hand Clin.* 1988;4:503–527.

47. Amadio PC. Epidemiology of hand and wrist injuries in sports. *Hand Clin.* 1990;6:379–381.

48. Stark HH, Jobe FW, Boyes JH, et al. Fracture of the hook of the hamate in athletes. *J Bone Joint Surg Am.* 1977;59:575–582.

49. Rettig ME, Dassa GL, Raskin KB, et al. Wrist fractures in the athlete: distal radius and carpal fractures. *Clin Sports Med.* 1998;17:469–490.

50. Bishop AT, Beckenbaugh RD. Fractures of the hamate hook. *J Hand Surg.* 1988;13A:135.

51. Nuber GW, McCarthy WJ, Yao JS, et al. Arterial abnormalities of the hand in athletes. *Am J Sports Med.* 1990;18:520–523.

52. Porubsky GL, Brown SI, Urbaniak JR. Ulnar artery thrombosis: a sports-related injury. *Am J Sports Med.* 1986;14:170–175.

53. Nuber GW, Assenmacher J, Bowen MK. Neurovascular problems in the forearm, wrist and hand. *Clin Sports Med.* 1998;17:585–610.

54. Nuber GW, Lowery CW, Chandwick RO, et al. Digital vessel trauma from repetitive impact in baseball catchers. *J Hand Surg.* 1976;1:236–238.

55. Itoh Y, Wakano K, Takeda T, et al. Circulatory disturbances in the throwing hand of baseball pitchers. *Am J Sports Med.* 1987;15:264–269.

56. Sugawara M, Ogino T, Minami A, et al. Digital ischemia in baseball players. *Am J Sports Med.* 1986;14:329–334.

Racket Sports Injuries

R acket sports such as tennis, squash, badminton, racquetball, and table tennis are some of the most popular activities worldwide. Tennis in particular has an exceedingly high level of participation in many countries and has a vast amount of scientific literature regarding benefits, injuries, and injury prevention. This chapter will provide an overview of the history of tennis, an understanding of the game, and an overview of the epidemiology, biomechanics, and treatment of tennis-related injuries. Squash and badminton will likewise be discussed.

HISTORY OF TENNIS

The original racket sport called "le jeu de paume" was played in 13th-century France on an indoor court where players used their hands.[1] Ultimately, badminton evolved in 1873 from the village of Badminton, England, as a popular lawn game using a soft shuttlecock. A few years later, squash evolved as an indoor game using a small, hard ball. An apparent hybrid of these sports, lawn tennis was invented in 1874; this new sport involved a racket length in between that used in badminton and squash, and a softer ball.

The first Wimbledon Championship was hosted in Wimbledon, England, on July 19, 1877 with 22 male players. The sport of lawn tennis was brought to the United States a few years after. The fledgling United States (lawn) Tennis Association (USTA) organized the first national tournament in Newport, Rhode Island, in 1881, and even had a women's event in Philadelphia in 1887. Professional and amateur tennis started increasing in popularity, until the Association of Tennis Players (ATP) was formed in 1972 for men. Meanwhile, Billie Jean King was instrumental in forming the Woman's Tennis Association (WTA) after defeating Bobby Riggs in the historic "Battle of the Sexes" match in 1973. Today there are more than 2 million men and women tennis players in the United States and many more worldwide, competing at all ages and skill levels.

THE GAME

Tennis can be played in singles or doubles format with the USTA having competitive age divisions for 8-year-olds to 85 and over. The game itself varies in physiologic demand based on skill level and competition level as well as age. The work-to-rest intervals vary between 1:2 and 1:5,[2] with average length of points lasting 6.36 seconds in high-level collegiate players.[3] VO_2 max ranges between 44 and 69 mL/kg/min in high-level tennis players, which would classify tennis players as being highly anaerobically trained.[4] The 36th Bethesda Conference Task Force classified tennis as a high dynamic (endurance), low static (strength) activity. However, several studies have demonstrated both concentric and eccentric left ventricular hypertrophy consistent with other high dynamic and high static sports.[5] Understanding these parameters is important when designing sports-specific training and conditioning programs for tennis players.

In a comprehensive review of health benefits, tennis was concluded to be beneficial in improving aerobic fitness, lowering body fat percentage, developing a more favorable lipid profile, reducing the risk for developing cardiovascular disease, and improving bone health.[6]

EPIDEMIOLOGY OF INJURIES

Adult Tennis Players

Tennis in general is considered a low-risk sport with regard to severe injuries. Injury patterns are generally different based on skill level and age. However, despite an exhaustive, systematic review of all 28 descriptive epidemiology articles related to tennis injury rates, no known epidemiologic interventional study has been performed to date.[7] Spreen[8] found the most common causes of withdrawal on the men's ATP tour to be injuries to the back, foot/ankle, and hip/thigh. In a retrospective cross-sectional survey of 529 USTA league players, the elbow, shoulder, and knee were the most commonly injured areas resulting in loss of an ability to play or practice for 7 days or more.[9] In this study, there were 52.9 injuries per 100 players, with a total of 299 injuries in 528 players (Fig. 8-1). Tennis players are not at a higher injury risk compared to other individual recreational sports. A retrospective cohort survey study in golfers reported 3.06 injuries per player in professional players and 2.07 injuries per player in amateur players, with a total of 637 injuries in 703 golfers.[10] In a retrospective survey of recreational runners, 45.8% of 4,358 male joggers sustained an injury.[11]

Junior Tennis Players

Competitive junior tennis players have a unique situation in that they are exposed to inordinately high volumes of tennis during some of their developing years. They may often play 10 to 30 hours/week of tennis, have fitness and conditioning, and also travel for numerous tournaments in a year. In designing injury prevention and training programs, Roettert et al.[12] found seven components of fitness to be the best predictors of a higher national ranking (Table 8-1). Despite these rigorous training and competition schedules, there is still no evidence to date that outlines the volume of tennis that junior players should play. The USTA Sport and Science Committee has recommendations for annual competitive match volumes, with admittedly little literature support (Table 8-2).[13] Hutchinson et al.[14] found an incidence of 21.5 injuries per 1,000 athletic exposures (AE) and 9.9 injuries per 100 players, where lower extremity injuries predominated.

KINETIC CHAIN AND STROKE EVALUATION

The tendency for developing upper extremity injuries is hypothesized to be a result of a breakdown of the kinetic chain and dysfunctional force transfer from

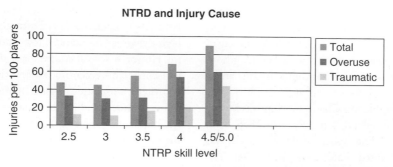

FIGURE 8-1 NTRP (National Tennis Rating Program) and Total Injury Prevalence. A nonstatistical trend is demonstrated toward more total injuries as the level of ability increases from 2.5 to 4.5/5.0. Overuse injuries predominate overall, with traumatic injuries more common in advanced players. (From Jayanthi NA, Sallay P, Hunker P. Skill level related injuries in competition tennis players. *Med Sci Tennis.* 2005;10:12–15.)

TABLE 8-1	Fitness Predictors for Higher USTA Junior National Ranking

1. Hexagon drills
2. Side shuffle (agility)
3. Push-ups
4. Dominant internal rotation range of motion
5. Dominant external rotation range of motion
6. Sit and reach
7. Sit-ups

From Roettert EP, McCormick TJ, Brown SW, et al. Relationship between isokinetic and functional strength in elite junior tennis players. *Isokin Exerc Sci.* 1996;6:15–20.

TABLE 8-2	USTA Sports and Science Committee Recommendations for Competitive Match Volume

- 12 years old and under: Up to 40 matches annually
- 14 years old and under: Up to 70 matches annually
- 16 years old and under: Up to 90 matches annually

From Riewald S. USTA junior tennis player injury risks. Paper presented at North American Regional Meeting of International Society for Tennis and Medicine Science, White Sulfur Springs, WV, August 10, 2006.

lower extremity, hip, and trunk to the terminal upper extremity. Isolated movements occur as a result. Fifty-four percent of force generation should ideally occur from the hip/pelvis during the serve (see below).[15] The subsequent upper extremity force generation is much less, with the shoulder at 21%, elbow at 15%, and wrist at 10%.[15]

Tennis strokes include the serve, ground strokes (forehand and backhand), and volleys (forehand and backhand). The serve occurs with sequential coiling of the lower extremity and pelvis to develop elastic

energy to uncoiling from counterrotation of the hips/trunk with the terminal upper extremity acting in a whip-like fashion (Fig. 8-2). Forehand and backhand groundstrokes typically involve preparation with hip/trunk rotation and shoulder turn approximately 90 degrees to the net, and again an uncoiling of the lower extremity with leg drive, trunk rotation, and finally shoulder rotation towards the target (Fig. 8-3). The elbow, forearm, and wrist act during the terminal portion of the stroke for control, not power. Tennis players become susceptible to injury with inciting events such as changes in play volume, stroke

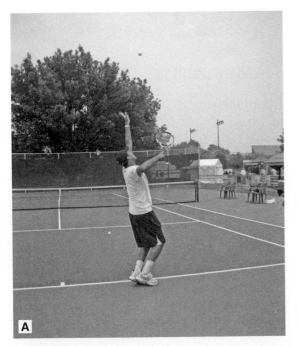
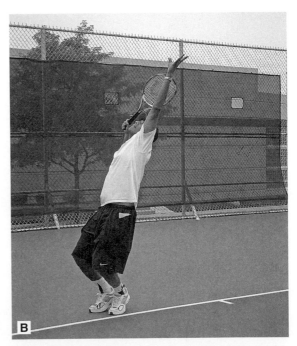

FIGURE 8-2 Serve employing kinetic chain with primary force generation from hips, pelvis, and knee bend with sequential coiling to develop necessary elastic energy for a powerful serve in a professional (ATP) tennis player. (Courtesy of Mahesh Bhupathi.)

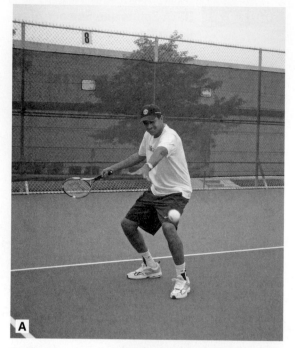 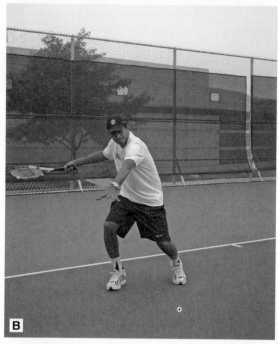

FIGURE 8-3 A. (*Left*). Traditional forehand with force generation from legs and pelvis in a neutral stance. **B.** (*Right*). Modern open stance forehand with increased abduction and hyperextension forces on right hip in a professional ATP tennis player. (Courtesy of Mahesh Bhupathi.)

adjustments, or technical flaws in a predisposed player who may be older, inflexible, or who had prior injuries (Fig. 8-4).

TENNIS-SPECIFIC ADAPTATIONS (ASYMMETRIC TENNIS PLAYER)

The unilateral nature of tennis creates certain adaptions over time. The significance of these adaptions as a way to improve performance, or a risk factor for injury, is debatable. Modification of the extremes of adaptations is a typical goal for injury-prevention programs and tennis-specific rehabilitation programs. The upper extremity, including the shoulder, elbow, and forearm, has some asymmetric differences that will be highlighted later in the chapter. Additionally, the contralateral rectus abdominus has been found to have asymmetric hypertrophy in asymptomatic high-level tennis players.

TENNIS INJURIES

Shoulder

The shoulder in some tennis players is considered susceptible to injury in some due to tennis-specific adaptions as well as a break in the kinetic chain transfer of energy. Lateral scapular slide with weak scapular stabilizers, strong internal rotation with weak external rotation, increased glenohumeral laxity, and a tight posterior capsule are all patterns seen in many overhead athletes. At 90 degrees of abduction, decreased internal rotation, increased external rotation, and a global loss of combined internal and external rotation, glenohumeral internal rotation deficit (GHIRD) was seen in 27 ATP tennis players (as had previously been noted in baseball players; Fig. 8-5).[16] A posterior capsule stretching program, "sleeper stretch" (Fig. 8-6) has been shown to reduce GHIRD[17]; however, no study has demonstrated its efficacy in reducing pain or improving function.

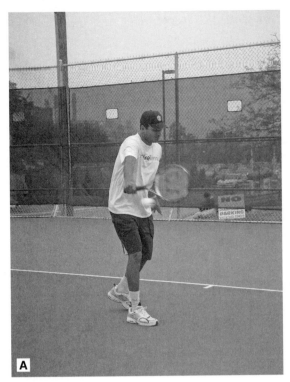
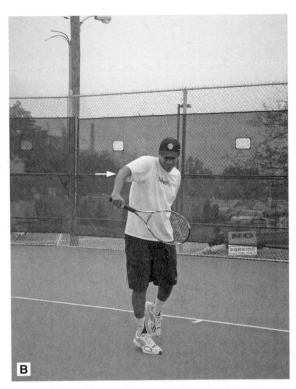

FIGURE 8-4 A. (*Left*). Correct technique at point of contact in one-handed backhand with force generation from leg drive, hip, pelvis, and linear momentum with shoulder, arm, and wrist. **B.** (*Right*). Incorrect technique (*arrow*), particularly with bent elbow and shoulder before point of contact. (Courtesy of Mahesh Bhuphathi.)

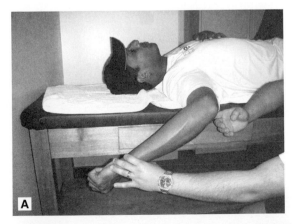
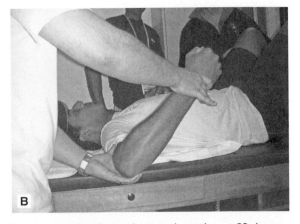

FIGURE 8-5 Glenohumeral internal rotation deficit (GHIRD) with increased glenohumeral external rotation at 90 degress (**A**, *left*) and decreased glenohumeral rotation at 90 degrees (**B**, *right*) in a professional ATP tennis player. This is a common adaptation pattern in experienced tennis players. (Courtesy of Mahesh Bhupathi.)

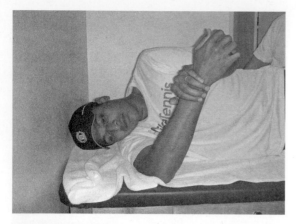

FIGURE 8-6 "Sleeper stretch," a posterior capsule stretch that can be done at night without assistance. It involves lying in the right lateral decubitis position and putting the shoulder and elbow at 90 degrees, while applying a downward force to improve internal glenohumeral rotation. (Courtesy of Mahesh Bhupathi.)

Common Shoulder Pathologies

1. Subacromial impingement with or without rotator cuff pathology/tear.
2. Superior labrum, anterior/posterior labral tears (SLAP).
3. Posterior (internal) impingement.

Subacromial impingement typically hurts with overhand motions such as the serve and/or overhead shots in the dominant shoulder. The pain pattern is typical of most impingement processes. SLAP tears usually cause discomfort in the follow-through phase of the serve or overhand in the dominant shoulder as it applies a traction force to the superior labrum (Fig. 8-7A). Posterior (internal) impingement will typically cause pain in the cocking phase of the dominant shoulder (Fig. 8-7B), where the supraspinatus tendon is impinged between posterosuperior glenoid and the greater tuberosity of the humeral head.

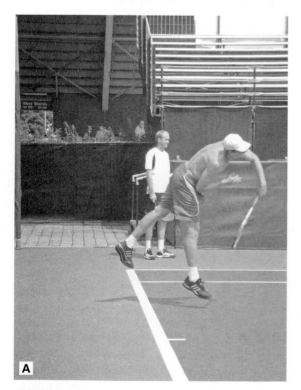

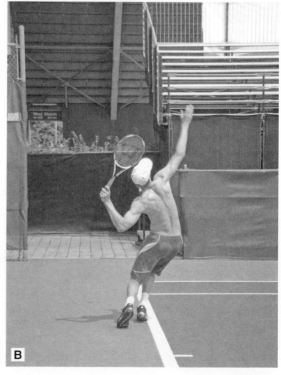

FIGURE 8-7 A. (*Left*). Follow-through on serve with elevation above the ground and in front of baseline. Pain in this portion of serve may represent a labral tear. **B.** (*Right*). Counterrotation of hip/pelvis and toss in front in serve of professional ATP player. (Courtesy of Eric Butorac.)

Tennis-Specific Tips

1. Perform deep knee bends during strokes (10 degrees or more).
   - Shoulder and elbow torque are significantly less with larger knee bends (>10 degrees).[18]
2. Increase counterrotation of hips/trunk.
   - To increase force transfer from hip/trunk up to 54%.[15]
3. Toss the ball in front of the body during serve.
4. Hit flat serves initally, before adding spin.
5. "Swing harder" is the *last* tip for a faster serve.

Rehabilitative Principles

Functional shoulder rehabilitation incorporates an acute phase, a recovery phase, and finally a functional phase prior to return to tennis.[19] The acute phase consists of shoulder motion in pain-free ranges, below 90 degrees of abduction and posterior capsule stretches when necessary to correct GHIRD. Additionally, maintenance of strength and scapular control consists of isometric and closed kinetic chain (CKC) exercises early in rehabilitation as well as introducing core strengthening. The recovery phase progresses to proprioceptive neuromuscular facilitation (PNF) patterns in diagonal shoulder movements, and CKC exercises above 90 degrees. Higher-level functional strengthening as well as continued kinetic chain and core strengthening should be incorporated. The functional phase of rehabilitation should progress to multiplanar motions in all directions as well as incorporating functional eccentric strengthening in 90-degree abduction with rapid movements (Fig. 8-8A). Proprioceptive shoulder training as well as integration of the kinetic chain should continue with all rehabilitative exercises until the tennis player can pass tennis-specific functional exercises.

Return to Tennis after Shoulder Surgery

In a retrospective review of 51 experienced tennis players with an average age of 51, 40 players returned to tennis after open or arthroscopic repair/debridement of the rotator cuff at an average of 9.8 months after surgery; there was no difference with open repair or arthroscopy.[20] The same group evaluated functional outcomes with 28 tournament players of average age 26.9 years after having appropriate rotator cuff and labral debridement for posterior impingement. Of 28 players, 22 were able to return to tennis, although 20 of those who returned still had some pain with tennis.[21]

Elbow

Typically, elbows in experienced tennis players have a loss of terminal extension, pronation, and supination as well as asymmetric hypertrophy of the forearm muscles. The elbow is also the most often injured area, particularly in recreational players. There is a 50% incidence of elbow injuries in club players 30 years or older,[22] with a fourfold increase in players over 40 years old.[23] The risk of elbow injury is also two to four times greater if playing more than 2 hours daily,[23] while overall injury risk is not increased up to 6 hours/week of playing.[9] Interestingly, only one case of lateral epicondylitis was reported in over 700 players

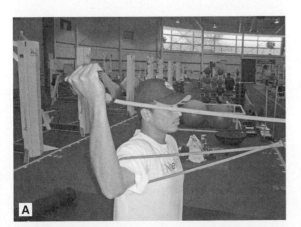
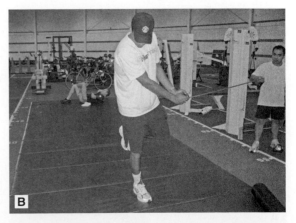

FIGURE 8-8 Functional strengthening of the upper extremity and shoulder in a tennis player. **A.** (*Left*). Eccentric strengthening of shoulder in 90–90 position. **B.** (*Right*). The same player incorporating core stability and functional eccentric strengthening of the upper extremity while recreating backhand stroke. (Courtesy of Mahesh Bhupathi.)

(including seniors) over 3 years at the French Open.[24] These data support the theory that tennis elbow is actually a rare problem in the advanced player, but much more common in the recreational player as a result of differences in technique.

Common Elbow Pathology

1. Lateral epicondylitis.
2. Medial epicondylitis.
3. Ulnar collateral ligament insufficiency, with or without ulnar nerve involvement.
4. Valgus extension-overload.

Symptoms of lateral epicondylitis, "tennis elbow," typically occur in the terminal eccentric phase of a one-handed backhand, particularly when there is excess uncontrolled wrist extension. Both medial and lateral epicondylitis can occur with forehands and serves. There is likely excess pronation on forehands and serves with tennis elbow, while traction on the medial epicondyle on extreme grips to develop more topspin (typically in advanced players) may result in medial epicondylitis. Additional medial elbow probems such as ulnar collateral

ligament insufficiency and ulnar neuritis may develop with progressive and excess valgus on serves, and again may involve some traction injury from forehand groundstrokes. Posterior valgus extension-overload typically is most painful in the posterior elbow from the terminal extension and snap at the elbow from serves and overhead shots. Tensile forces at the medial elbow lead to compression laterally, then stress posteriorly, occasionally resulting in osteophytes and impingement.

Tennis-Specific Tips

1. The player should be evaluated for a one-handed versus two-handed backhand.
   - There is no difference in wrist extensor activity with one- and two-handed backhands. However, the extra hand may act as a "check reign" to limit end ranges of motion to abnormal elbow/forearm movement patterns, and uncontrolled terminal wrist extension.
2. Grip moderately or lightly and only on contact.
3. Avoid early forearm pronation on forehands and serves, and terminal wrist extension on backhands.

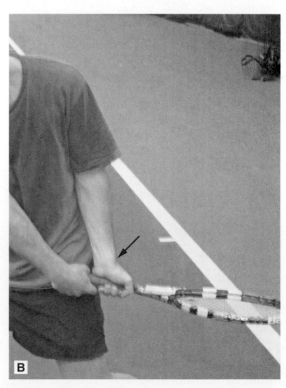

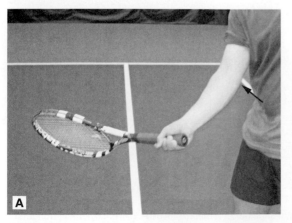

FIGURE 8-9 A. (*Left*). Semi-Western grip in an advanced player to generate more topspin, but putting traction on medial epicondyle (*red arrow*). **B.** (*Right*). Excess supination, dorsiflexion, and ulnar deviation of nondominant (left) wrist of a two-handed backhand (*red arrow*). (Courtesy of Steve Nudo.)

- Instruction on stroke modification (in office or 1 hour on court) and routine conservative therapy resulted in 90% resolution of elbow pain in tennis players with less than 6 months of pain, and obviated the need for surgery in any of the players.[25]
4. Do not lead with elbow (Fig. 8-4B).
5. Avoid extreme grips.
   - Limit semi-Western grip (Fig. 8-9A) in medial elbow pain.
6. Consider lowering string tension, and limit volume to less than 6 hours weekly.

Rehabilitative Principles

The three components of elbow rehabilitation are the acute phase, a strengthening phase, and a functional phase. The acute phase focuses on pain relief, reduction of tennis volume, resting volar splint, and use of a counterforce brace if necessary. An initial introduction of passive stretching and kinetic chain rehabilitation can be started. The strengthening phase involves continued upper extremity and core strengthening. Isometric strengthening and progressive eccentric strengthening of wrist extensors while incorporating the kinetic chain can then be added (Fig. 8-8B). The functional strengthening phase incorporates correction of biomechanical errors; functional eccentric wrist extensor strengthening, particularly for backhand; and modification of forearm pronation on forehands and serve. Functional return to tennis after upper extremity injuries is presented later in the chapter.

Return to Tennis after Elbow Surgery

Nonoperative treatment of ulnar collateral ligament insufficiency resulted in 42% improvement in throwing athletes. Good and excellent results have been seen in ulnar collateral ligament reconstruction in experienced hands. Arthroscopic drilling with surgical debridement resulted in improvement in 97% of patients in experienced hands.[26]

Wrist

Ulnar wrist injuries have become an increasingly common problem with tennis players. The modern game involves a higher combination of powerful serves and topspin forehands, accounting for 75% of all strokes. Muscular adaptions of the wrist were seen in a study of 32 female elite USTA junior tennis players who were found to have significantly greater dominant wrist and forearm pronation strength and also dominant forearm weakness in supination.[27]

At the French Tennis Federation National Training Center, 11.2% of reported injuries in men and 15.7% of reported injuries in women occurred at the wrist.[28] Injuries to the extensor carpi ulnaris (ECU) were the most common.

Common Wrist Pathology

1. Extensor carpi ulnaris injury.
   - Tendinosis, subluxation, rupture.
2. Triangular fibrocartilage complex (TFCC) injury.
   - Traumatic, nontraumatic.
3. Ulnar impaction.

Ulnar wrist injuries typically occur in the nondominant wrist of the player with a two-handed backhand or a dominant forehand due to a combination of ulnar deviation, supination, and dorsiflexion (Fig. 8-9B). This is usually an attempt by the player to generate high rotational forces to generate excess topspin. Traumatic injuries, including acute TFCC tears and ECU ruptures/subluxations, can result from excess, uncontrolled rapid radial deviation from the original position described above.

Tennis-Specific Tips

1. Limit excess movement of the following:
   - Ulnar deviation, supination, wrist extension.
2. Limit early/excess topspin.
   - Nondominant wrist (two-handed backhand), dominant (forehand).
3. Utilize core muscles and lower extremities in force generation.

Rehabilitative Principles

In a study of 28 elite players with ECU subluxations, ulnar gutter splints were prescribed for 3 to 4 months followed by serial ultrasounds with full return to play achieved in all players.[28] ECU tendinosis can be usually treated with a splint, a corticosteroid injection, and dedicated ECU tendon rehabilitation. ECU rupture should be treated operatively. Treatment of TFCC injuries varies depending on acuity of injury and location of the tear within the TFCC. Successful arthroscopy for erosions related to ulnar impaction syndrome have also been reported.

Functional Progression in the Rehabilitation of Upper Extremity Injuries

1. Mini-tennis from service line with swing from point of contact → follow through.
2. Mini-tennis from two-thirds court with progressively more backswing and gentle spin.

3. Full court with leg drive but no heavy spins or heavy pace.
4. Throwing tennis ball from baseline line to the other side.
5. Serves from baseline.
6. Full groundstrokes → full serves → competition.[29]

Back

Renkawitz[30] noted that more than 50% of amateur German tennis players suffer from low back pain during and after tennis, and 38% of players on a men's professional tour missed at least one tournament during the season due to low back pain. In fact, injuries to the back are the most common cause of withdrawal from the ATP tour.[8]

Common Back Pathology
1. Lumbar disc herniation (prolapse).
2. Lumbar facet syndrome.
3. Pars stress fracture/spondylolysis.
4. Sacroiliac joint dysfunction.

Junior tennis players, particularly those with hyperlordotic spines, may place themselves at risk for low back injuries that are typically extension-based, with hyperextension on serves (particularly heavy topspin). Additionally, lack of appropriate core stability in multiple planes makes the low back more susceptible to increased forces during the open stance forehand. The adult tennis player typically develops hip flexion contractures from repetitive flexion on serves and follow-through. The thoracic spine allows for 35 degrees of rotation whereas the lumbar spine allows for only 5 degrees of rotation. Therefore, abnormal forces of rotation on the lumbar spine that can occur with serves as well as groundstrokes (especially in multiplanar or combined motions) may also contribute to injury patterns.

Tennis Tips
1. Young tennis players should limit heavy topspin, or "kick" serves when they have extension-based low back pain.
2. Spinal rotation on groundstrokes and serve should occur primarily in the thoracic spine, while trying to maintain a neutral lumbar spine.
3. Limit multiplanar motions.
4. The adult player should try to develop as much hip extension as possible on serves to prevent progression of hip flexor contractures.

Rehabilitative Principles
A 7-week home back exercise program of 20 minutes daily was successful in improving pain ratings and also noting improvements in performance in 70 amateur German tennis players.[30] Electromyographic follow-up studies also demonstrated improvements in trunk extension strength.[30] Treatment programs should have specificity toward the condition involved. Posterior element problems such as facet syndrome and spondylolysis should initially limit extension, and flexion-based disorders such as discogenic pathology should limit initial flexion. Incorporation of eccentric abdominal control and overall core stability in sagital, coronal, transverse, and functional planes is the hallmark of treatment in tennis players.

Lower Extremity

Lower extremity injuries occur more frequently in advanced players due to the high amount of force generation and rapid directional changes. Traumatic injuries are generally more commonly reported in these players, which include ankle sprains, medial gastrocnemius strains (tennis leg), as well as knee ligament and meniscal injuries. Overload injuries such as Achilles tendonitis and sesamoiditis from loading the forefoot do also still occur in the lower extremity in these players. Maquirriain and Ghisi[31] noted a stress fracture incidence of 12.9% in elite tennis players with the majority being to the lower extremity (metatarsal, tarsal, navicular, and tibia). Typically training programs requiring high amounts of intensive training and competition may result in increased overload injuries to the lower extremity.

Tennis with an Anterior Cruciate Ligament-Deficient Knee
There is a 1.8% overall anterior cruciate ligament (ACL) rupture incidence from tennis-related injuries. Middle-aged recreational tennis players may continue to play tennis, even if ACL-deficient, if they have no history of recurrent subluxations or advancement of meniscal or articular cartilage abnormalities. Sixteen ACL-deficient tennis players with an average age of 39 were found to have lower postinjury function as well as performance ratings.[32] Tennis-specific limitations in these players included reduced rapid directional changes, playing a maximum of three sets of singles, and playing only on hard courts. Doubles play, clay courts, and side-to-side movement were not statistically different.

Tennis after Joint Replacement Surgery

Fifty-eight USTA members with a mean age of 70 were able to return to tennis after total hip replacement surgery, with only three revisions required at 7-year follow-up.[33] All players noted significant overall improvement in pain and function. General recommendations following total hip replacement are that doubles play is acceptable and singles play is not recommended. These recommendations may be modified based on the individual and level of play.

Thirty-three USTA members with a mean age of 57 were able to return to tennis after total knee replacement surgery. Twelve percent of players complained of pain and stiffness. General recommendations following total knee replacement are the same as for total hip replacement. These recommendations, however, may be modified based on the individual and level of play.[34]

Functional Progression in the Rehabilitation of Lower Extremity and Back Injuries (10 Minutes Each)

1. Side shuffle along service line and around court (preferably clay court).
2. Mini-tennis from service line in only one service box.
3. Mini-tennis from service line including both service boxes.
4. Two-thirds court adding more lateral movements (entire court width).
5. Full court with neutral spine and good leg drive with no heavy spins or pace.
6. Serves from baseline.
7. Full groundstrokes → full serves → competition.[29]

TENNIS EQUIPMENT

Tennis rackets and other tennis equipment were developed primarily to maximize performance while mitigating the chance for injury. Theoretically, an increase in vibration may lead to an increase in injuries, particularly to the upper extremity. The choice of tennis racket should be based on style of play. A head-light racket is more appropriate for the serve-and-volley player, while a head-heavy racket is more appropriate for powerful groundstrokes. Lower tennis string tension typically imparts more power with less control, while multifilament and natural gut strings anecdotally may give players a "softer," more comfortable feel. Injury-modifying equipment (tennis

elbow straps, vibration dampeners, wrist splints, knee braces) were found to be used more commonly in those players who were injured; however, no protective effect has been demonstrated.[9] Vibration dampeners are used to decrease string vibrations in the racket, but do not result in any reduced racket frame vibration to the forearm.[35] The strings only weigh 1/20th of the weight of the racket, and vibration reduction is overall negligible. Counterforce braces (tennis elbow straps) have been effective in decreasing forces to the extensor carpi radialis brevis (ECRB) in cadaver studies and to the forearms in tennis players, but are not necessarily effective in injury reduction.

Tennis-Specific Tips

1. Choose the heaviest racket that does not affect swing speed for style of play.
2. Vibration dampeners effect is negligible in mitigating forces to the upper extremity.
3. Tennis elbow straps may mitigate forces to ECRB but are not necessarily effective in reduction of injuries.
4. Lowering string tension with upper extremity injuries may allow for increased power, therefore requiring less force development from the upper extremity.
5. Players with lower extremity and knee injuries should consider clay court tennis.
   • Slower playing surface.
   • Knee pain ratings are much better on clay courts than hard courts.

SQUASH

Squash originated in the 19th century in England; however, the United States became the first nation to form a dedicated association and solidify the game in 1907. American-style squash uses a hard ball and a slightly larger court than the English style. Modern rackets are 70 cm long with a maximum string area of 500 cm² and weight between 110 to 200 g. Squash balls are made of rubber, with two pieces glued together to form a hollow sphere and buffed to a matte finish. The balls are marked with a small colored dot to indicate the level of bounce. During play, the ball may reach speeds in excess of 170 mph. The players are categorized into retrievers, shooters, power players, and "all rounders" depending on their style of play. Squash provides an excellent cardiovascular workout, 70% more than either tennis or racquetball.[36]

The majority of the injuries in squash are acute or traumatic events and a relatively small proportion are from overuse. Head and eye injuries are not uncommon. Eime et al.[37] studied the epidemiology of squash injuries requiring hospitalization between 2000 and 2001. They noted an overall injury rate of 35.5/100,000 players. Sixty-eight percent of the injuries involved the lower extremity; 80% were male, and eye injuries were the most common reason (32.7%) for presentation to the emergency department.

In a retrospective study of racket sport patterns of injuries, Chard and Lachmann[38] noted that squash players sustained more injuries, at 59% compared to 21% for tennis players and 20% for badminton players. Squash players sustained more knee, lumbar region, and ankle injuries, whereas upper extremity injuries were more common in tennis.

BADMINTON

Badminton was originally developed in India during the 18th century and was called "Poona." In 1893, the village of Badminton (England) formally developed rules of play. Badminton rackets are light, weighing between 70 and 100 g without strings. The string tension is normally in the range of 18 to 36 lb. The fastest recorded stroke in badminton is 206 mph, whereas that for the tennis stroke is only 153 mph. This is because badminton players use the terminal upper extremity like a whip during play to a greater extent than tennis players, accounting for faster racket-head velocity.

Kroner et al.[39] studied badminton injuries seen in a Denmark hospital during a 12-month period in 1986. A total of 217 injuries in 203 patients were seen, constituting 4.1% of all sports injuries seen during that period. Joints and ligaments were injured in 58.8% of badminton players/patients and were most frequently located in the lower extremities. They were significantly more common in patients younger than age 30. Muscle injury occurred in 19.8% of patients and was more frequent in older patients. Although most injuries were minor, 6.8% of patients did require hospitalization.

INJURY PREVENTION IN RACKET SPORTS

A majority of the literature regarding prevention has focused on proper eye wear for squash players. Such protection is obviously recommended.[40]

Players participating in all racket sports should participate in a comprehensive flexibility, strengthening, and fitness exercise program to enhance performance while mitigating chance of injury. Individuals with systemic illnesses and cardiopulmonary restrictions should have physician clearance before participating even in a recreational manner.

SUMMARY

- Overuse injuries are common in tennis, particularly in recreational players.
- Upper extremity injuries are likely a result of breakdown of the kinetic chain, particularly in recreational tennis players.
- Correction of biomechanical factors is helpful in preventing recurrence in all racket sports.
- Lower extremity and trunk injuries are more common in advanced tennis players.
- Quantity of play may be less of an issue than quality of play in recreational tennis players.
- Squash and badminton can be highly aerobic sports with rapid directional changes resulting in more lower extremity injuries.
- All racket sports discussed have cardiovascular benefit, and overall they have relatively low injury rates in comparison to other individual recreational sports.

REFERENCES

1. Kramer J, Sloane S, Campbel J, et al. *The Complete Guide to USPTA Membership*. Houston: U.S. Professional Tennis Association; 2005.
2. Kovacs MS. A comparison of work/rest intervals in men's professional tennis. *Med Sci Tennis*. 2004;9:10–11.
3. Kovacs MS, Strecker E, Chandler WB, et al. Time analysis of work/rest intervals in men's collegiate tennis. In: *National Strength and Conditioning Conference, 2004*. Minneapolis: NSCA; 2004;18:364.
4. Green JM, Crews TR, Bosak AM, et al. A comparison of respiratory compensation thresholds of anaerobic competitors, aerobic competitors and untrained subjects. *Eur J Appl Physiol*. 2003;90:608–613.
5. Pluim BM, Zwinderman AH, van der Laarse A, et al. The athlete's heart. A meta-analysis of cardiac structure and function. *Circulation*. 2000;101:336–344.
6. Pluim BM, Staal JB, Marks BL, et al. Heath benefits of tennis. *Br J Sports Med*. 2007. Available at: http://bjsm.bmj.com/cgi/content/abstract/bjsm.2006.034967v2. Accessed October 13, 2007.
7. Pluim BM, Staal JB, Windler GE, et al. Tennis injuries: occurrence, aetiology, and prevention. *Br J Sports Med*. 2006; 40:415–423.

8. Spreen D. Injury statistics and trends of ATP players. *Med Sci Tennis*. 2001;6. Available at: http://www.stms.nl/index. php?option=com_content&task=view&id=768&Itemid=263. Accessed October 13, 2007.

9. Jayanthi NA, Sallay P, Hunker P. Skill level related injuries in competition tennis players. *Med Sci Tennis*. 2005;10: 12–15.

10. Gosheger G, Liem D, Ludwig K, et al. Injuries and overuse syndromes in golf. *Am J Sports Med*. 2003;31: 438–443.

11. Marti B, Minder C, Abelin T. On the epidemiology of running injuries. The 1984 Bern Grand Prix study. *Am J Sports Med*. 1988;16:285–294.

12. Roettert EP, McCormick TJ, Brown SW, et al. Relationship between isokinetic and functional strength in elite junior tennis players. *Isokin Exerc Sci*. 1996;6:15–20.

13. Riewald S. USTA junior tennis player injury risks. Paper presented at North American Regional Meeting of International Society for Tennis and Medicine Science, White Sulfur Springs, WV, August 10, 2006.

14. Hutchinson MR, Laprade RF, Quinter MB, et al. Injury surveillance at the USTA boys' tennis championships: a 6-year study. *Med Sci Sports Exerc*. 1994;27:826–830.

15. Kibler WB. Clinical biomechanics of the elbow in tennis: implications for evaluation and diagnosis. *Med Sci Sports Exerc*. 1994;26:1203–1206.

16. Schmidt-Wiethoff S. 2002 kinematic analysis of internal and external rotation range of motion in professional tennis. *Med Sci Tennis*. 2003;8:18–19.

17. Kibler WB, Chandler TJ. Range of motion in junior tennis players participating in an injury risk modification program. *J Sci Med Sport*. 2003;6:51–62.

18. Fleisig G, Nicholls R, Eliot B, et al. Kinematics used by world class tennis players to produce high-velocity serves. *Sports Biomech*. 2003;2:51–64.

19. Kibler WB. Rehabilitation principles of injuries in tennis. In: Renstrom PA, ed. *Handbook of Sports Medicine and Science: Tennis*. Oxford: Blackwell; 2002:262–277.

20. Sonnery-Cottet B, Edwards B, Noel E, et al. Rotator cuff tears in middle-aged tennis players: results of surgical treatment. *Am J Sports Med*. 2002;30:558–564.

21. Sonnery-Cottet B, Edwards B, Noel E, et al. Results of arthroscopic treatment of posterosuperior glenoid impingement in tennis players. *Am J Sports Med*. 2002;30: 227–232.

22. Nirschl R. The etiology and treatment of tennis elbow. *Am J Sports Med*. 1974;2:308–323.

23. Gruchow HW, Pelletier D. An epidemiologic study of tennis elbow: incidence, recurrence, and effectiveness of prevention strategies. *Am J Sports Med*. 1979;7:234–238.

24. Montalvan B, Parier J, Gires A, et al. Results of three years medical surveillance at the international championships at Roland Garros: an epidemiological study in sports pathology. *Med Sci Tennis*. 2004;9:14–15.

25. Ilfeld FW. Can stroke modification relieve tennis elbow? *Clin Orthop Rel Res*. 1992;276:182–186.

26. Nirschl RP. Elbow tendinosis/tennis elbow. *Clin Sports Med*. 1992;11:851–870.

27. Ellenbecker TS, Roetert EP, Riewald S. Isokinetic profile of wrist and forearm strength in elite female junior tennis players. *Br J Sports Med*. 2006;40:411–414.

28. Montalval B, Parier J, Brasseur JL, et al. Extensor carpi unaris injuries in tennis payers: a study of 28 cases. *Br J Sports Med*. 2006;40:424–429.

29. Pluim BM. Modified from injury cards. Available at: http://www.stms.nl. Accessed August 2007.

30. Renkawitz T. Neuromuscular efficiency of erector spinae in high performance amateur tennis players. *Med Sci Tennis*. 2006;11:26–31.

31. Maquirriain J, Ghisi JP. The incidence and distribution of stress fractures in elite tennis players. *Br J Sports Med*. 2006;40:454–459.

32. Maquirriain J, Megey PJ. Tennis specific limitations in players with an ACL-deficient knee. *Br J Sports Med*. 2006;40:451–453.

33. Mont MA, LaPorte DM, Mulllick T, et al. Tennis after total hip arthroplasty. *Am J Sports Med*. 1999;27:60–64.

34. Mont MA, Rajadhyaksha AD, Marxen JL, et al. Tennis after total knee arthroplasty. *Am J Sports Med*. 2002;30:163–166.

35. Li FX, Fewtrell D, Jenkins M. String vibration dampers do not reduce racket frame vibration transfer to the forearm. *J Sports Sci*. 2004;22:1041–1052.

36. Bellamy R. *The Story of Squash*. London: Casell; 1978.

37. Eime R, Zazryn T, Finch C. Epidemiology of squash injuries requiring hospital treatment. *Int J Inj Contr Saf Promot*. 2003;10:243–245.

38. Lachmann SM, Chard MD. Racquet sports—patterns of injury presenting to a sports injury clinic. *Br J Sports Med*. 1987;21:150–153.

39. Kroner K, Schmdit SA, Neilson AB, et al. Badminton injuries: *Br J Sports Med*. 1990;24:169–172.

40. Eime R, Finch C, Wolfe R, et al. The effectiveness of a squash eye ware promotion strategy. *Br J Sports Med*. 2004; 39:681–685.

Golf Injuries

G olf is a sport that affords people of all ages and skill levels the opportunity to play. It is a relatively simple game to play, with its objective to hit a ball into a hole with a club, in as few strokes as possible. It has gained much popularity over the past few decades on account of advanced technologies, increased media attention, and dynamic golf personalities.[1] Today, there are approximately 28.7 million golfers in America.[1]

Golf is usually considered a very, low-impact, low-intensity sport, as there is no direct physical competition with other players. However, as with other sports, overuse and traumatic injuries are inherent to golf. Overuse injuries are usually related to excessive practice and reluctance to rest an injury, whereas traumatic injuries may occur from hitting fixed objects such as rocks.[2–4] Amateur golfers typically develop injuries related to poor swing mechanics.[2–4]

This chapter will focus on the biomechanics of the golf swing as well as several common golf-related injuries and their management.

THE GOLF SWING

The golf swing can be separated into five phases: backswing, downswing, impact, and follow-through. Each phase of the swing should be performed in a coordinated, fluid movement. It must be stressed that the following description is for the right-handed golfer.

Preparation

The golf swing begins with the golfer addressing the ball. At address, the feet are spread shoulder width apart with the ball placed at the center of the stance (Fig. 9-1A). The spine is relatively neutral, though the position of the arms will naturally introduce a slight

increased thoracic kyphosis. The hands should hang immediately below the shoulders with both elbows straight, which typically introduces roughly 30 to 45 degrees of shoulder flexion, depending on the golfer's stance. Both wrists are pronated approximately 45 degrees so that the palmar surfaces are facing and the hands can grip the golf club (Fig. 9-1B). The grip should be held primarily in the fingers of both hands. For a right-handed golfer, the left hand should grip the club with approximately 1 inch of the butt end of the grip extending above the hypothenar eminence[3]; the right hand should be placed lower on the club overlapping the first two to three digits of the left hand (Fig. 9-1C). The hands should be placed on the grip so that both thumbs are on the superior aspect of the club. The golfer's grip on the club should be firm enough so the club is secure in both hands. Excessive grip pressure can result in elbow and wrist injuries, which are described later in the chapter.

Backswing

The backswing begins with the takeaway (sometimes considered a separate phase of the golf swing). The takeaway involves "hinging" the wrists, which is a coordinated movement of radial deviation of both wrists coupled with the extension of the right wrist and pronation of the left wrist (Fig. 9-2A). This movement is coupled with shoulder abduction and elbow flexion of the right arm and adduction of the left arm. The left elbow is maintained in a relatively straight position. Weight is then shifted from a central position to almost entirely on the right leg while rotating or "coiling" the trunk, hips, and shoulders to the right (Fig. 9-2A). The flexed knee position is maintained throughout the backswing and the left knee is adducted without picking the foot off of the

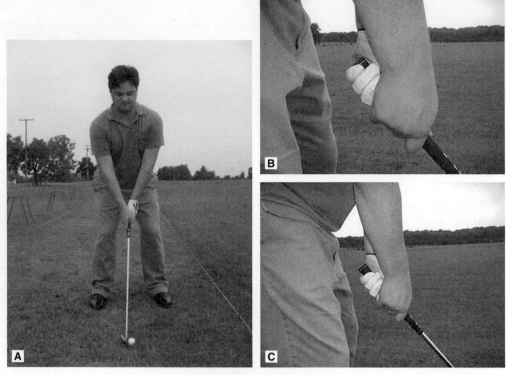

FIGURE 9-1 Preparation. Notice that the feet are shoulder width apart, and the hands are facing each other with the butt end of the club approximately 1 inch above the hypothenar eminence.

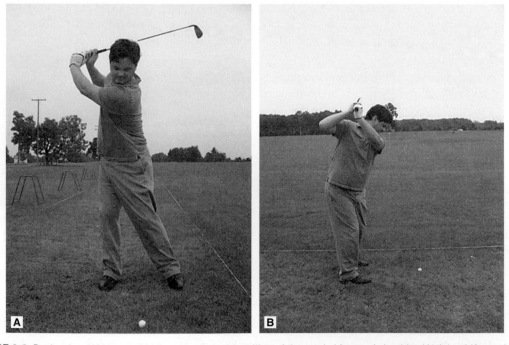

FIGURE 9-2 Backswing. Wrists are hinging, coupled with coiling of the trunk, hips, and shoulder. Weight shifts to the right leg for a right-handed golfer. Notice that the shaft of the club is parallel to the ground, pointing toward the intended target.

ground (Fig. 9-2B). Once the club is at the top of the swing with the shaft of the club approximately parallel to the ground and pointing toward the intended target, the backswing is complete (Fig. 9-2B). Excessive length or rotation of the backswing can lead to back pain, which is discussed later.

Downswing

The downswing is essentially the reverse of the backswing, but at an increasing velocity. After a slight pause at the top of the backswing, the downswing begins with an uncoiling of the trunk, while shifting the weight back to the left side so that it is equally distributed between the feet at impact (Fig. 9-3). During this motion, the left arm actively abducts, while the right arm adducts to stabilize the club. Before impact the left wrist supinates and ulnarly deviates while the right wrist flexes and ulnarly deviates back to the initial position. The swing accelerates throughout the downswing and reaches a maximal velocity at impact.

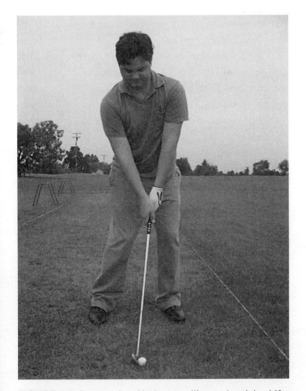

FIGURE 9-3 Downswing. Notice uncoiling and weight shifts during impact.

Impact

Impact is the point between the downswing and the follow-through when the club head makes contact with the golf ball (Fig. 9-3). Although the weight is being shifted to the left side of the body, and the trunk, hips, and shoulders are rotating left, weight should actually be equally dispersed between both legs and the golfer should be square to the ball during impact. The arms, wrists, and hands should return to the initial address position and the club head should be square to the target at impact. Ideally, the ball is struck first during impact and the *divot is taken during the follow-through*. A divot is a piece of turf, which is sometimes taken before or after impact. Taking the divot before the ball may cause hand, wrist, and shoulder injuries, which are described later.[2,3]

Follow-Through

The follow-through is the deceleration part of the swing, beginning with impact and ending at the completion of the golf swing. During this phase the hips extend and the shoulders and trunk complete the rotation to the left until the golfer is facing the intended target (Fig. 9-4). The weight continues to shift to the left foot until almost all of the body weight is over the left leg, allowing the right heel to come off the ground and the right knee to adduct. The arms continue on the arc of the downswing with the left shoulder abducting while the left elbow flexes and the left wrist supinates. Meanwhile, the right shoulder is adducting while the right wrist pronates. The club comes to rest over the left shoulder with the club head pointing down toward the ground (Fig. 9-4).

COMMON GOLF-RELATED INJURIES

According to the Consumer Product Safety Commission, golf-related emergency room visits totaled 50,160 in 2003.[5] Similarly, all medically treated golf injuries totaled 140,810 or 4.1% of the total reported medically treated sports injuries in 2003.[5] There are differences in experience levels of golfers in regard to anatomic region injured. Professional golfers have a higher overall prevalence of injury and have a tendency to sustain injuries to the low back and wrist compared to amateur golfers, who tend to injure the elbow more frequently (Table 9-1).[4,6,7] Additionally, women have significantly more wrist

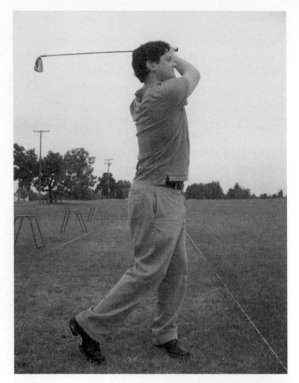

FIGURE 9-4 Follow-through. Notice weight shift to the left and deceleration completing the golf swing, until the golfer is facing the intended target and the head of the club pointing towards the ground.

injuries than men.[4,6,7] Table 9-2 lists the average time lost from sports for various body injury sites.

Back Injuries

The majority of back injuries related to golf are mechanical in nature (Table 9-3).[7] The inherent forces that are produced by a golf swing make back injuries

common, particularly during impact, follow-through, and backswing (Table 9-4).[8] The lateral bending, rotational, and compressive forces placed on the spine during the golf swing may lead to injuries including muscle strains, facet arthropathy, disc herniation, compression fracture, and spinal stenosis.[7] Furthermore, increased age and multiple comorbidities can place golfers at greater risk for compression fractures, lumbar degenerative disk disease, and spinal stenosis.[9]

The repetitive forces of flexion, rotation, and compression that the golf swing puts on the spine may put the golfer at risk of developing degenerative disc disease. Over time, this may lead to bulging of the disc and radial tears of the annulus fibrosis.[7] Golfers between the ages of 20 and 35 are at greatest risk.[7] Most often, herniation of the nucleus pulposus occurs with combined movements of flexion and rotation with compression.[9]

Patients with herniated discs generally complain of gradually worsening back pain with radicular symptoms. Pain and spasm are generally worsened with forward flexion and relieved with extension of the spine. Neurologic findings, such as weakness, parasthesia, and depressed deep tendon reflexes in a nerve root pattern, are suggestive of a herniated disc that is impinging on or irritating a nerve root. Signs and symptoms are usually unilateral, although they can occur bilaterally. A positive straight leg raise and dermatomal distribution of neurologic deficit is suggestive of radiculopathy; however, patients may display varying degrees of signs and symptoms. A variety of diagnostic studies can be used to determine the presence and degree of disc pathology. Electrodiagnostics (EDX) is the best test to demonstrate nerve injury as it is a test of nerve function. Radiographs can demonstrate joint space narrowing and bony pathology, whereas magnetic resonance imaging (MRI) can

TABLE 9-1	Prevalence Range of Golf-Related Injuries in Recent Literature			
Region	Amateur (%)	Professional (%)	Male (%)	Female (%)
Low Back	15–34	22–24	25–36	22–27
Shoulder	8–12[a]	8–12[a]	NA	NA
Elbow	25–33	7–10	8–33	6–50
Wrist	13–20	20–27	18–33	12–36

[a] Shoulder data listed includes injuries for all golfers.[4]

TABLE 9-2	Average Time Lost from Sport Due to Injury[6]
Region of Injury	**Average Time Lost (Days)**
Thoracic spine	137.4
Lumbar spine	69.0
Shoulder	36.1
Elbow	73.8
Wrist/hand	55.9

visualize disc and nerve involvement. However, MRI may have high false positives, as high as 66%.[10,11] Significant central herniation impinging on the cauda equina can lead to bowel and bladder retention or incontinence and is a medical emergency.

Muscle strains can occur along either side of the paraspinal musculature and are often aggravated by repetitive activity, particularly eccentric muscle contraction.[7] There is usually an acute onset of localized pain, sometimes associated with muscular spasm. The neurologic exam should be normal.

Mechanical back pain can often be treated successfully with conservative treatment and rest from exacerbating activities. Nonsteroidal anti-inflammatory drugs (NSAIDs), pain medication, and short-term use of muscle relaxants may be beneficial to treat acute low back pain.[12] Core muscles include transversus abdominis, internal obliques, external obliques, rectus abdominis, erector spinae, iliopsoas, quadratus lumborum, and gluteal muscles. Strengthening these muscles both concentrically and eccentrically can help golfers with low back pain better control their trunk

and pelvis during the golf swing and may help prevent recurrences of back injury.[7] Golfers should return to their sport only after they have regained full pain-free range of motion, strength and endurance, and can swing pain-free.[7] Golfers may often benefit from working with a Professional Golfers' Association (PGA) professional to improve swing biomechanics, synchronize rotation of the hips with the shoulders to reduce rotational stress, and decrease spine extension and lateral bending during the follow-through. Some physical therapists also specialize in golf-related injuries and golf rehabilitation.

There are few reports of vertebral compression fractures related to golf in the literature.[7] Golf is not a predisposing factor for compression fractures. However, with the large population of aging golfers, compression fractures are in the differential diagnosis for back pain. Patients with a history of osteoporosis or cancer are at greatest risk for developing compression fractures of the vertebrae.[7] Patients with compression fractures usually present with central, localized pain over the spine that improves with rest.[7] Lateral spine films can be helpful in diagnosing a compression fracture. Clinicians must consider pathologic fractures in patients with a history of cancer, as further diagnostic studies and treatments may be necessary. Treatment for compression fractures may include pain control, a rigid brace, and activity modification. Additional treatment options include vertebroplasty and kyphoplasty, both of which have been shown to significantly reduce pain with vertebral compression fractures as well as improve mobility.[13] A return to golf is not recommended until after the fracture is completely healed.[7]

TABLE 9-3	Common Low Back Injuries Among Golfers[7]			
Injury	**Mechanism**	**Risk Factors**	**Signs & Symptoms**	**Treatment**
Low back strain/sprain	Overuse, muscle imbalance	Poor swing biomechanics, inflexibility	Localized back pain, pain increased with activity, pain improved with rest	Activity modification, pain control, core strengthening and stretching regimen, swing modification
Disc herniation	Rotation with axial loading	Age 20–35, degenerative disc disease	Radiating low back pain, radicular-dermatomal pain, neurological defect	Activity modification, pain control, injections, core strengthening and stretching regimen
Compression fracture	Axial load with forward flexion	Osteoporosis	Localized midline back pain, kyphosis, pain improved with rest	Activity modification, rigid brace

TABLE 9-4	Injuries during Each Phase of the Golf Swing	
Swing Phase	**Location of Injury**	**Injuries (%)**
Backswing		20.8 (Total)
	Back	7.8
	Wrist	6.9
	Elbow	2.5
	Hand	1.9
	Shoulder	1.7
Downswing/impact		49.7 (Total)
	Wrist	20.3
	Back	13.9
	Elbow	6.1
	Hand	4.4
	Shoulder	2.5
	Knee	1.9
	Upper back	0.5
Follow-through		29.4 (Total)
	Back	11.9
	Shoulder	5
	Ribs	3.3
	Knee	2.8
	Wrist	2.5
	Neck	1.7
	Hand	1.1
	Elbow	1.1

Data adapted from McCarroll.[8]

TABLE 9-5	Shoulder Injuries of the Lead Arm Related to Swing Phase
Backswing[a]	**Follow-Through[a]**
Subacromial impingement	Subacromial impingement
Rotator cuff disease	Rotator cuff disease
Acromioclavicular joint disease	Anterior instability
Posterior glenohumeral instability	Biceps tendonitis

[a]Symptoms typically occur at the extremes of the motion (at the top of the backswing or the end of the follow-through).[8]

Shoulder Injuries

Shoulder injuries make up a significantly smaller proportion of golf-related injuries than do injuries to the back.[14] The repetitive nature of the golf swing causes most shoulder injuries. The lead shoulder in the golf swing is usually the symptomatic side, as often as 90% of the time.[14] A detailed history, including the location of pain and the phase of the golf swing that aggravates the pain, is important in determining the diagnosis (Table 9-5). It is also important to exclude causes of referred shoulder pain, particularly in patients with a complex medical history.[14]

The most common shoulder pathologies among golfers are rotator cuff disease and subacromial impingement (Table 9-6).[15,16] Both of these injuries are aggravated at the top of the backswing or at the end of the follow-through, the extremes of the shoulder's range of motion. In addition to pain, golfers with rotator cuff disease can also have weakness during the backswing.[14] Provocative shoulder maneuvers

can be used to differentiate between shoulder pathologies (Table 9-7). Treatment options usually begin with conservative treatment, including physical therapy and relative rest, progressing to active range of motion to strength training.[14] Additionally, swing modification to improve the backswing and downswing is recommended to prevent recurrences.[14]

Among professional and amateur golfers, acromioclavicular (AC) joint disease is one of the leading causes of shoulder pain.[16] It usually affects the lead arm at the top of the backswing, when the acromioclavicular joint is under maximal force.[17] Treatment has a high success rate and includes rest, physical therapy, and swing modification.[14] An AC joint corticosteroid injection can also be considered. When conservative treatment fails, distal clavicle excision is the recommended treatment.[14]

Posterior and anterior glenohumeral instability in elite golfers has been described in the literature. While both usually affect the lead shoulder, posterior instability typically occurs during the backswing, while anterior instability is usually seen during the follow-through.[18] Furthermore, posterior instability predisposes the golfer to secondary subacromial impingement.[15] The literature regarding treatment outcomes demonstrates similar outcomes between conservative and surgical treatment.[14] Patients who fail conservative treatment should be referred to a surgeon to explore other treatment options.

With the large percentage of older players, degenerative joint disease of the shoulder is a significant problem among senior golfers. Many of these golfers are limited by their pain and impaired range of motion. Recent literature suggests that glenohumeral arthroplasty is a successful treatment option

TABLE 9-6	Shoulder Injuries Related to Age[8]		
Younger Golfers	**Middle-Aged Golfers**		**Older Golfers**
Instability	Subacromial impingement		Rotator cuff disease
Trauma	Rotator cuff disease		Arthrosis of the
	Acromioclavicular disease		glenohumeral joint

for symptomatic glenohumeral arthritis.[19] Almost all of the golfers who undergo such procedures are able to return to the sport.[14]

Elbow Injuries

Elbow pain is a common complaint among golfers of all abilities, but is more prevalent among amateur golfers (Table 9-1). The two most common injuries sustained at the elbow are medial and lateral epicondylitis. Lateral epicondylitis, or "tennis elbow," is actually more common among golfers than medial epicondylitis, or "golfer's elbow."[20] The motion of the left arm of a right-handed golfer is similar to the backhand of a tennis player, and therefore repetitive action makes the golfer prone to lateral epicondylitis.[20] Patients typically describe pain in the left forearm or elbow during impact. Physical exam usually reveals tenderness just distal to the lateral epicondyle and increased pain with resisted wrist extension and passive wrist flexion. Medial epicondylitis is more common among amateurs who try to "cast" and unhinge their wrists at the beginning of the downswing (Fig. 9-5). This mechanism of prematurely ulnarly deviating the right wrist of the right-handed golfer at the initiation of the downswing often introduces excessive valgus stress on the elbow at impact. Patients often complain

of an aching pain around the medial epicondyle that may radiate into the forearm.[21,22] Treatment for epicondylitis is initially rest, ice, NSAIDs, and splinting.[22] Alternatively, corticosteroid injections may be used for more immediate relief. Once asymptomatic, it is important to correct poor swing mechanics (Fig. 9-6) and consider interventions such as increasing the grip size and use of a counterforce brace during play. Although some literature finds no significant change in muscle activity from altering grip size or using a counterforce brace,[23] such interventions may still be attempted at relatively little cost.[21,22]

Wrist and Hand Injuries

Injuries to the hand are relatively rare in golf. When they do occur, they are most common during impact (Table 9-4).[24] A fracture to the hook of the hamate during impact has been well-described in the literature, particularly with golfers who grip the butt end of the club with direct contact with the hook.

A variety of wrist conditions can be aggravated or caused by golf, including carpal tunnel syndrome, ulnar compression neuropathy at the wrist, and symptomatic ganglion cysts. Recent studies by McHardy et al. found that patients with preexisting conditions of the wrist have increased pain with golfing, whereas

TABLE 9-7	Provocative Tests for Diagnosing Shoulder Pathology[21]
Provocative Test	**Shoulder Pathology**
Neer test	Subacromial impingement syndrome
Hawkin test	Subacromial impingement syndrome
Empty-can test	Supraspinatus tendonitis/impingemement/tear
Yergason test	Subluxation/inflammation of long head of biceps tendon
Speed test	Biceps tendonitits
Drop-arm test	Large rotator cuff tears
Cross-over test	Acromioclavicular joint pathology
Apprehension test	Glenohumeral instability

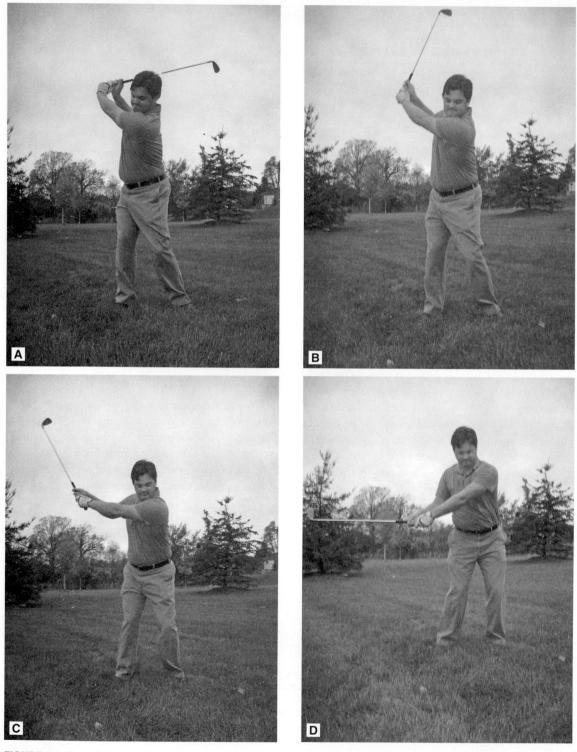

FIGURE 9-5 Casting. Premature ulnar deviation at the wrist during downswing, which may cause elbow pain.

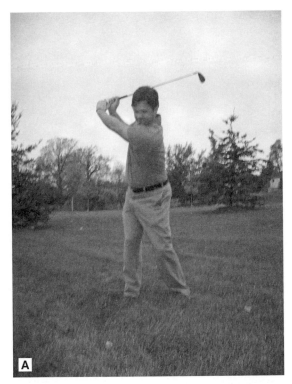
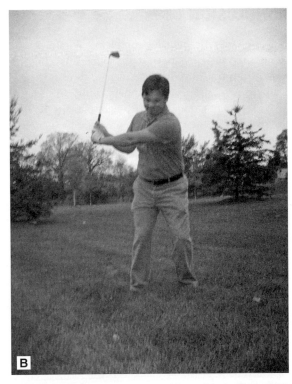

FIGURE 9-6 Proper correction of casting seen in Figure 9-5. Note the difference in club position and the wrists in Figure 9-5B compared to Figure 9-6A.

patients with preexisting musculoskeletal conditions of all other body regions report decreased pain with golfing.[2,4] Golf patients with identified wrist dysfunction should therefore be forewarned that playing golf may exacerbate their condition. The repetitive nature of the golf swing places a significant stress on the wrist,[25] particularly during the end of the downswing and through impact. To minimize risk of wrist injury, proper swing biomechanics must be reviewed and emphasized to decrease stress placed on the wrists, including minimizing wrist movement in the golf swing.

The most common injury to the wrist and hand is tendonitis.[26] Involvement of the extensor carpi ulnaris, extensor carpi radialis longus, extensor carpi radialis brevis, flexor carpi ulnaris, and flexor carpi radialis have been described in the literature.[22] Patients often present with an aching, burning pain that gets worse with repetitive activity. Upon examination, the patient may have tenderness and crepitus over the involved tendons and pain with flexion and extension of the wrist. A positive Finklestein test is suggestive of DeQuervain Tenosynovitis (Fig. 9-7).

Conservative treatment with NSAIDs, immobilization, and activity modification, followed by a stretching and strengthening regimen, is recommended. Patients may benefit from formal physical therapy or a golf-specific rehabilitation program.[22,27]

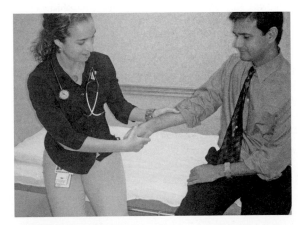

FIGURE 9-7 Finklestein test. Thumb in palm with passive ulnar wrist deviation reproducing pain.

CONCLUSION

Although golf is generally considered a "safe" sport, injuries can and do happen to the golfer. These injuries range from mild overuse tenindopathies to fractures. Knowledge of the more common injuries in golf is useful for the practitioner to help guide patients through the recovery process. Utilizing a team approach with PGA professionals or physical therapists who specialize in golf is essential to the management of golf-related injuries, since one of the eventual goals is usually to return to playing golf. This, combined with injury prevention techniques, will help ensure lifelong and safe enjoyment of the sport.

REFERENCES

1. National Golf Foundation. New Report: Number of Core Golfers Higher Than Previously Reported According to the New NGF Golf Research. Available at http://www.ngf.org/ cgi/whonews.asp?storyid=196. Accessed May 30, 2007.
2. McHardy A, Pollard H, Luo K. One-year follow-up study on golf injuries in Australian amateur golfers. *Am J Sports Med*. 2007;35:1354–1360.
3. Parziale JR, Mallon WJ. Golf Injuries and rehabilitation. *Phys Med Rehabil Clin N Am*. 2006;17:589–697.
4. McHardy A, Pollard H, Luo K. Golf injuries: a review of the literature. *Sports Med*. 2006;36:171–187.
5. Consumer Product Safety Commission. Hazardous Screening Report: Sports Activities and Equipment (Excluding Major Team Sports). Available at http://www.cpsc. gov/LIBRARY/hazard_ sports.pdf. Accessed May 30, 2007.
6. Gosheger G, Liem D, Ludwig K, et al. Injuries and overuse syndromes in golf. *Am J Sports Med*. 2003;31:438–443.
7. Baker RJ, Patel D. Lower back pain in the athlete: common conditions and treatment. *Prim Care Clin Office Pract*. 2005;32:201–229.
8. McCarroll JR. Overuse injuries in the upper extremity. *Clin Sports Med*. 2001;20:469–479.
9. Kirkaldy-Willis WH, Wedge JH, Yong-Hing K, et al. Pathology and pathogenesis of lumbar spondylosis and stenosis. *Spine*. 1978;3:319–328.
10. Atlas SJ, Nardin RA. Evaluation and treatment of low back pain: an evidence-based approach to clinical care. *Muscle Nerve*. 2003;27:265–284.
11. Jensen MC, Brant-Zawadzki MN, Obuchowski N, et al. Magnetic resonance imaging of the lumbar spine in people without back pain. *N Engl J Med*. 1994;331:69–73.
12. Deyo RA. Drug therapy for back pain. Which drugs help which patients? *Spine*. 1996;21:2840–2849.
13. De Negri P, Tirri T, Paternoster G, et al. Treatment of painful osteoporotic or traumatic vertebral compression fractures by percutaneous vertebral augmentation procedures: a nonrandomized comparison between vertebroplasty and kyphoplasty. *Clin J Pain*. 2007;23:425–430.
14. Kim DH, Millett PJ, Warner JJ, et al. Shoulder injuries in golf. *Am J Sports Med*. 2004;32:1324–1330.
15. Hovis WD, Dean MT, Mallon WJ, et al. Posterior instability of the shoulder with secondary impingement in elite golfers. *Am J Sports Med*. 2002;30:886–890.
16. Mallon WJ, Colosimo AJ. Acromioclavicular joint injury in competitive golfers. *J South Orthop Assoc*. 1995;4:277–282.
17. Bell R, Acus R, Noe D. A Study of acromioclavicular forces. *J Shoulder Elbow Surg*. 1993;2(suppl 1-2):S24:2.
18. Jobe FW, Pink MM. Shoulder pain in golf. *Clin Sports Med*. 1996;15:55–63.
19. Jensen KL, Rockwood CA. Shoulder arthroplasty in recreational golfers. *J Shoulder Elbow Surg*. 1998;7:362–367.
20. McCarroll JR, Retting AC, Shelbourne KD. Injuries in the amateur golfer. *Phys Sports Med*. 1990;18:122–126.
21. McShane JM, Graveley MJ, Hopper BD. Physical examination of the shoulder in the primary care setting. *Prim Care Clin Office Pract*. 2004;31:783–788.
22. McCarroll JR. Overuse injuries in the upper extremity. *Clin Sports Med*. 2001;20:469–479.
23. Hume PA, Reid D, Edwards T. Epicondylar injury in sport: epidemiology, type, mechanism, assessment, management and prevention. *Sports Med*. 2006;36:151–170.
24. Murray PM, Cooney WP. Golf-induced injuries of the wrist. *Clin Sports Med*. 1996;15:85–109.
25. Golfers' wrist. *BMJ*. 1977;2:1622.
26. Clancy WG Jr., Hagan SV. Tendinitis in golf. *Clin Sports Med*. 1996;15:27–35.
27. Hong E. Hand injuries in sports medicine. *Prim Care Clin Office Pract*. 2005;32:91–103.

Swimming and Diving Injuries

Swimming is a relatively nonweight-bearing sport that provides excellent cardiopulmonary benefits. Its popularity, both nationally and internationally is on the rise. The first edition of this text listed the participation in U.S. Masters Swimming (USMS) in 1989 at 28,600.[1] As of 2007, the enrollment in USMS was more than 40,000.[2] Likewise, participation in competitive swimming has seen a similar trend in popularity. The history of modern competitive swimming began in Europe around the turn of the 19th century and primarily utilized the breaststroke. Competitive swimming as we know it today was included in the first modern Olympiad in Athens in 1896.

Refinements of stroke techniques, training regimens, and new technologies have allowed swimmers to achieve maximal performances and thus to break records. It has been widely recognized that elite-level swimmers train at extremely high intensity, with regimens calling for up to 20,000 yards of lap swimming per day, 6 days per week. Training often occurs year-round with little downtime. A training regimen with extensive, dry-land work has become the norm for the elite-level swimmer. These athletes endure a tremendous amount of physical stress; the average collegiate swimmer performs more than 1 million strokes per arm annually.[3] This physical strain on the body can lead to various musculoskeletal problems. This chapter will focus on the hydrodynamics and various strokes in swimming, as well as review common musculoskeletal disorders seen in the sport. A similar review of diving is also included.

HYDRODYNAMICS AND BIOMECHANICS

Swimming can be most simply explained as the propulsion of the body through water using the arms and legs to catch, pull, and push water to gain forward momentum. A basic understanding of the physics of swimming can aid in the understanding of the sport and the treatment of its athletes. *Hydrodynamics* is the science of movement of bodies within a fluid medium. The goal of the swimmer is to overcome the various forms of *drag* within the water that reduce his or her speed. *Form drag* is water resistance that is dependent on body position. The more horizontal the body in water, the less form drag encountered by the swimmer. Thus, a streamlined position (see below) of the swimmer is important to reduce form drag. *Wave drag* is caused by turbulence at the water surface by the moving swimmer. Wave drag can be dissipated by adding more lane lines, as is seen in high-level competition, or by swimming in a deep pool. *Frictional drag* originates from the contact of the skin and hair with water. Swimmers often shave their body hair or wear newly designed swimsuits in competition to reduce this form of drag. *Sculling* describes the use of the hands to push large amounts of water quickly with small movements. *Pulling* refers to the use of the arms only and consists of the upper extremity motion of swimming without lower extremity kicking. *Kicking* can be used alone to propel the body through water. This utilizes the legs and feet to push water efficiently while the upper body is either in streamline position or stationary with the aid of a kickboard. The *streamline* position is the most aerodynamically efficient position for the swimmer to glide through water. This position is achieved by fully abducting the arms, placing one hand firmly in the palm of the other, with elbows in full extension against the head, and scapulae retracted. With the hands firmly together there is a smaller surface area to cut the water, and with arms fully abducted and elbows pressed against the head, drag is reduced, and the swimmer continues forward motion as effortlessly as possible.

Strokes

Four main strokes are recognized in competition: freestyle, backstroke, butterfly, and breaststroke. Freestyle is the most commonly learned stroke by swimmers, and most competitive swimmers are able to proficiently swim freestyle. In freestyle, 80% to 90% of the propulsive force is derived from the arms, while just 10% to 20% is from the kick. Grossly, this stroke is performed by sweeping the arms out of the water at opposite times. As the arm exits the water, the elbow is in a high position with hand and forearm relaxed; this is known as the recovery phase (Fig. 10-1). After the recovery phase is the entry or catch phase. During this phase, the athlete extends the hand out on top of the water and then with a pulling motion propels himself or herself through the water. The arm then continues laterally to clear the body and finishes the sweeping motion to enter the recovery phase again. While swimming freestyle, the athlete performs a *flutter* kick. The knees flex and extend and the feet move quickly back and forth to break the water and assist in forward propulsion.

In backstroke, the athlete utilizes the upper body to propel the body forward, but the flutter kick is more pronounced than it is in freestyle. While some freestylers will not use a kick at all (such as for long distance), all backstrokers work on developing a strong flutter kick for propulsion. In backstroke, the athlete initiates the recovery phase by allowing the arm to come out of the water, thumb facing up, and fully flexes the shoulder so the arm is pointing straight up. The arm then moves above the head, coming within about 4 inches from the water, when it is externally rotated so the ulnar side of the hand

enters the water first. With the hand slightly cupped, the swimmer catches the water during the pull phase of the stroke. While the swimmer sweeps the arm through the water, the arm begins in an abducted position and is then adducted to pull the water and create movement. As the athlete's arm nears the body, it must internally rotate again at the shoulder and the hand is used to push "down" along the body with the palm facing the bottom of the pool. This allows the current of water to propel the body forward. The arm is then in a fully extended position and is in position to enter the recovery phase.

In both freestyle and backstroke, body rotation is an important component of the stroke. Coaches often ask their athletes to envision that they are attached at each hip and each shoulder with a metal rod that forces simultaneous and similar movements to occur at the shoulder and ipsilateral hip. This makes the torso hard and rigid, which can only be achieved by adequate lumbar and core strength. The importance of core strength is highlighted here, as adequate core strength will assist the athlete in attaining a good streamlined position.

During the butterfly, the arms are no longer acting cyclically but instead are timed together and the kick is completed in the "off" count. The butterfly can consume a large amount of energy if not completed efficiently. While the kick in this stroke does not propel the body as much as in the backstroke, it is extremely important to achieve proper positioning in the water to alleviate stress placed on the upper body. The two-legged kick in the butterfly is called a *dolphin* kick. The dolphin kick is also used in other strokes as a mean of underwater propulsion immediately after a turn. The swimmer is in the prone position at the start of the kick, and it is most effective if the athlete's feet clear the water and are visible. Then with forceful and rapid hip extension and slight knee flexion, followed immediately by hip flexion and knee extension, the athlete pushes down on the water with the dorsum of the foot creating a large splash. The arms in this stroke go through a series of movements in which the athlete's torso rises out of the water, the arms swing from an extended position into a flexed position and into the water beyond the swimmer's head. As the athlete cups the water, the dolphin kick is performed. Once the athlete pulls the water, the arms move laterally to push water down and away from the body so the athlete can propel forward, ending in a position with the palms facing the athlete's legs.

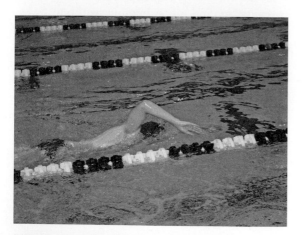

FIGURE 10-1 High elbow recovery technique.

During the breaststroke, the majority of the power is derived from the legs. Like the butterfly, the timing of the kick with the arm cycle is critical to the forward momentum of the swimmer. The kick utilized in this stroke is appropriately named breaststroke kick. It is initiated by internally rotating the hips, flexing the knees, externally rotating the lower leg, and dorsiflexing the foot in the first phase of movement. The athlete must first extend the hips and the knees, and push both feet forcefully into plantar flexion. The arms during this stroke mostly scull and set up the upper body for proper positioning to glide through the water. The arms in the recovery phase have the hands meeting in a "prayer position" in the middle of the sternum and come out over the water together with the arms fully extending at the elbow. The hands then move laterally to catch the water and pull straight back toward the feet. They then rotate in toward the torso to start to push the upper body toward the surface of the water. It is at this time that the legs flex and prepare for the kick.

Both freestyle and backstroke swimmers complete flip turns at the end of each length of the pool. Traditionally, backstrokers were required to use a turn in which the arm was fully extended, and using the hand as a point of contact on the wall to turn. The repetitive axial impact created by this maneuver often leads to problems with anterior instability (see below) (Fig. 10-2). Current rules allow backstrokers and freestylers alike to do a flip turn in which the swimmer is allowed to rotate onto the stomach one stroke prior to reaching the wall. While in the tuck position of the flip turn, the feet are used to push off the wall, and the athlete resumes the streamlined position.

Muscular Activity during Swimming

The freestyle swim arm cycle consists of four phases: early pull-through, late pull-through, early recovery, and late recovery (Fig. 10-3). Early pull-through is defined as the time from the beginning of hand entry to the time when the humerus is perpendicular to the axis of the torso. The late pull-through phase begins at the completion of early pull-through and ends as the hand exits the water. The entire pull-through phase of the swim cycle represents approximately 65% to 70% of the time spent in the freestyle stroke.[4] The hand and arm follow an S-shaped pattern in order to provide additional lift during this phase. Early recovery begins at hand exit and ends when the humerus is perpendicular to the water. Late recovery begins at the completion of early recovery and ends at hand entry.[5]

Because of the specific muscular requirement of the pull-through phase of the swim cycle, shoulder adduction and internal rotation muscle strength are proportionately stronger than the antagonistic motion. McMaster et al. have shown increases in adductor:abductor strength ratios and decreases in external rotation:internal rotation ratios in swimmers compared to nonswimmers.[6,7]

SHOULDER PATHOLOGY

Most injuries experienced by swimmers are due simply to overuse. While common sites of overuse injury include the knee and the back, shoulder problems prevail over other musculoskeletal problems seen by competitive swimmers. The prevalence of shoulder complaints in swimmers has been reported to approach 80%.[3,8] Age and level of training seem to influence the presence of shoulder complaints. McMaster and Troup surveyed swimmers at various age groups and found a prevalence of current shoulder pain of 10% in the national age group, 13% in senior elite development swimmers, and 26% in the U.S. National Swim Team.[9] Additionally, the authors found a lifetime history of shoulder pain in 47%, 66%, and 73% of athletes respectively, with the incidence of shoulder pain increasing with years of participation.[9]

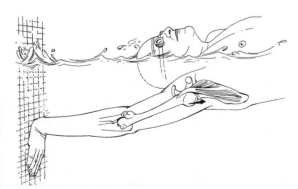

FIGURE 10-2 The impact sustained during the turn of backstroke can lead to anteroinferior instability. (From Rodeo SA. Swimming. In: Krishnan SG, Hawkins RJ, Warren RF, eds. *The Shoulder and the Overhead Athlete*. Philadelphia: Lippincott Williams & Wilkins; 2004:349–362. Reproduced with permission of Lippincott Williams & Wilkins.)

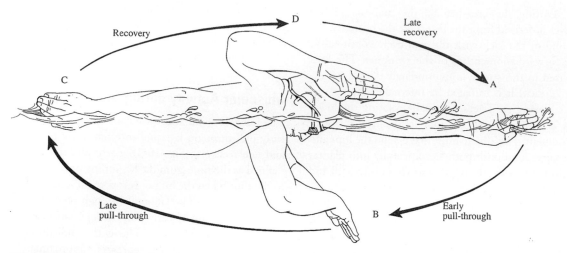

FIGURE 10-3 The swim cycle. (From Rodeo SA. Swimming. In: Krishnan SG, Hawkins RJ, Warren RF, eds. *The Shoulder and the Overhead Athlete*. Philadelphia: Lippincott Williams & Wilkins; 2004:349–362. Reproduced with permission of Lippincott Williams & Wilkins.)

While the speed of arm revolution during swimming is less than that of a baseball pitcher (approximately 80 degrees/second compared to 6,000 degrees/second),[10] the number of repetitive arm revolutions far exceeds that of the baseball pitcher. Thus, the shoulder problems seen in swimmers are unique and deserve special attention. Table 10-1 lists the various muscles around the shoulder and their actions.

Impingement

First coined in 1974, the term "swimmer's shoulder" describes the pain about the shoulder related to the act of swimming.[3] More specifically, it refers to the clinical condition known as subacromial impingement and can involve inflammation of local tissue within the subacromial bursa, rotator cuff tendons, and long head of the biceps tendon. In fact, swimmers usually have a nonoutlet impingement as a result of abnormal shoulder kinematics rather than classic impingement of the rotator cuff against acromial osteophytes or the coracoacromial ligament.

The microvascular anatomy of the rotator cuff tendons was described in 1970 by Rathbun and Macnab.[11] A zone of hypovascularity exists within the tendon approximately 1 cm proximal to the tendon insertion on the greater tuberosity. Furthermore, these vessels arise from both the insertion and myotendinous junction and run the length of the tendon.[11] Compression of these vessels may occur with the arm in adduction. The hypovascular "watershed area" of the rotator cuff may be predisposed to degenerative changes, which may occur first within the substance of the tendon.[11–13] Bigliani et al. described three types of acromial shape (type I: flat, type II: curved, type III: hooked) and noted higher incidence of rotator cuff pathology in patients with type III acomial shapes.[14] Neer and Welsh[15] classified impingement into three clinical stages. Stage I involves the development of reversible edema and hemorrhage within the rotator cuff. Patients in stage II present clinically with tears of the rotator cuff tendon. Stage III describes tears of the rotator cuff associated with acromial osteophytes and is commonly seen in the elderly population.[15,16]

Utilizing video analysis to document impingement during the freestyle swimming stroke, Yanai and Hay reported that impingement occurred when the hand entered the water and in the mid-aspect of the recovery phase.[17] They identified three factors related to the presence of shoulder impingement in swimmers: large amount of internal rotation during the pulling phase, delayed initiation of external rotation of the arm during the recovery phase, and decreased upward scapular rotation.[18]

TABLE 10-1	Muscles of the Shoulder Girdle and Their Actions

Muscles Acting on the Shoulder Complex

Muscle	Action
Latissimus dorsi	Depression of the shoulder girdle. Humeral extension, internal rotation, and adduction.
Levator scapulae	Elevation and downward rotation of the scapulae, extension and rotation of the cervical spine.
Rhomboid major	Scapular retraction, elevation, and downward rotation.
Rhomboid minor	Scapular retraction and elevation.
Serratus anterior	Scapular upward rotation, protraction, depression, elevation, and fixation to the thorax.
Upper trapezius	Scapular elevation, upward rotation, and extension and rotation of the cervical spine.
Middle trapezius	Scapular retraction and fixation to the thorax.
Lower trapezius	Scapular depression, retraction, and fixation to the thorax.
Pectoralis major	Depression of the shoulder girdle. Humeral adduction, horizontal adduction, flexion, and internal rotation.
Pectoralis minor	Scapular anterior tilting.
Biceps brachii	Humeral flexion and wrist supination.
Coracobrachialis	Humeral flexion and adduction.
Anterior deltoid	Humeral flexion, horizontal adduction, and internal rotation.
Middle deltoid	Humeral abduction and flexion.
Posterior deltoid	Humeral extension and external rotation.
Infraspinatus	Humeral external rotation, horizontal abduction, and humeral head stabilization.
Subscapularis	Humeral internal rotation and humeral head stabilization.
Supraspinatus	Humeral abduction, external rotation, and humeral head stabilization.
Teres major	Humeral extension, internal rotation, and adduction.
Teres minor	Humeral external rotation and horizontal abduction.
Triceps brachii	Humeral extension and adduction.

Glenohumeral Instability

Some degree of glenohumeral instability is acceptable in competitive swimmers and is considered normal. Indeed, it has been speculated that shoulder instability may be actually be beneficial to the swimmer in order to achieve a streamlined body position to best overcome drag in the water. McMaster and Troup have found instability of the shoulder in 15% of elite female swimmers.[9,19,20] Additionally, Zemek and Magee have noted generalized laxity in addition to anterior laxity in elite swimmers compared to recreational swimmers.[21]

In a review of 22 national elite level swimmers, Rupp et al.[22] found signs of anterior instability in 50% of athletes and impingement in 50%. There was a high incidence of scapular dyskinesis with scapular winging noted in 23% and scapular protraction in 55%. Isokinetic testing demonstrated lower external rotation:internal rotation ratios in swimmers compared to controls, thus emphasizing the presence of muscular imbalances in swimmers.[22] Bak et al. evaluated 36 competitive swimmers with shoulder pain. Fifty-one percent of these shoulders had concomitant

signs of impingement and increased glenohumeral translation. Furthermore, 22% of patients met criteria for generalized joint hypermobility.[23,24] Clearly, swimmer's shoulder is a result of some degree of glenohumeral instability that predisposes the shoulder to altered mechanics in the presence of muscular fatigue. The swimmer is particularly prone to this problem because of competitive selection for glenohumeral laxity, muscle imbalance due to the demands of the stroke, and fatigue based on training requirements.

Clinical Evaluation of the Shoulder

The history should include the current training regimen including yardage, types of strokes, the use of hand paddles, and any dry-land work that is being performed. Just as in the throwing athlete, the phase of the swimming stroke that exacerbates pain needs to be elucidated. Shoulder injuries in swimmers have been graded as evolving in stages. Stage 1 entails pain only after swimming; stage 2 pain occurs during and after a workout and is not disabling; stage 3 is disabling pain during and after a workout; and stage 4 describes pain with normal activities of daily living or pain interfering with competition.[25,26] Night pain can be a major component of subacromial impingement and rotator cuff pathology, as lying on one's side tends to exacerbate pain of the decubitus shoulder. Feelings or sensations of instability need to be explored.

The physical examination should include inspection and should be done on an exposed shoulder. Women should wear a halter top with the shoulders fully exposed as straps from a bra, swimsuit, or sports bra may obscure subtle abnormalities (Fig. 10-4). Visible deformities should be documented, including possible acromioclavicular (AC) joint enlargement and rotator cuff muscle atrophy. Previous operative scars should be documented. The point of maximal tenderness should be elicited with palpation throughout the shoulder. Shoulder range of motion should be documented in the standing position and includes forward flexion, abduction, internal rotation in adduction and abduction, and external rotation in adduction and

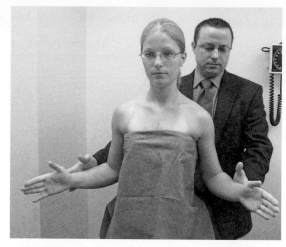

FIGURE 10-5 Rotator cuff strength is assessed in the standing position. The external rotation strength of the infraspinatus is assessed with the shoulder in neutral abduction in approximately 15 degrees of external rotation.

abduction. Strength in abduction, and internal and external rotation, should also be determined during this portion of the examination (Fig. 10-5).

Special tests for the presence of specific shoulder pathology should be performed. The Hawkin and Neer impingement signs are performed with the shoulder in abduction and various degrees of forward flexion and internal rotation (Fig. 10-6). Yergason

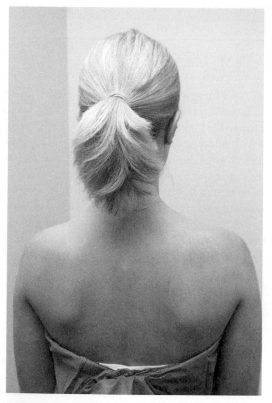

FIGURE 10-4 Visualization of the shoulder musculature is greatly enhanced if the examinee is wearing a halter top or a similar gown and positioned under the room lights.

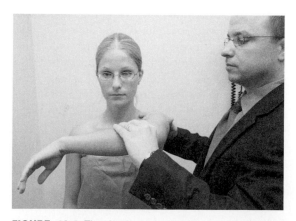

FIGURE 10-6 The impingement sign as described by Hawkins is performed with the patient's shoulder at 90 degrees of forward elevation and internal rotation. The examiner's contralateral hand can be used to stabilize the scapula and palpate subacromial crepitation.

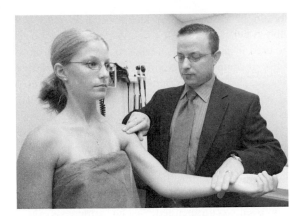

FIGURE 10-7 Speed test is performed to assess biceps tendon pathology with the shoulder in 90 degrees of forward flexion and full external rotation. Pain will be generated at the biceps tendon and will reproduce symptoms.

and Speed tests are done to illicit the presence of proximal biceps pathology (Fig. 10-7). Labral tests such as the O'Brien maneuver can identify superior labral tears (Fig. 10-8). AC joint pathology is identified by a cross-arm adduction test and AC joint compression test.

Next, the patient is moved to the sitting position and the stability of the shoulder is assessed. An anterior drawer test is performed with the arm adducted to the side and an anteriorly directed force is applied

to the shoulder (Fig. 10-9). The amount of anterior translation is subjectively assessed and graded, as outlined in Table 10-2. Inferior translation is graded as a "sulcus sign" and distance of inferior translation in centimeters.

The patient is then moved to the supine position and the examination continued. Range of motion in abduction is documented. Any loss of internal rotation is noted, as this could be a sign of posterior capsular tightness and a condition known as glenohumeral internal rotation deficit (GIRD). Instability examination continues with posterior translation testing while crepitation, symptoms, and apprehension are noted. Finally, apprehension in abduction and external rotation is noted. A relocation test is positive if symptoms resolve after a posteriorly directed force is applied to the shoulder (Fig. 10-10).

Management

Injuries in swimmers usually result from cumulative, repetitive trauma. Conservative management of shoulder problems in swimmers is generally the basis of initial treatment. Unlike many other sports, however, the initial treatment of shoulder injuries in swimmers does *not* entail complete elimination of the offending activity—swimming. Several authors have advocated a period of relative rest.[27–33] Temporary avoidance of certain strokes or positions

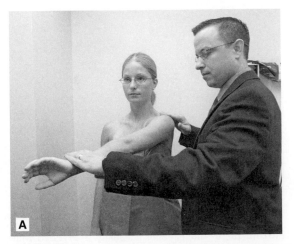
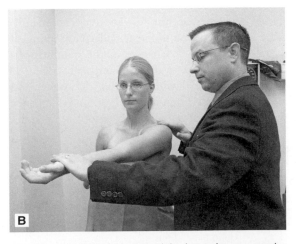

FIGURE 10-8 Several labral tests have been described to determine the presence of a superior labral anterior to posterior (SLAP) lesion. The O'Brien maneuver is performed with the shoulder in 90 degrees of forward flexion and 15 degrees of adduction. The arm is fully internally rotated to place the biceps on tension and resisted forward flexion is performed. If pain is present in this position and relieved in the externally rotated position, the test is positive and indicative of a SLAP tear.

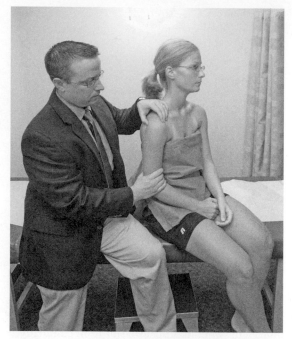

FIGURE 10-9 Instability is assessed initially in the sitting position with the shoulder in neutral abduction and hand relaxed and sitting on the patient's lap. Anterior drawer is performed with the contralateral hand stabilizing the scapula and the ipsilateral hand grasping the humeral head and applying an anteriorly directed force to the head. The degree of translation is assessed and recorded (see text). Inferior translation and posterior translation can also be assessed in the seated position.

should be eliminated. A kickboard held with the elbows bent to avoid the impingement position may be used if the athlete is unable to swim comfortably without shoulder pain. During this period of relative rest, ice should be used judiciously and a short course of nonsteroidal anti-inflammatory drugs (NSAIDs) is recommended.

The precise duration of relative rest has not been established; however, resumption of training should be gradual and closely monitored by athletic trainers and medical personnel. If pain persists, a 3-day period of absolute rest with adjunctive high-dose NSAIDs has been recommended.[25] The athlete is then reassessed prior to return to the water, and if pain persists upon the resumption of training, the athlete should be evaluated by a physician. Rehabilitation should strongly be considered.

should be suggested, but absolute rest is rarely indicated and often results in rapid deconditioning of the elite swimmer.[34] Changes in the training regimen are the first line of treatment and should be closely coordinated with the athlete's coaches and athletic trainers. Intensity, yardage, and frequency should be reduced initially. The use of hand paddles

TABLE 10-2	Anterior Shoulder Translation Grading System	
Grade	**Meaning**
0	No anterior translation
I	Up to glenoid rim
II	Over the glenoid rim, but spontaneously reduced
III	Over the glenoid rim, but not spontaneously reduced

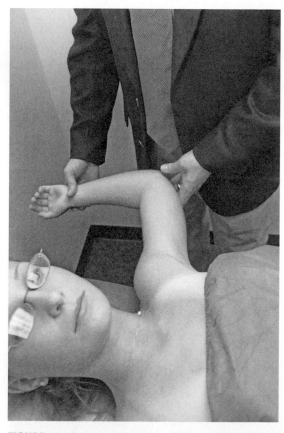

FIGURE 10-10 Anteroinferior instability is assessed with the apprehension test. In the abducted externally rotated position, a feeling of uneasiness or pain is felt by the patient. A relocation test is positive when a posteriorly directed force is applied and the feeling is resolved.

Shoulder Rehabilitation in the Swimmer

In the face of recalcitrant shoulder pain, a rehabilitation program should be designed to fit the patient's individual pathology. The services of a physical therapist or athletic trainer familiar with the unique problems seen by swimmers should be employed. Below is a general treatment algorithm for patients to follow while in rehabilitation.

Phase I

- **Goal: pain modulation, inflammation control, increase range of motion, improve periscapular strengthening.**
- Application of ice three to four times daily for 10 to 20 minutes at a time.
- Modalities such as electrical stimulation, ultrasound, phonophoresis, or iontophoresis may be beneficial.
- Cross-friction massage early to decrease inflammation.
- Postural awareness to include shoulder shrugs/depression, retraction, circles, etc.
- Functional range of motion should be returned through stretching exercises and joint mobilization, progressing from passive range of motion to active range of motion in multiple planes (Figs. 10-11 and 10-12).
- Gentle isometric exercises below the level of the shoulder in order to avoid aggravating positions, followed by variable resistance tubing exercises then isotonic and isokinetic exercises (Fig. 10-13).[35]
- Eccentric strengthening with resistance tubing is utilized for shoulder girdle strengthening.

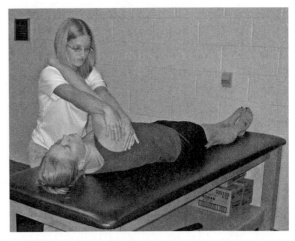

FIGURE 10-12 A partner stretch for posterior capsular tightness is performed with the patient in the supine position stabilizing the shoulder with the weight of the body providing a capsular stretch.

Phase II

- **Goal: increase strength and end-range flexibility.**
- Continued use of modalities, cross-friction massage, and postural awareness as needed.
- Stretching exercises continued.
- Internal rotator strengthening exercises emphasized if shoulder is still painful.[23,24]
- External rotation with elastic bands with the scapulae retracted once pain-free.
- Eccentric exercises advanced to include concentric strengthening while increasing repetitions and resistance.
- Above-shoulder exercises introduced.

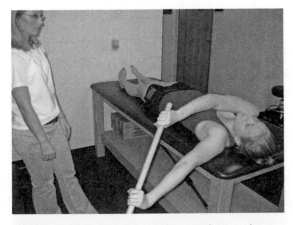

FIGURE 10-11 In the presence of a posterior capsular contracture, a posterior capsular stretch can be included in the rehabilitation protocol.

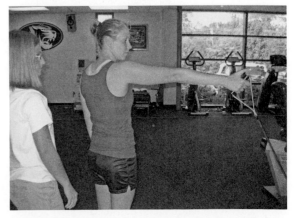

FIGURE 10-13 Resistance tubing exercise emphasizing supraspinatus strength.

Phase III
- **Goal: increase functional strength.** Specific exercises include the following.
- "Seated rows" for scapular stabilization with elastic bands and scapulae retracted, and standing scapular retraction with the shoulders flexed (Figs. 10-14 to 10-16).
- The "hitchhiker" is performed lying prone while extending and abducting the shoulders with the elbow in full extension.
- "Push-up with a plus"—essentially a classic push-up with continuation and protraction of the scapulae, emphasizing the serratus anterior musculature.
- "Dead bug" exercise performed with the swimmer in the supine position and the back flat on the ground; arms and legs are brought off the ground in an alternating fashion.

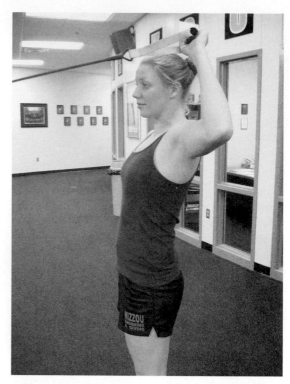

FIGURE 10-15 As shoulder pain resolves, the shoulder is strengthened in a functional position of abduction.

- "Quadruped" emphasizes the lower back and is performed with the athlete on all fours while lifting the right leg and left arm alternatively.
- Strengthening program includes resistance and dumbbell work. Begin to include strengthening in functional positions.

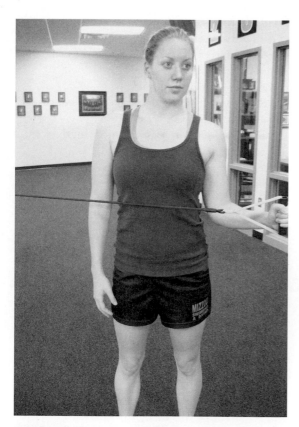

FIGURE 10-14 Swimmers often have relative weakness of the shoulder external rotators. Resistance tubing is often used to rehabilitate such weakness and is performed initially in the adducted position.

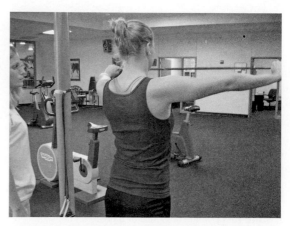

FIGURE 10-16 Resistance tubing exercises are used as a part of an individualized rehabilitation program.

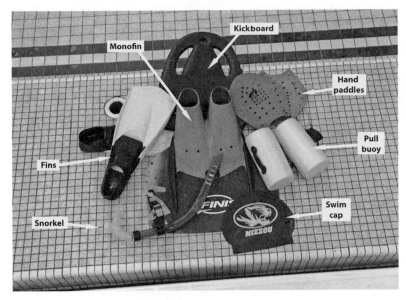

FIGURE 10-17 The common equipment used during training and rehabilitation.

In the figure, the labeled equipment includes: Monofin, Kickboard, Hand paddles, Pull buoy, Fins, Snorkel, Swim cap.

Phase IV

- **Goal: core strengthening and functional return to prior activities.**
- Core stability, specifically the muscles of the low back, abdomen, and pelvis.[36]
- Shoulder strength should be restored through full range of motion and into the end range of motion.
- Completion of a functional progression (see below) prior to return to sports.

Stroke mechanics while in the water should also be observed as part of the rehabilitation program, as subtle alterations may be evident in the injured athlete. For example, a dropped elbow should be recognized and corrected, whereas a high elbow during the recovery phase may help prevent impingement by limiting excessive abduction.[27,37] Another example is increasing body roll to the side of injury, which may aid in limiting abduction of the shoulder. Normal body roll is between 70 and 100 degrees and allows easier recovery.[38]

After the athlete has completed a successful rehabilitation program, a functional progression to return to activity is performed. The goal of a swimming functional progression is to safely recondition the athlete to his or her previous level of participation. The progression should be designed to gradually increase the intensity and duration of swimming over a given period of time. Sample guidelines are presented below:

- The athlete should experience pain-free swimming and only progress yardage if asymptomatic.
- The coach and trainer should supervise stroke drills and mechanics in the early phases of the functional progression.
- Butterfly stroke is avoided if possible.
- Paddles and pull-buoys are avoided if possible (Fig. 10-17).
- Breaststroke or simple kicking with a kickboard can be utilized if tired or sore.
- Fins can be used to increase speed and relieve stress on shoulders.
- Home exercises should be continued throughout the season.
- If previously swimming less than 7,000 yards per day, the athlete should begin swimming 1,000 to 1,500 yards per day, and increase 500 yards every other day until reaching full yardage.
- If previously swimming more than 7,000 yards per day, the athlete should begin swimming 2,000 to 2,500 yards per day and increase 1,000 yards every other day until reaching full yardage.

OTHER MUSCULOSKELETAL PROBLEMS IN THE SWIMMER

Knee pain in swimmers, often termed breaststroker's knee, is a common manifestation of overuse in the breaststroker.[8,39] Overuse pain is typically in a medial peripatellar location, specifically along the medial patellar retinaculum. Anterior knee pain has a variety of causes including patellofemoral malalignment, patellar or femoral trochlear cartilage damage, medial retinacular strain, neuroma of the infrapatellar branch of the saphenous nerve, lateral retinacular tightness, or iliotibial (IT) band tightness. Evaluation of anterior knee pain should include an examination of the entire extremity from the hip to the foot. Rotational malalignment of the femur and/or tibia can lead to abnormal patellar stresses. The tibiofemoral quadriceps (Q)-angle is measured in 30 degrees of knee flexion with the patella engaged in the trochlear groove. The Q-angle is the angle subtended between the quadriceps vector (often from the anterior superior iliac spine to the center of the patella) and the patella tendon (from the center of the patella to the center of the tibial tubercle). Abnormal Q-angle is greater than 15 degrees in females and greater than 12 degrees in males. Other factors contributing to patellofemoral pain include knee and ankle valgus, pes planus, and a pronated forefoot. Structural abnormalities might be addressed in the initial treatment of anterior knee pain. Additionally, IT band tightness and vastus medial obliquus (VMO) weakness should be assessed and treated if necessary.

Back pain in the swimmer can occur as a result of muscular strain from the flip turn or from the repetitive hyperextension of the butterfly stroke.[27–32,40] Less commonly, stress fractures of the pars interarticularis (spondylolysis) can occur.[28,41] In swimmers, most pars defects are discovered incidentally and may not be symptomatic.[28,41] Thorough physical examination, radiographic examination, and occasionally magnetic resonance imaging (MRI) or bone scan are required to develop a complete diagnosis. Treatment should be individualized to the patient's needs and expectations.

DIVING

The evolution of diving as a sport has been traced to the 17th century, when German and Swedish acrobats moved equipment to the beaches to perform over and into water.[42] In the 1904 Olympic Games in St. Louis, competitive diving was included in the swimming program, thus beginning the traditional grouping of these two sports despite their distinctly different physical characteristics.

Understanding the unique injuries seen in competitive divers requires basic knowledge of the sport of competitive diving. Diving is divided into springboard and platform competitions. There are 77 springboard and 97 platform dives possible. The format of the Olympic diving competition involves 3-meter springboard and 10-meter platform events for men and women. The competitor is graded on proficiency in forward, backward, reverse, inward, and twisting dives, and male divers must perform one dive from a handstand starting position (Fig. 10-18). Dives are performed in the straight, pike, tuck, or twist positions (Fig. 10-19). Half of the dives performed in competition are required ("compulsory"), while the other half are optional and are declared prior to competition. Each dive is assigned a degree

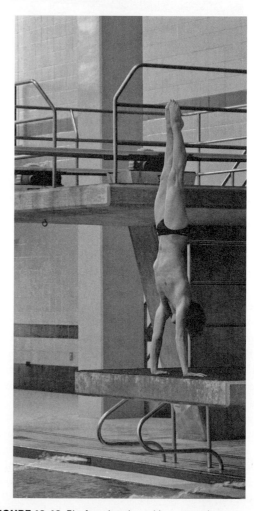

FIGURE 10-18 Platform handstand is a compulsory component of men's diving.

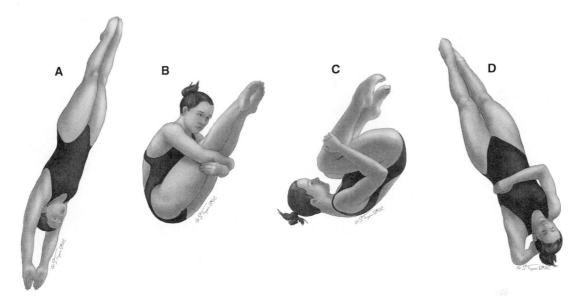

FIGURE 10-19 Four positions can be assumed during the flight phase of the dive: **(A)** straight, **(B)** pike, **(C)** tuck, and **(D)** twist.

of difficulty ranging from 1.2 to 3.6. Dives are scored by a panel of judges based on the approach, take-off, elevation, technique, grace exhibited in the air, angle of entry, and amount of splash (Fig. 10-20).[42]

The incidence of injury in competitive diving is difficult to ascertain in the current medical literature. Most of the reports describing injuries in diving are related to recreational diving. These reports depict diving as a sport with a high rate of head and neck injuries; however, the same rates do not apply in the sport of competitive diving. Very few reports exist regarding the true incidence of injuries in competitive diving.[42,43] When an injury is defined as the inability to train at least 1 week, it has been estimated that the incidence of injury in competitive diving is between 92% and 100%.[42] Males and females tend to be injured at the same rate and there are trends toward higher incidence of injury with more years of training. The number of dives performed over a career may not be as important as the difficulty of the dives performed.[42]

Pathomechanics of Injury

Diving injuries usually occur by two basic mechanisms: repetitive microtrauma or rapid macrotrauma. The most common sites of injury in divers are the spine, shoulder, elbow, wrist, and hand. While abundant references to catastrophic injuries to the spine

are available in the medical literature, there is not a reported incidence of this in organized diving. In competitive divers, however, injuries to the spine are often related to repetitive overuse and hyperextension within the lumbar segments. Hyperextension of the back can occur in various parts of the dive including take-off for a back or reverse dive, coming out of a rotation, or "saving" a dive that is not vertical. As seen with other athletes performing repetitive hyperextension, such as gymnasts and football linemen, divers are prone to posterior-element lumbar spine pathology. Spondylolysis, spondylolisthesis, and facet arthropathy can also occur, but it must be noted that the incidence is much lower in divers than in gymnasts.

As in swimmers, shoulder injuries in divers can be a significant source of time lost from competition or practice. Rubin[42] surveyed the U.S. National Diving Team and found 80% to have had shoulder injuries that precluded training for at least 1 week. They found no relationship to premorbid range of motion, lateral scapular slide, direction of twisting, or hand position on impact. Injured extremities did, however, demonstrate a reduction in peak torque and peak torque/body weight in external rotation. Like swimmers, a majority of divers have subtle (and sometimes marked) multidirectional instability. Rubin has stated that almost all platform divers demonstrate a sulcus sign.[42] Furthermore, a variety of shoulder pathologies can be seen with divers secondary to

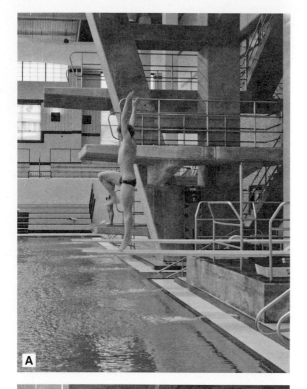
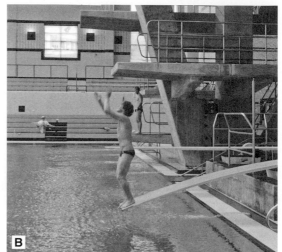
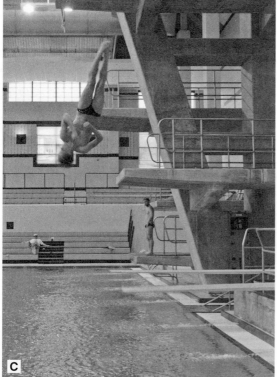
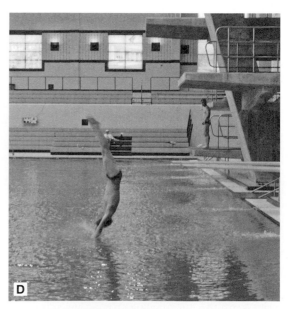

FIGURE 10-20 The phases of the dive include the **(A)** approach, **(B)** take-off, **(C)** flight, and **(D)** entry.

repetitive microtrauma, but the potential for a single traumatic event is present in this sport.

The rehabilitation of shoulder injuries in divers is similar to that of swimmers. The practitioner and therapist should construct a rehabilitation program that is individualized to the injured athlete's strength needs. Particular emphasis is placed on optimizing strength of scapular stabilizing muscles and core strengthening and stability. One difference that is not intuitive is that scapular stabilizers should be strengthened in a functional position in divers. Following a traditional strengthening program, the shoulder should be strengthened in the abducted overhead position similar to the entry position.

The elbow, wrist, and hand are subject to high stresses during the dive. It has been suggested that during the entry phase, hyperextension of the elbow can lead to injury to the ulnar collateral ligament of the elbow and ulnar neuritis.[42] Additionally, triceps tendonitis at the myotendinous junction may be encountered in divers unable to maintain the elbow in full extension during entry. Injuries to the wrist and hand are usually a result of repetitive impact and forced dorsiflexion at entry. The most common injuries are subtle carpal instability, dorsal impaction syndrome, sprains, and flexor carpi ulnaris tendinitis.[44] A variety of other types of injuries have been reported in divers and the practitioner should be aware that these can occur.[45–47] It should also be noted that many divers start off as gymnasts. They may bring a history of gymnastics-related injuries to their new sport.

CONCLUSION

Swimming and diving are gaining in popularity, and the demographics of these athletes are changing. Practitioners should be familiar with the sport-specific needs of these athletes and the unique demands of the sport. Shoulder pathology is quite common in both of these groups of athletes. Pathology is often related to subtle glenohumeral instability and muscular imbalance. Recognition of these issues can help guide the treatment program while maintaining the athlete's fitness. With the assistance of athletic trainers, therapists, coaches, and athlete compliance, many shoulder problems can be successfully treated nonoperatively. Furthermore, prevention of injury is particularly important because of the highly repetitive stress experienced by these athletes in normal competition preparation.

REFERENCES

1. Wei F. In: Buschbacher RM, Braddom RL., eds. Swimming Injuries. *Sports Medicine and Rehabilitation: A Sport-Specific Approach.* 1st ed. Philadelphia: Hanley & Belfus; 1994:67–94.
2. U.S. Masters Swimming. 2007 Statistics. http://www.usms.org. Accessed September 21, 2007.
3. Richardson AB, Jobe FW, Collins HR. The shoulder in competitive swimming. *Am J Sports Med.* 1980;8:159–163.
4. Nuber GW, Jobe FW, Perry J, et al. Fine wire electromyography analysis of muscles of the shoulder during swimming. *Am J Sports Med.* 1986;14:7–11.
5. Scovazzo ML, Browne A, Pink M, et al. The painful shoulder during freestyle swimming. An electromyographic cinematographic analysis of twelve muscles. *Am J Sports Med.* 1991;19:577–582.
6. McMaster WC, Long SC, Caiozzo VJ. Isokinetic torque imbalances in the rotator cuff of the elite water polo player. *Am J Sports Med.* 1991;19:72–75.
7. McMaster WC, Long SC, Caiozzo VJ. Shoulder torque changes in the swimming athlete. *Am J Sports Med.* 1992;20:323–327.
8. Kennedy JC, Hawkins R, Krissoff WB. Orthopaedic manifestations of swimming. *Am J Sports Med.* 1978;6:309–322.
9. McMaster WC, Troup J. A survey of interfering shoulder pain in U.S. competitive swimmers. *Am J Sports Med.* 1993;21:67–70.
10. Pappas AM, Zawacki RM, McCarthy CF. Rehabilitation of the pitching shoulder. *Am J Sports Med.* 1986;13:223–235.
11. Rathbun JB, Macnab I. The microvascular pattern of the rotator cuff. *J Bone Joint Surg Br.* 1970;52:540–553.
12. Macnab I. The painful shoulder due to rotator cuff tendinitis. *RI Med J.* 1971;54:367.
13. Macnab I. Rotator cuff tendinitis. *Ann R Coll Surg Engl.* 1973;53:271–287.
14. Bigliani LU, Ticker JB, Flatow EL, et al. The relationship of acromial architecture to rotator cuff disease. *Clin Sports Med.* 1991;10:823–838.
15. Neer CS II, Welsh RP. The shoulder in sports. *Orthop Clin North Am.* 1977;8:583–591.
16. Sigholm G, Styf J, Korner L, et al. Pressure recording in the subacromial bursa. *J Orthop Res.* 1988;6:123–128.
17. Yanai T, Hay JG. Shoulder impingement in front-crawl swimming: II. Analysis of stroking technique. *Med Sci Sports Exerc.* 2000;32:30–40.
18. Yanai T, Hay JG, Miller GF. Shoulder impingement in front-crawl swimming: I. A method to identify impingement. *Med Sci Sports Exerc.* 2000;32:21–29.
19. McMaster WC. Anterior glenoid labrum damage: a painful lesion in swimmers. *Am J Sports Med.* 1986;14:383–387.
20. McMaster WC. Swimming injuries. An overview. *Sports Med.* 1996;22:332–336.
21. Zemek MJ, Magee DJ. Comparison of glenohumeral joint laxity in elite and recreational swimmers. *Clin J Sport Med.* 1996;6:40–47.
22. Rupp S, Berninger K, Hopf T. Shoulder problems in high level swimmers—impingement, anterior instability, muscular imbalance? *Int J Sports Med.* 1995;16:557–562.
23. Bak K, Fauno P. Clinical findings in competitive swimmers with shoulder pain. *Am J Sports Med.* 1997;25:254–260.

24. Bak K, Magnusson SP. Shoulder strength and range of motion in symptomatic and pain-free elite swimmers. *Am J Sports Med.* 1997;25:454–459.

25. Johnson JE, Sim FH, Scott SG. Musculoskeletal injuries in competitive swimmers. *Mayo Clin Proc.* 1987;62:289–304.

26. Fowler P. Symposium: Shoulder problems in overhead-overuse sports. Swimmer problems. *Am J Sports Med.* 1979;7:141–142.

27. Fowler PJ, Regan WD. Swimming injuries of the knee, foot and ankle, elbow, and back. *Clin Sports Med.* 1986;5: 139–148.

28. Goldstein JD, Berger PE, Windler GE, et al. Spine injuries in gymnasts and swimmers. An epidemiologic investigation. *Am J Sports Med.* 1991;19:463–468.

29. Hunter LY, Andrews JR, Clancy WG, et al. Common orthopaedic problems of female athletes. *Instr Course Lect.* 1982;31:126–151.

30. McLean ID. Swimmers' injuries. *Aust Fam Physician.* 1984;13:499–502.

31. Richardson AB. Orthopedic aspects of competitive swimming. *Clin Sports Med.* 1987;6:639–645.

32. Wilson FD, Lindseth RE. The adolescent "swimmer's back." *Am J Sports Med.* 1982;10:174–176.

33. Weldon EJ, 3rd, Richardson AB. Upper extremity overuse injuries in swimming. A discussion of swimmer's shoulder. *Clin Sports Med.* 2001;20:423–438.

34. Costill DL, Kovaleski J, Porter D, et al. Energy expenditure during front-crawl swimming: predicting success in middle-distance events. *Int J Sports Med.* 1985;6:266–270.

35. Scott SG. Current concepts in the rehabilitation of the injured athlete. *Mayo Clin Proc.* 1984;59:83–90.

36. U.S. Swimming. Core stabilization. Available at: www.usa-swimming.org. Accessed September 21, 2007.

37. McMaster WC. Shoulder injuries in competitive swimmers. *Clin Sports Med.* 1999;18:349–359.

38. Counsilman JE. *The Science of Swimming.* Englewood Cliffs, NJ: Prentice-Hall; 1968.

39. Stulberg SD, Shulman K, Stuart S, et al. Breaststroker's knee: pathology, etiology, and treatment. *Am J Sports Med.* 1980;8:164–171.

40. Kenal KA, Knapp LD. Rehabilitation of injuries in competitive swimmers. *Sports Med.* 1996;22:337–347.

41. Keene JS, Drummond DS. Mechanical back pain in the athlete. *Compr Ther.* 1985;11:7–14.

42. Rubin BD. The basics of competitive diving and its injuries. *Clin Sports Med.* 1999;18:293–303.

43. Mutoh YTM, Miyashita M. Chronic injuries in elite swimmers, divers, water polo players, and synchronized swimmers. In: Ungerechts BE, Wilke K, Reischle K, et al., eds. *International Series on Sports Sciences,* vol. 18. *Swimming Science.* Champaign, IL: Human Kinetics; 1988:333–337.

44. le Viet DT, Lantieri LA, Loy SM. Wrist and hand injuries in platform diving. *J Hand Surg Am.* 1993;18:876–880.

45. Albrand OW, Corkill G. Broken necks from diving accidents: a summer epidemic in young men. *Am J Sports Med.* 1976;4:107–110.

46. Albrand OW, Walter J. Underwater deceleration curves in relation to injuries from diving. *Surg Neurol.* 1975;4: 461–464.

47. Shinozaki T, Kondo T, Takagishi K. Olecranon stress fracture in a young tower-diving swimmer. *Orthopedics.* 2006; 29:693–694.

Road Cycling Injuries

Road cycling as a sport has increased in popularity in recent years in the United States in part due to Lance Armstrong's run of seven consecutive Tour de France victories. As other forms of cycling, including mountain biking (discussed in the next chapter) and track racing (time trials, sprints), increase in popularity, so too do the number of injuries associated with road cycling. In a study of 518 recreational cyclists, 85% reported one or more chronic overuse injuries during the past year; within that same group approximately 10% had injuries severe enough to stop cycling for greater than 1 month and 3% stopped cycling completely.[1] The typical cyclist averages over 5,400 revolutions per hour and achieves approximately 30,000 revolutions in 100 miles, which has been shown to predispose the cyclist to overuse injuries.[2] This chapter will review the proper fit of the cyclist to the bike frame, biomechanics of cycling, and common cycling injuries.

PROPER FIT OF THE CYCLIST TO THE BIKE FRAME

A proper fit of the cyclist to the bike frame is important for the comfort of the cyclist, to prevent chronic overuse injuries, and for optimal performance (Fig. 11-1). In general, the size of the bicycle frame must first be addressed, with measurements taken from the top tube of the bicycle to the cyclist's pubic symphysis. Burke suggested that there should be a 1- to 2-inch space between the top tube and pubic symphysis when the cyclist stands astride the frame.[3]

Pelvis to saddle, shoe to pedal, and hands to handlebar are three areas of the greatest contact between the cyclist and the bicycle. The pelvis-to-saddle contact is addressed via saddle height, saddle fore/aft position, and saddle tilt. Although multiple formulas have been suggested for the optimal saddle height, Lemond et al. suggested measurement from the pubic symphysis to the floor (in cm) multiplied by a factor of 0.883 to obtain this value.[4] If clipless pedals are used, another 3 mm is then subtracted.[4] Additionally, adjusting the saddle forward lowers the height, and vice versa. Saddle tilt is important, as approximately 60% of the cyclist's weight rests on the center of the saddle. Ideally, the saddle should be parallel to the ground; women, however, may prefer their saddle maintained at slightly downward tilt to reduce perineal pressure. Improper tilt and saddle width can place the cyclist at risk for perineal sores and other urogenital problems, including erectile dysfunction and impotence, as discussed later.[2,5]

In regard to the shoe-to-pedal contact, many cyclists use toe clips that lock the shoe to the pedal for maximal energy transfer; the ideal position is with the first metatarsal aligned over the pedal axle (Fig. 11-2).[2,6] Ironically, such "clips" are called "clipless" pedals, because they were an advance over previous toe cages, called "clips."

Contact between the hands and the handlebar requires optimal positioning of the torso and shoulders over the handlebars. Ideally, the cyclist's torso is flexed to approximately 45 degrees while the hands are in the drops (curved part of the handlebars). The elbows are flexed approximately 60 to 70 degrees, and the wrists are in neutral. Adjustments of the torso can be made through changes to the stem length. With respect to the handlebar tilt, many cyclists tend to have the handlebars rotated slightly elevated/upward, as too far of a downward tilt may cause the athlete to stretch further, creating an overreach.

Ideally, cyclists should have multiple fittings to their bike frame. Initial settings are typically established in a static position (without addressing the dynamic position while spinning). The cyclist's personal

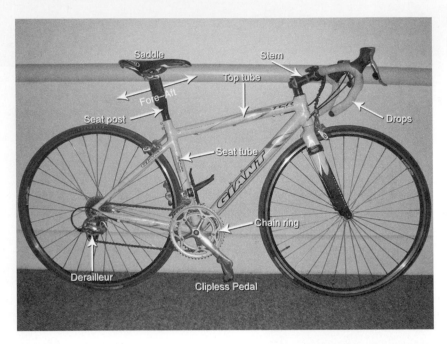

FIGURE 11-1 The road bicycle with components labeled.

biomechanics and aerodynamics can then be evaluated and adjustments made based on dynamic fittings. Any adjustments should be relatively small, and completed with one component at a time. Once adjusted, the cyclist should then complete several training rides to determine whether the new position is more desirable.[2]

BIOMECHANICS OF CYCLING

Road cycling is most readily thought of as the ability to overcome the physical forces that slow the bike, including wind resistance, tire-terrain resistance, and gravitational forces. Propulsion of the bike requires the cyclist to utilize a wide range of muscles to complete rotation of the pedal 360 degrees in a push-and-pull motion to gain forward momentum. The road cycling stroke can be divided into the following phases: propulsion, bottom dead center, and recovery.

During the road cycling stroke, the greatest force generation occurs during the *propulsion phase*, or the force that propels the bicycle forward. This phase begins at the top of the 360-degree arc and ends at the bottom. Muscles primarily used in the propulsive phase include gluteus maximus and hamstrings (hip extension), quadriceps (knee extension), iliotibial band (lateral stabilization), gracilis (medial stabilization), and

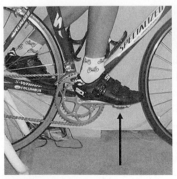
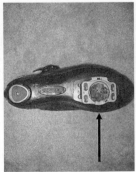
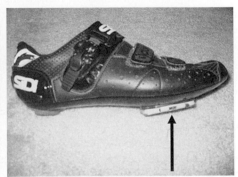

FIGURE 11-2 Cleat positioned so first metatarsal is aligned over the pedal axle.

gastrocnemius (plantar flexion). Following the propulsion phase is the *bottom dead center*, which involves continued plantar flexion via the gastrocnemius and knee flexion via the hamstrings.[7] Finally, in the *recovery phase* the tibialis anterior (dorsiflexion), quadriceps, hamstrings, gracilis, and iliotibial band are engaged to return the pedal to the top of the stroke to complete the cycle. Throughout the cycling stroke, the trunk is flexed in a range of 20 to 35 degrees, with erector spinae and the abdominal muscles maintaining this posture.

It should be noted that the efficiency can be improved by utilizing toe clips and cleated shoes (Fig. 11-2), which prevent the side-to-side and back-and-forth sliding motion of the foot.[8,9] Some clipless systems allow internal/external rotation movement of the foot; others are truly rigid and allow no such movement. The latter may transfer more force up the kinetic chain.

Table 11-1 outlines some common injuries or complaints by cyclists that can be alleviated by adjustments of the aforementioned bike components.

ACUTE INJURIES

Acute injuries can be categorized into major (due to trauma) or minor (due to abrasions) injuries. Traumatic injuries are often the result of collision with motor vehicles. Of these, 50% are due to loss of control of the bike after the collision, with subsequent falls; and 17% are due to direct collision with

TABLE 11-1 Overuse Injuries Due to Posture with Recommended Bicycle Adjustments

Ailment	Contributing Position	Bicycle Adjustment
Posterior neck pain, scapular pain for clarity	Too great of a reach, handlebars too low, too stretched out	1. Ride more upright, shorten reach 2. Raise stem height 3. Shorten stem length 4. Ride with hands on hoods or tops of bars
Hand neuropathy (cyclist's palsy, ulnar nerve)	Too much pressure on bars, handlebars too low, saddle too far forward, excessive downward saddle tilt	1. Increase padding on bars and gloves 2. Avoid prolonged pressure, change hand position often 3. Raise stem height 4. Move saddle back if too far forward 5. If saddle is tilted down, position it level
Low back pain	Too stretched out	1. Ride more upright, shorten reach 2. Raise stem height 3. Shorten stem length
Tibialis anterior tendonopathy	Saddle height too high	Lower saddle height
Achilles tendonopathy	Saddle height too high (excessive stretch)	Lower saddle height
	Saddle height too low (with concomitant dropping of heel to generate more power)	Raise saddle height
Morton neuroma/foot pain/numbness	Cleat position	Usually, move cleat back, but may be forward
	Irregular sole	Check sole for inner wear or cleat bolts pressing inward
	Shoes too tight	Wider shoes, loosen Velcro straps/shoe buckle
Perineal numbness	Saddle too high	Lower saddle height
	Tilt angle excessively up or down	Adjust angle closer to level with the ground

From Silberman MR, Webner D, Collina S, et al. Road bicycle fit. *Clin J Sport Med.* 2005;5:271–276.

the motor vehicle.[10–12] The majority of acute injuries are abrasions, or "road rash," lacerations, and contusions.[10–12] Management of these acute injuries is largely dependent on the severity of the injury and can range from local wound care to emergency department referral.

CHRONIC/OVERUSE INJURIES TO THE UPPER EXTREMITY

Ulnar Neuropathy at the Wrist

Ulnar neuropathies are commonly attributed to increased pressure or weight distribution on the handlebars. Ulnar neuropathy at the wrist is due to entrapment or compression of the ulnar nerve in relation to the Guyon canal. The cyclist may complain of numbness and tingling of the 4th and 5th digits, as well as difficulty in opening jars or turning doorknobs if there is atrophy of the instrinic hand muscles. Sensation on the dorsum of the hand is typically spared, since this area is innervated by the dorsal ulnar cutaneous nerve, which branches proximal to the Guyon canal. This can help differentiate proximal from distal injury. There may also be weakness of hand intrinsic muscles; the Froment sign (Fig. 11-3) is a test where the patient is asked to grasp a sheet of paper between the first two digits. The patient who has ulnar neuropathy at the wrist will substitute the flexor policis longus muscle (an anterior interosseous/median innervated muscle) for the ulnar-innervated

adductor policis, with flexion of the first distal interphalangeal joint. Diagnosis is made with electrodiagnostic studies, and sensitivity can approach 95%.[13] Treatment initally begins with relative rest, ice, compression, and elevation (RICE). A wrist splint may be utilized to relieve pressure off the Guyon canal and to help protect the nerve from further compression. Ergonomic correction of the bicycle, such as adjustments to the saddle position so that less body weight is distributed over the hands, may be helpful. In addition, alterations to the stem length and decreasing the handlebar angle may also help decrease stress on the wrists. Surgical consultation may be considered if the above treatments fail.

Median Neuropathy at the Wrist

Median neuropathy at the wrist, or carpal tunnel syndrome (CTS), occurs due to compression of the carpal tunnel over long periods of time in the cyclist. CTS typically presents with pain and paresthesias in the distribution of the median nerve distal to the carpal tunnel, particularly at night. Patients may feel the need to shake out their hands while symptomatic, called a positive "flick" maneuver, though this finding has limited clinical value in diagnosing CTS.[14] Patients may also complain of dropping objects due to hand weakness. On exam, patients typically have sensory impairment in the first 3½ digits, weakness in thumb abduction, and positive Phalen and Tinel signs. Electrodiagnostic studies are the diagnostic modality of choice, with sensitivity approaching 85%

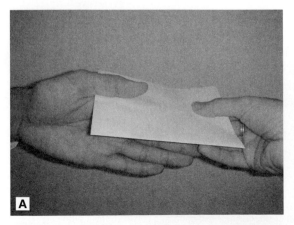 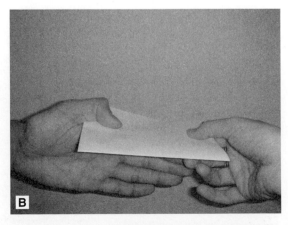

FIGURE 11-3 A. Negative Froment sign with intact ulnar nerve. Note neutral position of thumb distal interphalangeal joint. **B.** Positive Froment sign, indicating ulnar neuropathy. Note flexion of the thumb distal interphalangeal joint.

and specificity 95%.[15] Treatment begins with wrist splints for protection and rest, stretching of the transverse carpal ligament, and stretching of the median nerve longitudinally, called a median nerve glide.[16] Corticosteroid injection into the carpal tunnel can be done in refractory cases. Surgical consultation is indicated if the aforementioned treatments fail.

De Quervain Tenosynovitis

De Quervain tenosynovitis occurs as a result of continuous, tight grip as well as frequent gear shifting (sharp, frequent wrist movements), causing repetitive, chronic stress and vibration. There is inflammation of the extensor pollicis brevis and abductor pollicis longus tendons, resulting in pain and swelling in the first dorsal wrist compartment (Fig. 11-4). Patients may have a positive Finklestein maneuver (Fig. 11-5), which is passive ulnar deviation of the thumb-in-palm. Rest, ice, and anti-inflammatory medication are the initial treatments. A thumb spica orthotic as well as modalities such as ultrasound and iontophoresis

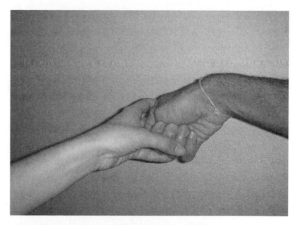

FIGURE 11-5 Finkelstein maneuver to elicit de Quervain stenosing tenosynovitis, an inflammation of extensor pollicis brevis and abductor pollicis longus tendons.

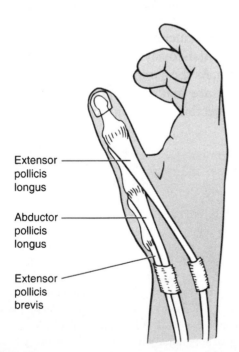

Extensor pollicis longus

Abductor pollicis longus

Extensor pollicis brevis

FIGURE 11-4 Extensor pollicis brevis and abductor pollicis longus sharing the same tendon sheath. These tendons are involved in de Quervain stenosing tenosynovitis. (From Anderson MK, Hall SJ, Martin M. *Sports Injury Management.* 2nd ed. Philadelphia: Lippincott Williams & Wilkins; 2000.)

can be employed to relieve pain and inflammation. Direct corticosteroid injection into the tenosynovium can be done for refractory cases. Preventive strategies include changing the gear-shifting mechanism to an alternate position on the handlebars.[17]

CHRONIC/OVERUSE INJURIES TO THE LOWER EXTREMITY

Most overuse injuries in cyclists tend to occur in the lower extremity compared to the upper. Many of these injuries involve the knee and are primarily are due to misalignment of the athlete to the bike.

Patellar Tendonitis

Patellar tendonitis, or jumper's knee, is technically a misnomer, since tendonitis implies a muscle-to-bone injury, whereas this disorder affects bone-to-bone (patella to tibia). Patellar tendonitis is due to significant angular traction on the insertion of the tendon (technically a ligament) at the inferior pole of the patella, or near its insertion onto the tibial tubercle. Pain typically presents at the inferior pole of the patella and is exacerbated with negotiating stairs. Increased mileage, hill workouts, and a seat that is too low may contribute to the development of patellar tendonitis. Examination may reveal tenderness to palpation at the inferior pole of the patella and pain reproduction on knee extension with the knee fully flexed. Tightness in the hamstrings, quadriceps, and tendo-Achilles may also be noted.[18] Initial treatment includes RICE, anti-inflammatory medications, and stretching of tight hamstrings. Therapeutic modalities such as iontophoresis can also be used to decrease inflammation. Once inflammation subsides, quadriceps strengthening can be implemented to balance forces across the knee. Orthotics such as a neoprene knee sleeve (soft knee orthotic) can be used to prevent recurrent inflammation and reduce patellar excursion during movement. Integration of plyometric exercises can be gradually implemented. These exercises involve jumping or single- and double-leg hopping to incorporate both concentric and eccentric strengthening exercises. Bike adjustments to prevent recurrence may include saddle elevation or backward saddle adjustment to reduce angular traction on the patellar tendon. Likewise a *floating cleat system* may be added, which allows for a small amount (ideally 5 degrees) of foot rotation through the pedaling cycle.[19]

Patellofemoral Pain Syndrome

Patellofemoral pain syndrome occurs as a result of synovial inflammation or wearing of the articular cartilage between the patella and femur. Friction produced by repetitive flexion and extension of the knee can lead to a cycle of inflammation and subsequent softening of the retropatellar cartilage (chondromalacia patella). Patellofemoral pain syndrome occurs most commonly when the cyclist is utilizing larger gears on the ride, pedaling with too slow of a cadence, or after a hilly ride, which all can increase resistance and friction on the knee. Common complaints may include retropatellar knee pain, as well as a "grating" or "grinding" sensation upon knee extension. Pain with prolonged sitting is called a positive "theatre sign." Increased Q-angle (Fig. 11-6), femoral anteversion, and excessive foot pronation can increase risk of developing patellofemoral pain.[20] Anterior joint line tenderness of the knee may be noted along with joint crepitus and lateral patellar tracking. Hip abductor weakness and inflexibility of the hip flexors is commonly seen in chondromalacia.[21] The patellofemoral grind test involves asking the patient to contract the quadriceps mechanism while the examiner applies downward pressure, reproducing pain. False positives are common, however. Radiographs with a "sunrise" view of the patella

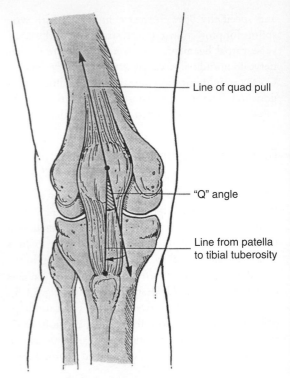

FIGURE 11-6 The Q-angle is measured between the quadriceps and a line from center of the patella to the tibial tubercle. (From Anderson MK, Hall SJ, Martin M. *Sports Injury Management.* 2nd ed. Philadelphia: Lippincott Williams & Wilkins; 2000.)

may demonstrate lateral patellar tilt. Treatment typically begins with rest, ice, and anti-inflammatory medications. A physical therapy program should be implemented that incorporates strengthening weak hip abductors, knee extensors, and core stabilizers,[22] and stretching of tight hip flexors. McConnell taping can be implemented if maltracking is found on exam. This involves taping the patella to replicate correct biomechanical patellar tracking, combined with multiplanar, closed and open kinetic chain exercises, and has been showed to achieve improvement rates of greater than 90%.[23] Additionally, if pain from excessive patellofemoral joint reactive forces prevent optimal quadriceps strengthening, short-arc (less than 45 degrees) closed kinetic chain exercises can be implemented to incur the least joint reactive force.[24] Surgical referral may be needed for refractory cases. Cycling-specific treatment includes similar bike adjustments as mentioned in patellar tendonitis.

Iliotibial Band Friction Syndrome

The iliotibial band (ITB) originates from the tensor fascia late and inserts on the Gerdy tubercle on the tibia. Functionally, the band moves posterior to the lateral femoral condyle in knee flexion and moves anteriorly during knee extension. During cycling, increased cadence can result in increased friction of the IT band against the lateral femoral condyle, causing significant irritation. It is also commonly attributed to cleats that are rotated too far medially, a saddle that is too high or positioned too far back, or due to excessive internal tibial rotation. Predisposing factors for developing ITB syndrome include genu varus, excessive foot pronation, leg-length discrepancy, prominence of the greater trochanter of the femur, and training errors.[25] Patients typically present with lateral knee pain as well as pain around the greater trochanter of the femur. The Noble compression test (Fig. 11-7) may be positive.[26] Management of ITB syndrome consists of RICE and the use of anti-inflammatory medications until acute symptoms subside. A rehabilitation program consisting of stretching the ITB, hip flexors, and glutei should be considered. Strengthening hip adductors, glutei, and tensor fascia lata is stressed. Leg length discrepancies and foot pronation problems should be corrected with appropriate foot orthotics. Corticosteroid injection, either at the greater trochanter or lateral femoral condyle, can also be useful. Cycling-specific recommendations include modification of seat height to an ideal knee flexion of 25 to 30 degrees at the bottom dead center of the stroke cycle, which has been suggested to reduce pressure on the knee joint.[3]

Plica Syndrome

Plica are remnants of embryologic walls of the knee, which normally remain asymptomatic, but can become inflamed if injured. The medial plica is the most commonly cited cause of plica syndrome in the literature, as the medial plica functions to passively restrict patellar excursion.[19,27] Overuse is typically the cause of inflammation as the plica bowstrings across the femoral condyle (Fig. 11-8).[18] Injury occurs in

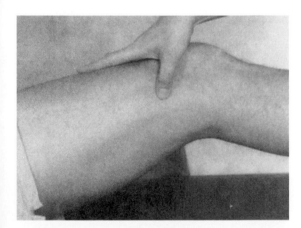

FIGURE 11-7 The Noble test for ITB friction syndrome. The patient is supine and the knee is flexed 90 degrees. The clinician then palpates the lateral epicondyle of the femur while extending the knee; pain on extension is a positive finding as the iliotibial band crosses the lateral femoral epicondyle. (From Anderson MK, Hall SJ, Martin M. *Sports Injury Management*. 2nd ed. Philadelphia: Lippincott Williams & Wilkins; 2000.)

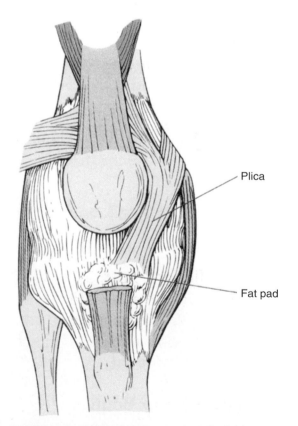

FIGURE 11-8 Medial plica. Overuse is typically the cause of inflammation as the plica bowstrings across the femoral condyle. (From Anderson MK, Hall SJ, Martin M. *Sports Injury Management*. 2nd ed. Philadelphia: Lippincott Williams & Wilkins; 2000.)

cyclists when traction is placed on the medial plica, particularly while the patella is deviating laterally.[19] Additional causes of medial plica injury in cyclists occur if cleats are too far externally rotated and if the saddle is elevated too high or set too far backwards.[19] Patients typically present with anteromedial knee pain, as the plica is impinged in the patellofemoral joint for the first few steps after walking, and then abates. Pseudolocking may be present, mimicking a torn meniscus.[18] Cyclists may describe a "popping" feeling while pedaling. Exam may reveal a joint effusion, medial joint line tenderness and a hypertrophied membrane may be palapated.[27] Magnetic resonance imaging provides little diagnostic value, as direct arthroscopy is considered the standard for diagnosis. [27] Treatment focuses on reducing inflammation with ice, anti-inflammatory medications, and relative rest. Bike adjustments should be made accordingly. Modalities such as phonophoresis can be used to reduce pain, along with a neoprene knee sleeve to help prevent bowstringing of the plica. Surgery to remove the plica may be warranted if conservative measures fail; the success rate of surgery is greater than 80%.[27]

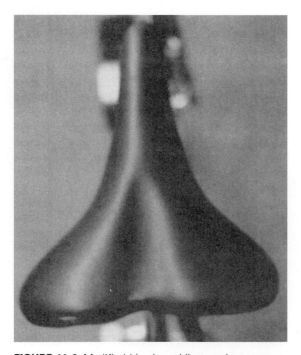

FIGURE 11-9 Modified bicycle saddle to reduce pressure on the pudendal nerve. (From Fu FH, Stone DA. *Sports Injuries: Mechanisms, Prevention, Treatment.* 2nd ed. Philadelphia: Lippincott Williams & Wilkins; 2000.)

INJURIES ASSOCIATED WITH THE GROIN/BUTTOCKS

The most commonly reported groin injury is genital numbness.[28] The course of the pudendal nerve makes it susceptible to compression against the bike saddle, especially when riding for long periods of time. This causes increased perineal pressure and results in a compression neuropathy.[5] Another source of genital numbness may be due to arterial insufficiency, as penile blood flow dramatically decreases during cycling. In this condition, blood flow can be restored by standing up intermittently while cycling.[29] The recommended strategy of decreasing genital numbness revolves around encouraging the cyclist to include frequent standing during a long workout and changing to a different saddle design (Fig. 11-9) that shifts the weight to a wider area of the buttocks and ischial tuberosities.[5] If the cyclist has extended duration of genital numbness, it is recommended to refrain from cycling until normal sensation returns and numbness regresses.[5]

CONCLUSION

Cycling is a recreational, competitive, and at times rehabilitative form of exercise. Its increased popularity over the past decade has led to an increased susceptibility to injury, particularly among recreational cyclists, who may present to sports medicine professionals for evaluation. An understanding of the most common cycling injuries will assure continued growth and enjoyment of this form of exercise.

REFERENCES

1. Wilber CA, Holland GJ, Madison RE, et al. An epidemiological analysis of overuse injuries among recreational cyclists. *Int J Sports Med.* 1995;16:201–206.
2. Silberman MR, Webner D, Collina S, et al. Road bicycle fit. *Clin J Sport Med.* 2005;5:271–276.
3. Burke ER. *Serious Cycling.* 2nd ed. Champaign, IL: Human Kinetics; 2002.
4. LeMond G, Gordis K. *Greg LeMond's Complete Book of Bicycling.* 2nd ed. New York: Pedigree Books; 1990.
5. Leibovitch I, Mor Y. The vicious cycling: bicycling related urogenital disorders. *Euro Urol.* 2005;47:277–287.
6. Sanderson DJ. The biomechanics of cycling shoes. *Cycling Sci.* 1990;2:27–30.
7. De Vey Mestdagh K. Personal perspective: in search of an optimum cycling posture. *Appl Ergon.* 1998;29:325–334.

8. Ericson MO, Nisell R, Nemeth G. Joint motions of the lower limb during ergometeric cycling. *J Orthop Sports Phys Ther*. 1988;9:273.

9. O'Brien T. Lower extremity cycling biomechanics: a review and theoretical discussion. *J Am Podiatr Med Assoc*. 1991;81:585–592.

10. Kronisch RL, Chow TK, Simon LM, et al. Acute injuries in off-road bicycle racing. *Am J Sports Med*. 1996;24:88–93.

11. Powell B. Medical aspects of racing. In: Burke ER, ed. *Science of Cycling*. Champaign, IL: Human Kinetics; 1986:185.

12. Weiss BD. Bicycle-related head injuries. *Clin Sports Med*. 1994;13:99–112.

13. Cowdery SR, Preston DC, Herrmann DN, et al. Electrodiagnosis of ulnar neuropathy at the wrist: conduction block versus traditional tests. *Neurology*. 2002;59:420–427.

14. Hansen PA, Micklesen P, Robinson LR. Clinical utility of the flick maneuver in diagnosing carpal tunnel syndrome. *Am J Phys Med Rehabil*. 2004;83:363–367.

15. Norvell JG, Steele M. Carpal tunnel syndrome. E-medicine. Available at: http://www.emedicine.com/emerg/topic83.htm. Accessed December 3, 2007.

16. Gronseth G. Your questions answered: exercise for carpal tunnel. *Neurology Now*. 2007;3:37.

17. Richmond DR. Handlebar problems in bicycling. *Clin Sports Med*. 1994;13:165–173.

18. Anderson MK, Hall SJ, Martin M. *Sports Injury Management*. 2nd ed. Philadelphia: Lippincott Williams & Wilkins; 2000.

19. Holmes JC, Pruitt AL, Whalen NJ. Lower extremity overuse in bicycling. *Clin Sports Med*. 1994;13:187–205.

20. Hilyard A. Recent developments in the management of patella-femoral pain: the McConnell programme. *Physiotherapy*. 1990;76:559–565.

21. McConnell J. The management of chondromalacia patellae: a long-term solution. *Aust J Physiother*. 1986;32:215–219.

22. Kibler WB, Press J, Sciascia A. The role of core stability in athletic function. *Sports Med*. 2006;36:189–198.

23. McConnell J. The physical therapists approach to patellofemoral disorders. *Clin Sports Med*. 2002;21:363–388.

24. Steinkamp LA, Dillingham MF, Markel MD, et al. Biomechanical considerations in patellofemoral joint rehabilitation. *Am J Sports Med*. 1993;21:438–444.

25. Messier SP, Pittala KA. Etiologic factors associated with selected running injuries. *Med Sci Sports Exerc*. 1988;21:501–505.

26. Noble CA. Iliotibial band friction syndrome in runners. *Am J Sports Med*. 1980;8:232–234.

27. Bigelow TL. Plica syndrome. Available at: http://www.emedicine.com/orthoped/topic543.htm. Accessed December 3, 2007.

28. Schwarzer U, Weigand W, Bin-Saleh A, et al. Genital numbness and impotence rate in long distance cyclists. *J Urol*. 2004;172:637–641.

29. Nayal W, Schwarzer U, Klotz T, et al. Transcutaneous penile oxygen pressure during bicycling. *BJU Int*. 1999;83:623–625.

CHAPTER 12

Matthew Smuck

Mountain Biking Injuries

T he story of mountain biking begins one century before it was included as a full medal event in the 1996 summer Olympic Games. In 1896, a group of infantrymen called the "Buffalo Soldiers" were ordered to test the bicycle for military use in the mountains. To accomplish this, they rode customized bikes on dirt roads and trails from Missoula, Montana, to Yellowstone and back. In the decades that followed, isolated groups and certain individuals pursued off-road cycling on modified bikes. Then in the 1970s the modern sport of mountain biking was set into motion by a group of cycling enthusiasts in Marin County, California, including racer Gary Fisher and frame builder Tom Ritchey. A combination of their enthusiasm in venturing off-road and their ability to build and sell customized bikes led to an explosion of the sport's popularity.

Because mountain biking is popular in many nonmountainous regions, the term "off-road" biking is also used. Although the latter description is more accurate, the former is more popular. The challenges of the sport remain even in the absence of mountains. For instance, many popular biking trails on Midwest river bluffs are more challenging than actual mountain trails. Although the length of climbs and descents are shorter on river bluff trails, they can be steeper, narrower, and strewn with more natural obstacles.

Since this book contains a chapter on road cycling (Chapter 11), one might ask why a separate chapter on mountain biking is necessary. The simple answer is that the types of injuries, rates of injuries, and their associated risk factors differ.[1–3] Furthermore, mountain biking is no longer a minor cycling subcategory. It has been the largest area of growth in cycling over the past two decades. And for over a decade mountain bikes have accounted for more annual sales than any other single category of bicycles.[4] Therefore, knowledge of the specifics of mountain biking injury

is important for anyone who treats musculoskeletal disorders.

DEMOGRAPHICS

Following its rapid growth in the 1980s and 1990s, participation in mountain biking has reached a plateau. The National Sporting Goods Association reports that 8.5 million Americans rode bikes off-road in 2006.[5] This is equivalent to the number of Americans who participated in tennis, volleyball, or alpine skiing. Mountain biking appeals to a wide range of individuals, from children to octogenarians, and is most popular among males aged 20 to 39.[2,3,6–8] Injury reporting reflects this age and sex distribution (Fig. 12-1), with males accounting for around 80% of all mountain biking injuries.[3,8,9,10]

Mountain bikers spend more time riding off-road in the warmer months, when most injuries occur.[3,11] Studies of competitive mountain bikers show that pro/elite-level racers spend 10 hours per week training off-road, and up to 2 hours per week racing.[10] Less is known of the varied riding patterns of recreational mountain bikers. One survey found that recreational cyclists spend on average 5 hours per week off-road.[6] Compared to recreational road cyclists, mountain bikers are less likely to cycle daily but ride a similar number of miles per week.[3]

ERGONOMICS, GEOMETRY, AND MECHANICS

Currently, every mountain bike manufacturer offers several models to satisfy a wide range of riding styles, including bikes designed solely for downhill riding. The geometry of the frame and the components fitted

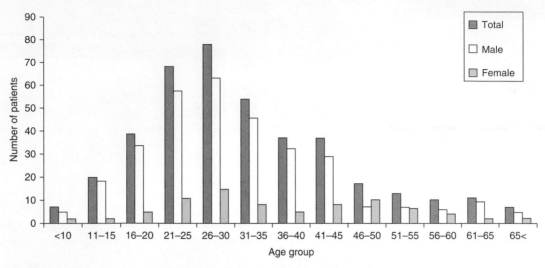

FIGURE 12-1 The number of patients admitted with mountain biking injuries to regional trauma centers in Southwest British Columbia during a 10-year study period. (From Kim PT, Jangra D, Ritchie AH, et al. Mountain biking injuries requiring trauma center admission: a 10-year regional trauma system experience. *J Trauma*. 2006;60:312–318.)

to a bike change drastically depending on its purpose (Fig. 12-2). Consumer demand for lighter, stronger materials and a softer ride has fueled progressive development of mountain bikes and their components.[12] Standard equipment on high-end mountain bikes includes clipless pedals (cycling shoes attach to the pedal by a cleat and release by ankle rotation), hydraulic disc brakes, and suspension systems (Fig. 12-2). These design and mechanical improvements have increased the efficiency, speed, and abilities of mountain bikes. Thus they also present additional hazards.

Mountain bikers are subject to repeated external forces such as impacts and vibration. These repeated stresses can increase the risk of repetitive use injuries. One study demonstrated the importance of reducing these forces by finding a lower incidence of wrist and neck pain in mountain bikers riding with suspension systems.[13] Despite these forces, mountain bikers have a lower risk of repetitive use injuries compared to road bikers. While these injuries are among the most common in road cyclists, they account for only 10% of mountain biking injuries.[9] Several ergonomic factors are likely responsible for this. For example, mountain bike geometry places the rider in a more upright and natural position, reducing the amount of flexion in the hips and the lumbar spine. This position also reduces the amount of cervical lordosis required to see ahead. Also, the varied terrain inherent

to mountain biking causes the rider to frequently change position, avoiding the prolonged postures maintained during road riding.

Cycling with a lowered seat has been linked to knee injuries in road cyclists. Mountain bikers often lower their seats during downhill riding. This allows the center of gravity to be lowered and shifted toward the rear of the bike, a position that is necessary to prevent the rear wheel from lifting while braking and causing a forward fall. While riding uphill or on trails with gentle slopes, the ideal seat position on a mountain bike is similar to that on a road bike, providing similar lower extremity ergonomics. Overuse knee injuries are known to occur in mountain bikers,[9,10,13] but the incidence is unknown and may be greater than or less than that observed in road cyclists.

EPIDEMIOLOGY

Mountain biking is often perceived to be a dangerous sport. This perception is fueled by video clips featuring top-level riders performing amazing stunts. But, is mountain biking riskier than other forms of bicycling? According to the existing research, it is not. While it is true that mountain biking produces more injuries than road riding, the majority are minor injuries such as skin lacerations or contusions.[3,9,10,13] Compared to cyclists injured while riding on paved

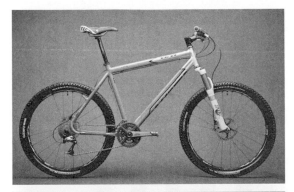

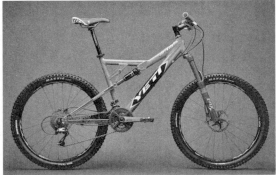

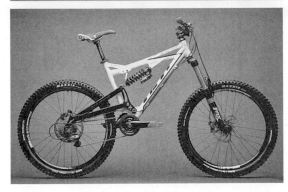

FIGURE 12-2 Mountain bike geometry by type. Progressing from cross-country bike *(top)*, to trail bike *(middle)*, and downhill bike *(bottom)*, the frame is made more sturdy, the seat is lowered, the amount of suspension travel increases, and the head angle (the angle between the front fork and the ground) is less horizontal.

surfaces, injured mountain bikers are less likely to require the care of a physician or need hospitalization.[3,6] So despite the higher incidence of injuries, the overall risk profile of mountain biking is similar to that of road biking.[3,6]

Injury rates are best known in competitive cyclists since the organized structure allows for better study designs. These studies provide no details about injuries that occur with training or recreational riding.

However, they most likely represent injury information in the worst-case scenario. This is because competitive mountain bikers are up to four times more likely to be injured during a race than they are during training.[9,10] And mountain bikers involved in competition are more likely to be injured compared to purely recreational riders.[9]

Several prospective studies show that approximately 0.5% of all participants (including cross country, downhill, and dual slalom racers) were injured while racing.[7,8,14,15] Although the overall injury rates were similar between the different events, they were substantially different if calculated according to the time spent racing. It takes a few minutes for downhill racers to complete an obstacle-strewn course at speeds sometimes exceeding 45 mph, while cross-country racers zigzag up and down mountain trails for hours. So it is no surprise that downhill racing produced more injuries when standardized by time. In downhill racing there were 43.4 injured cyclists/1,000 hours of racing time versus 3.7 injured cyclists/1,000 hours racing time in cross-country.[15]

Information about injuries in recreational mountain bikers comes from one of two sources: surveys and reviews of hospital records. The former is limited by a responder bias and relies on the memory of the respondents. The latter is limited to information on the most serious injuries only. Of all the survey studies, the most extensive was conducted in Germany. Out of the 3,873 mountain bikers who responded, 3,474 reported some type of injury related to the sport.[2] Most injuries were mild, such as superficial skin lesions. Only 10% of reported injuries were severe, and half of the respondents consulted a physician after an injury. Overall, the injury risk rate was 0.6% per year, or 1 injury/1,000 hours of biking. Excluding the minimal severity injuries, the risk rate dropped to 0.15% per year.

For many years the overall number of serious mountain biking injuries has steadily increased (Fig. 12-3).[12] Early on this finding was attributed to the sport's expanding popularity. However, since participation has stabilized one would expect injury rates to follow. The authors of one study suggest that recent trends in mountain biking account for the continued increases in rates of serious injuries, with riding shifting from cross-country to the more aggressive downhill style, particularly in certain regions.[12] This is likely due to a combination of factors, including improved bike and suspension designs, interest of new participants, experienced riders seeking new

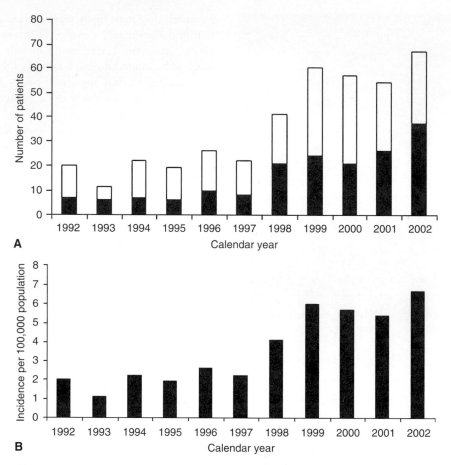

FIGURE 12-3 Annual number of patients with mountain biking injuries admitted to regional trauma centers in Southwest British Columbia. The top chart shows the total number of admissions with the most serious injuries indicated by the black bars. On the bottom chart the annual incidence of admissions is adjusted per 100,000 of the total population in the catchment area. Charts reflect a threefold increase in admissions/incidence over the study period. (From Kim PT, Jangra D, Ritchie AH, et al. Mountain biking injuries requiring trauma center admission: a 10-year regional trauma system experience. *J Trauma*. 2006;60:312–318.)

challenges, and improved access to downhill trails (many ski resorts have opened mountain bike parks with chairlift access to trails). Since risk of injury is greater with downhill riding,[15] future increases in injury rates are expected if this trend continues.

INJURY SPECIFICS

Severity

It is no surprise that injuries occur in mountain biking. Challenging terrain maneuvered at high speed seems a fine recipe for accidents and injuries, and

leads many to believe it is a dangerous sport. In this regard, mountain biking is like alpine skiing decades ago, a young sport viewed as extreme by the mainstream. As occurred with alpine skiing over time, an increasing number of participants with continually improved trail access may tame the sport's reputation.

As in alpine skiing, in mountain biking severe injuries do occur, but with less frequency than often assumed. One large study of seven Seattle-area hospitals and local coroner records found only one death related to biking off-road.[3] Although unreported cases likely exist, at the time this chapter was written only one other report of death from a mountain biking injury has been published.[12] Other reports of significant morbidity from mountain biking injuries include small bowel evisceration,[16] brain injury,[3,17] and tetraplegia.[12,18] Still, the majority of mountain biking injuries are mild, requiring no treatment or only self-treatment.[6]

An avid mountain biker in a pair of shorts can often be identified by small lacerations on the lower legs caused by twigs or brush on the sides of narrow trails. These are rarely sufficient to label as an injury. As this example highlights, a discussion of injuries requires some context in terms of severity. Validated and standardized methods of grading injury severity exist, but these measures are not used in many studies. Therefore, when compiling information from many sources, a more simple mechanism is required. In this chapter, injuries will be discussed in terms of severity as follows. *Mild* indicates superficial injuries that are often self-treated and cause little or no interruption in sporting activity, including small skin lacerations, abrasions, and contusions. *Moderate* refers to injuries such as muscle strains or ligament sprains that often cause interruption of sports activity and may or may not require medical attention. *Severe* injuries are those that typically require medical care and cause major disruptions in sports activities and normal daily activities. These include fractures, dislocations, ligament tears, concussions, and internal organ injuries.

As stated before, when it comes to mountain biking, the majority of injuries are of mild severity. Surveys of recreational mountain bikers found that 75% of injuries were mild.[2,6] Musculoskeletal injuries accounted for another 20%, with one-fourth moderate and three-fourths severe. Head and facial injuries accounted for a very low 0.5%.[2] When recreational cyclists were injured, 70% required no treatment or were self-treated, and 26% were seen by a physician.[6]

Differences are observed in competitive mountain bikers. One survey of elite-level competitive cyclists found that nearly half of them had experienced a "major" injury related to the sport.[10] At racing events, musculoskeletal injuries, both moderate and severe, occurred in 35% of injured cross-country racers and 55% of injured downhill racers.[15] Abrasions, contusions, and lacerations, or other mild injures, occurred in 95% of injured cross-country racers and 73% of injured downhill racers.[15]

A better look at the serious injuries related to mountain biking is available in studies conducted from emergency rooms and orthopedic trauma services.

These studies provide few details about the more common and less severe injuries, while providing important information about the most dangerous injuries faced by mountain bikers. Fortunately, the majority of injured mountain bikers seen in emergency rooms are able to go home, with only 6% requiring hospital admission.[3] Obviously, hospitalization is needed in only the most serious injuries. In a study of 84 hospitalized mountain bikers in a single orthopedic trauma unit, 5% had potentially life-threatening injuries.[11] These included one person with a head injury, one with a C2/3 fracture dislocation, one with intra-abdominal bleeding, and one with hemothorax. Another study of injured mountain bikers admitted to three trauma centers in Southwest British Columbia found that 66% required surgery.[12] In long-term follow-up, 86% were discharged home without any aid, 5% went home with outpatient rehabilitation or home nursing care, and 5% went to a rehabilitation facility (4% were sent to another hospital and lost to follow-up).[12]

Injury Risk

The challenges created by riding a bike over irregular terrain is part of the appeal of mountain biking. Since automobiles are not involved in mountain biking injuries, and repetitive use injuries are uncommon, the primary determinate of injury risk is the rider's ability to avoid an accident. In this matter, several factors come into play including those related to the rider, to the bike, and to the terrain (Table 12-1).

As for the rider, one research team found over 90% of injuries were attributed to failures of judgment.[2] Injured mountain bikers are less likely to blame external factors and are more apt to accept blame for their injuries, citing the following reasons: 36% excessive speed, 35% unfamiliar terrain, 23% inattentiveness, and 20% riding beyond one's ability.[6]

Mechanical failure accounted for 5% to 16% of injuries in four different studies,[6–8,15] and is more likely to cause serious injuries (Table 12-2).[15] In the largest study of competitive downhill racing injuries, a staggering 36% of downhill accidents were caused by mechanical failures, with flat tires being the most frequently sited problem.[8] Other components whose failure led to injury included brakes, chains, forks, handlebars, pedals, cranks, and suspension parts.[14]

Terrain has a substantial impact on injury risk, second only to rider judgment, with approximately 80% of injuries incurred while riding downhill.[6–8,15]

TABLE 12-1	**Mechanisms of Injury at a Large Annual Mountain Bike Racing Event over 8 Consecutive Years. Data combine injured racers from all three categories: cross-country, dual slalom, and downhill.**

	Women (n = 22)		Men (n = 71)	
	No.	%	No.	%
Loss of control	12	54.5[a]	20	28.2
Loss of traction	2	9.1	7	9.9
Collision with object	2	9.1	5	7.0
Collision with rider	2	9.1	11	15.5
Mechanical problem	0	0	15	21.1[b]
Trail surface irregularity (1998–2001)	3	13.6	10	14.1
Other	0	0	3	4.2
Unknown	1	4.5	0	0

[a]$p = 0.04$ for percentage of female vs. male subjects reporting loss of control as the cause of injury.
[b]$p = 0.02$ for percentage of male vs. female subjects reporting mechanical problem as the cause of injury.
From Kronisch RL, Pfeiffer RP, et al. Gender differences in acute mountain bike racing injuries. *Clin J Sport Med.* 2002;12:158–164.

During cross-country racing, all fractures and over 90% of concussions occur while riding downhill.[8] Racers in downhill events are prone to more severe injuries compared to cross-country racers (Table 12-3).[8,15] In addition to increasing the risk of an injury, the higher velocities while riding downhill increase the forces of collision, thus raising the potential severity of an injury. Earlier in this chapter, several cases of tetraplegia and death were cited. Each occurred while riding downhill.

The mechanism of a fall also influences injury risk. In mountain biking, forward falls are known to

TABLE 12-2	**Mechanisms of Injury and Resulting Severity at Three Major Race Events during 1 Year. Data from all cross-country and downhill racers. Mean *injury severity score* is a standardized rating where a score between 1 and 3 represents mild injury, 4 to 15 moderate injuries, and >15 severe injury.**

	No. Injured Cyclists	No. Treated in Emergency Room	Mean Injury Severity Score
Mechanism of Injury			
Loss of traction	10	3	1.5
Loss of control	6	5	3.7
Mechanical failure	5[a]	4	3.8
Collision with another rider	4	0	1.0
Collision with a stationary object	3[b]	2	4.3
Unknown	3	1	1.3
Total	31	15	2.5

[a]3 tires, 1 handlebar, 1 suspension fork.
[b]1 pole, 1 barrier, 1 rock.
From Kronisch RL, Pfeiffer RP, Chow TK. Acute injuries in cross-country and downhill off-road bicycle racing. *Med Sci Sports Exerc.* 1996;28:1351–1355.

TABLE 12-3	Differences in Injury Severity Comparing Cross-Country and Downhill Racers. Injury severity is indicated on the right by the mean *injury severity score,* a standardized rating where a score between 1 and 3 represents mild injury, 4 to 15 moderate injuries, and >15 severe injury.
Cross-country	2.15
Men	2.00
Women	2.50
Downhill	3.27
Men	3.00
Women	4.50

From Kronisch RL, Pfeiffer RP, Chow TK. Acute injuries in cross-country and downhill off-road bicycle racing. *Med Sci Sports Exerc.* 1996;28:1351–1355.

occur more frequently and they are more likely to cause serious injury.[7] Well over half of mountain biking injuries are related to forward falls.[7,8] It is the most likely mechanism to result in fractures,[8] shoulder injury,[2] cervical spine injuries,[18] and concussions.[8,15]

Gender plays a role in mountain biking injury. Compared to other injured cyclists, injured mountain bikers are older and more often male.[1,3] The different participation rates between the sexes explains this male predominance. However, injury risk is actually higher in female mountain bikers.[8,15] A study conducted during 8 consecutive years at one race event found that women sustain nearly twice as many injuries as men during competition, 0.77% versus 0.40%, and that they were more than twice as likely to have a fracture when injured, 46% versus 21%.[8] Odds ratios indicate that women racers were 1.94 times more likely to be injured and 4.17 times more likely to sustain a fracture than men. For a detailed view of fractures incurred by men and women racers, see Table 12-4.

There are many reasons for the increased risk in women. First, female mountain bike racers have

TABLE 12-4	Number of Fractures Observed by Location in Male and Female Competitors at a Single Annual Mountain Bike Racing Event during 8 Consecutive Years. Data combines injured racers from all three categories: cross-country, dual slalom, and downhill.

	Women	Men
Finger(s)	0	2
Metacarpal	4	2
Carpal	1	1
Distal radius	1	3
Clavicle	4	6
Scapula	0	1
Rib(s)	1	3
Lumbar body	2	0
Pelvis	0	1
Facial	0	1
Total	13[a]	20[a]

[a] Some subjects had fractures in more than one location.
From Kronisch RL, Pfeiffer RP, et al. Gender differences in acute mountain bike racing injuries. *Clin J Sport Med.* 2002;12:158–164.

fewer years of riding experience than males racing at the same level.[10] Next, women are more likely to fall forward over the handlebars.[15] Finally, significantly more women reported "loss of control" as the cause of their accident.[8] Some have suggested that differences in body mass and upper body strength account for these last two factors. For instance, as the downhill slope of a trail increases, a larger portion of the cyclist's gravitational force serves to move the bicycle downhill while a lower portion holds the cyclist to the seat. Although heavier male riders produce a stronger downhill force vector, lighter women riders are more easily ejected from the bicycle seat by an external force, such as a bump in the trail.[8] In addition, less upper body strength reduces one's ability to maintain control of a bike in a difficult situation.[14] Both of these factors may contribute to a greater chance of losing control when traveling at high speed on challenging terrain. This theory is supported by finding that significantly more women cite loss of control of the bike as a cause of injury.[8]

Another factor related to injury risk is level of experience. One would expect less experienced riders to have more accidents, but one large survey found that riders with more than 4 years experience had a higher incidence of joint and bone injuries than first-year cyclists.[2] Studies of competitive mountain bikers found no difference in injury rates between pro and amateur cross-country racers, but in downhill racers the injury rate was 2.7 times higher in the pro racers. Since the average professional racer is more experienced than the average amateur racer, this study suggests that experience actually increases the risk of injury. The same is true when comparing recreational mountain bikers to the typically more experienced competitive cyclists. In a large survey study, mountain bikers who compete are more likely to be injured than those who only ride recreationally.[9] Most likely this is due to the increased risk of injury during competition. In fact, this same study found a fourfold increase in injury risk during competition. This comes as no surprise, since in competition bikers ride more aggressively and at greater speeds while more fatigued.

Injury Type

Injuries requiring admission to a regional trauma center occurred with the following frequencies: 47% musculoskeletal, 12% head, 12% spine, 10% chest, 10% facial, 5% abdominal, and 2% genitourinary.[12] In a fall, the elbow or shoulder is most often the site of initial impact, and the upper extremity is the most common region involved in musculoskeletal injuries (Fig. 12-4).[11] When clavicle fractures, acromioclavicular separations, and shoulder dislocations are considered together, the shoulder becomes the single site most prone to serious injury.[14] As many as one-fourth of all serious injuries occur at the shoulder,[9] with clavicle fractures the most common type of serious injury.[11] Other studies show a similar distribution[2,15]; however, there are two minor subgroups in which

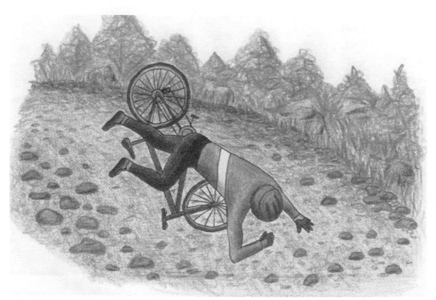

FIGURE 12-4 Diagram of a biker falling forward over the handlebar with elbow striking the ground. Forward falls are the most common mechanism resulting in serious injury from mountain biking, and the shoulder is the single most commonly injured site. (Artwork by Andrea Parsons, MD.)

lower extremity injuries occur with slightly greater frequency.[10,12] First, in a study limited to the most seriously injured bikers admitted to regional trauma centers, upper extremity fractures were observed in 25% and lower extremity fractures in 29%.[12] Second, a study limited to competitive cyclists at the pro/elite level found that lower extremity injuries accounted for 53% of all musculoskeletal injuries, with the knee being the single most commonly injured site.[10]

Another important but less common location for musculoskeletal injures is the spine. Forward falls where the head strikes first, instead of the shoulder, can result in neck injuries from compression, hyperflexion, hyperextension, or lateral bending. Several studies have noted acute neck pain following injury in mountain bikers.[7,11] And the neck is the most common site for an acute muscle injury.[7] Of course, catastrophic neck injuries also occur, with several reported cases of tetraplegia resulting from mountain bike crashes.[12,18] Lumbar fractures have been observed[8]; otherwise little is known about low back injuries in mountain biking.

Following injuries to the extremities, and excluding all mild injuries, the head is the next most commonly injured site, accounting for about 10% of all injuries.[2,11,15] Differences are observed based on the style of riding. More concussions are suffered by injured cross-country racers than injured downhill racers, 15% and 9%, respectively.[15] Facial injuries are more common in the severely injured.[1,12]

Finally, and to be complete, reported mountain biking injuries not discussed elsewhere in this article include pancreas transection,[16] unlar artery occlusion,[19] dislocation of the incus,[20] scrotal abnormalities,[21] and injuries to the spleen, liver, small bowel, adrenal gland, pancreas, mesentery, colon, omentum, kidney, uterus, and testicles.[12]

EVALUATION AND TREATMENT OF THE INJURED MOUNTAIN BIKER

The most severe injuries including internal organ damage, serious brain injury, and spinal cord injury often require surgery and extensive rehabilitation. Treatment of these injures is beyond the scope of this chapter. Mild injuries, such as skin abrasions or contusions, require simple first aid. Since acute muscle injuries are more common than chronic repetitive injuries in mountain bikers,[9] the reader is referred to Chapter 11 for a discussion of repetitive use injuries.

In the field, or in the acute setting, it is important to gather information about the mechanics of an injury. If possible, protective equipment such as the helmet, gloves, and body armor should be inspected for signs of damage. Witnesses should be interviewed if they are available. In cases of an apparent mild injury, the examination should focus on the area of injury and the most immediate proximal and distal regions. A neurovascular check of the injured limb must be completed. Inspection of the injured area to look for deformity, swelling, and skin wounds is important, since these findings can be signs of more serious underlying injuries. Palpation for swelling, tenderness, and crepitus should precede range-of-motion testing. If there is apparent deformity, significant tenderness, or loss in range of motion, the injured area needs to be immobilized until examined radiographically.

In more serious injuries it is best to have a low level of suspicion for cervical spine fractures and head injury, especially with forward falls. Loss of consciousness, even for a brief time, should trigger transport to an emergency room for further evaluation. The cervical spine should be immobilized, even if there is no pain or tenderness. The victim should be monitored for changes in mental status and neurologic status.

As for the more common musculoskeletal injuries that occur in mountain biking, treatment depends on the location of injury and the severity of injury. Fractures and ligament tears require immobilization for between 2 to 6 weeks, and sometimes need surgery. For most other injuries, the focus is on rehabilitation. Early mobilization is desired whenever possible since immobilization leads to contractures and muscle atrophy. An acutely inflamed joint or tendon, or a sprained ligament, should not be immobilized for more than a few days. Ice is generally applied for 15 minutes every hour for the first few days after the injury and can be used in conjunction with anti-inflammatory medication to control inflammation and pain.

Once inflammation and pain have subsided, range-of-motion exercises should begin. Movement through normal range of motion allows the injured tissues to heal properly and maximizes the strength of repair. Isometric exercises are used for strengthening when full range of motion is not possible or needs to be avoided. Isotonic strengthening may begin when there are no limits in range of motion.

The final phase of rehabilitation is retraining on a bike. This is a critical step in healing and helps reduce risk of further injury. It begins with short rides on a stationary bike, increasing resistance and duration gradually over a few weeks. With each increase in activity, signs of recurring pain or weakness should trigger a reversal to a tolerable level of activity. Once aggressive riding on a stationary bike is tolerated, gradually replace it with road riding. If this is tolerated, then off-road riding is allowed. During this time, cross-training is encouraged, especially with activities that do not produce any symptoms from the injury.

PREVENTION

Injury prevention in mountain biking, as in other sports, is mostly common sense. Although helmet use is more common with mountain bikers than with other cyclists, compliance is not 100%.[3] By reducing potential injury from an impact, simply wearing a helmet reduces the risk of head injury by 6.6-fold, and risk of brain injury by 8.3-fold.[22] Other protective equipment is also available, but has not been studied.

The single best way to reduce mountain biking injuries is to avoid a fall. Therefore, mountain bikers must assess their abilities honestly and ride accordingly. It is important to maintain good physical condition, develop good riding skills, and obtain adequate training before trying more difficult trails or tricks. Before every ride it is important to become familiar with the terrain and use extra caution in downhill sections. Female riders may want to perform an upper body strengthening program. Furthermore, prevention requires attention to the ride, not just the rider. Regular bike inspections and maintenance are a necessary part of the sport. And when possible, selecting a bike with a lower head angle (the angle between the front fork and the ground) may reduce the chance of a forward fall. Finally, it is important to educate mountain bikers about injury risk factors and measures they can use to prevent future injuries.

REFERENCES

1. Gassner RJ, Hackl W, Tuli T, et al. Differential profile of facial injuries among mountain bikers compared with bicyclists. *J Trauma*. 1999;47:50–54.
2. Gaulrapp H, Weber A, Rosenmeyer B. Injuries in mountain biking. *Knee Surg Sports Traumatol Arthrosc*. 2001;9:48–53.
3. Rivara FP, Thompson DC, Thompson RS, et al. Injuries involving off-road cycling. *J Fam Pract*. 1997;44:481–485.
4. Bicycle Retailer and Industry News. Available at: www.bicycleretailer.com. Accessed June 29, 2007.
5. Ten-Year History of Selected Sports Participation. Available at: http://www.nsga.org/public/pages/index.cfm?pageid=153. Accessed June 29, 2007.
6. Chow TK, Bracker MD, Patrick K. Acute injuries from mountain biking. *West J Med*. 1993;159:145–148.
7. Chow TK, Kronisch RL. Mechanisms of injury in competitive off-road bicycling. *Wilderness Environ Med*. 2002;13:27–30.
8. Kronisch RL, Pfeiffer RP, Chow TK, et al. Gender differences in acute mountain bike racing injuries. *Clin J Sport Med*. 2002;12:158–164.
9. Kronisch RL, Rubin AL. Traumatic injuries in off-road bicycling. *Clin J Sport Med*. 1994;4:240–244.
10. Pfeiffer RP. Off-road bicycle racing injuries: the NORBA pro/elite category. *Clin Sports Med*. 1994;13:207–217.
11. Jeys LM, Cribb G, Toms AD, et al. Mountain biking injuries in rural England. *Br J Sports Med*. 2001;35:197–199.
12. Kim PT, Jangra D, Ritchie AH, et al. Mountain biking injuries requiring trauma center admission: a 10-year regional trauma system experience. *J Trauma*. 2006;60:312–318.
13. Frobose I, Lucker B, Wittmann K. Overuse symptoms in mountain bikers: a study with an empirical questionnaire [in German]. *Dtsch Z Sportmed*. 2001;52:311–315.
14. Kronisch RL, Pfeiffer RP. Mountain biking injuries. *Sports Med*. 2002;32:523–537.
15. Kronisch RL, Pfeiffer RP, Chow TK. Acute injuries in cross-country and downhill off-road bicycle racing. *Med Sci Sports Exerc*. 1996;28:1341–1355.
16. Lovell ME, Brett M, Enion DS. Mountain bike injury to the abdomen, transection of the pancreas and small bowel evisceration. *Injury*. 1992;23:499–500.
17. Chow TK, Corbett SW, Farstad DJ. Do conventional bicycle helmets provide adequate protection in mountain biking? *Wilderness Environ Med*. 1995;6:385–390.
18. Apsingi S, Dussa CU, Soni BM. Acute cervical spine injuries in mountain biking: a report of 3 cases. *Am J Sports Med*. 2006;34:487–490.
19. Applegate KE, Spiegel PK. Ulnar artery occlusion in mountain bikers. *J Sports Med Phys Fitness*. 1995;35:232–234.
20. Saito T, Kono Y, Fukuoka Y, et al. Dislocation of the incus into the external auditory canal after mountain biking accident. *ORL J Otorhinolaryngol Relat Spec*. 2001;63:102–105.
21. Frauscher F, Klauser A, Stenzl A, et al. US findings in the scrotum of extreme mountain bikers. *Radiology*. 2001;219:427–431.
22. Zentner J, Franken H, Lobbecke G. Head injuries from bicycle accidents. *Clin Neurol Neurosurg*. 1996;98:281–285.

CHAPTER 13

Gerard A. Malanga, Jason Peter,
and Dennis A. Bandemer, Jr.

Football Injuries

The origins of American football come from the European game of rugby, which originated at the Rugby Boy's School in England.[1] Football has since progressed from its humble beginnings to a nationally and internationally recognized sporting event. Athletes of all ages participate in organized football games, from the peewee to the professional levels. The ability to diagnose and treat football-related injuries requires a firm understanding of the musculoskeletal system and exposure to common football problems. Often the greatest experience is acquired directly on the playing field. This chapter will focus on football injuries that are commonly treated by sports clinicians on and off the playing field.

TRAUMATIC BRAIN INJURY

Concussion

Football players are at high risk for significant head trauma, which may result in a concussive injury. A concussion results in altered brain functioning that can have both short- and long-term sequelae. An estimated 300,000 concussions occur annually in the United States, with an occurrence rate from 0.25 to 23.0 per 1,000 athletes.[2] Prior to 2001, the diagnosis of sports concussion and determining when an athlete should return to play were complicated by conflicting guidelines. Since 2001 there have been two international symposia on sports concussion. A significant result of these symposia was the acceptance of a unified concussion grading scale and the development of the Sports Concussion Assessment Tool (SCAT); (Fig. 13-1). The SCAT is intended to be used by sideline physicians, athletic trainers, and coaching staff to aid the diagnosis of sports concussions. The SCAT evaluates cognitive features, physical signs, and typical concussion symptoms, and provides a basic neuropsychological assessment (memory and attention). More in-depth neuropsychological testing may be needed to detect the presence of cognitive deficits, and can help manage a safe return to play. Common impairments are retrograde amnesia, memory difficulties, decreased reaction time, and decreased processing speeds.[3–6] Following an acute concussion, the athlete should be removed from the game and evaluated by medical personal, and the athlete should not be allowed to return to a game. The Prague symposium (the Second International Symposium on Sports Concussions) recommended that each athlete progress through a series of steps prior to return-to-play. Each step lasts a minimum of 24 hours, and the athlete must remain symptom free. If symptoms reoccur, the athlete should return to the previously asymptomatic level. The steps are the following: physical/cognitive rest, light aerobics, sport-specific exercises, noncontact activities, full-contact activities, and full return to competitive play.

Concussion versus Postconcussion Syndrome

Concussion problems can be categorized into two groups: acute and postconcussive. In acute concussions, the most common symptoms are headache, dizziness, and blurred vision. The most common signs are deficits in immediate recall, retrograde amnesia, and difficulty with processing information.[7] Additional findings may include loss of consciousness, nausea, attention deficit, disorientation, confusion, tinnitus, slurred speech, inappropriate behavior, irritability, altered taste, altered smell, impact

[Sport Concussion Assessment Tool (SCAT)]

This tool represents a standardized method of evaluating people after concussion in sport. This tool has been produced as part of the Summary and Agreement Statement of the Second International Symposium on Concussion in Sport, Prague 2004

Sports concussion is defined as a complex pathophysiological process affecting the brain, induced by traumatic biomechanical forces. Several common features that incorporate clinical, pathological and biomechanical injury constructs that may be utilized in defining the nature of a concussive head injury include:

1. Concussion may be caused either by a direct blow to the head, face, neck or elsewhere on the body with an 'impulsive' force transmitted to the head.
2. Concussion typically results in the rapid onset of short-lived impairment of neurological function that resolves spontaneously.
3. Concussion may result in neuropathological changes but the acute clinical symptoms largely reflect a functional disturbance rather than structural injury.
4. Concussion results in a graded set of clinical syndromes that may or may not involve loss of consciousness. Resolution of the clinical and cognitive symptoms typically follows a sequential course.
5. Concussion is typically associated with grossly normal structural neuroimaging studies.

Post Concussion Symptoms

Ask the athlete to score themselves based on how they feel now. It is recognized that a low score may be normal for some athletes, but clinical judgment should be exercised to determine if a change in symptoms has occurred following the suspected concussion event.

It should be recognized that the reporting of symptoms may not be entirely reliable. This may be due to the effects of a concussion or because the athlete's passionate desire to return to competition outweighs their natural inclination to give an honest response.

If possible, ask someone who knows the athlete well about changes in affect, personality, behavior, etc.

Remember, concussion should be suspected in the presence of ANY ONE or more of the following:
- Symptoms (such as headache), or
- Signs (such as loss of consciousness), or
- Memory problems

Any athlete with a suspected concussion should be monitored for deterioration (i.e., should not be left alone) and should not drive a motor vehicle.

For more information see the "Summary and Agreement Statement of the Second International Symposium on Concussion in Sport" in the April, 2005 edition of the Clinical Journal of Sport Medicine (vol 15), British Journal of Sports Medicine (vol 39), Neurosurgery (vol 59) and the Physician and Sportsmedicine (vol 33). This tool may be copied for distribution to teams, groups and organizations.
©2005 Concussion in Sport Group

The SCAT Card
(Sport Concussion Assessment Tool)
Athlete Information

What is a concussion? A concussion is a disturbance in the function of the brain caused by a direct or indirect force to the head. It results in a variety of symptoms (like those listed below) and may, or may not, involve memory problems or loss of consciousness.

How do you feel? You should score yourself on the following symptoms, based on how you feel now.

Postconcussion Symptom Scale	None		Moderate			Severe	
Headache	0	1	2	3	4	5	6
"Pressure in head"	0	1	2	3	4	5	6
Neck pain	0	1	2	3	4	5	6
Balance problems or dizzy	0	1	2	3	4	5	6
Nausea or vomiting	0	1	2	3	4	5	6
Vision problems	0	1	2	3	4	5	6
Hearing problems / ringing	0	1	2	3	4	5	6
"Don't feel right"	0	1	2	3	4	5	6
Feeling "dinged" or "dazed"	0	1	2	3	4	5	6
Confusion	0	1	2	3	4	5	6
Feeling slowed down	0	1	2	3	4	5	6
Feeling like "in a fog"	0	1	2	3	4	5	6
Drowsiness	0	1	2	3	4	5	6
Fatigue or low energy	0	1	2	3	4	5	6
More emotional than usual	0	1	2	3	4	5	6
Irritability	0	1	2	3	4	5	6
Difficulty concentrating	0	1	2	3	4	5	6
Difficulty remembering	0	1	2	3	4	5	6
(follow up symptoms only)							
Sadness	0	1	2	3	4	5	6
Nervous or anxious	0	1	2	3	4	5	6
Trouble falling asleep	0	1	2	3	4	5	6
Sleeping more than usual	0	1	2	3	4	5	6
Sensitivity to light	0	1	2	3	4	5	6
Sensitivity to noise	0	1	2	3	4	5	6
Other: _____	0	1	2	3	4	5	6

What should I do?
Any athlete suspected of having a concussion should be removed from play, and then seek medical evaluation.

Signs to watch for:
Problems could arise over the first 24-48 hours. You should not be left alone and must go to a hospital at once if you:
- Have a headache that gets worse
- Are very drowsy or can't be awakened (woken up)
- Can't recognize people or places
- Have repeated vomiting
- Behave unusually or seem confused; are very irritable
- Have seizures (arms and legs jerk uncontrollably)
- Have weak or numb arms or legs
- Are unsteady on your feet; have slurred speech

Remember, it is better to be safe. Consult your doctor after a suspected concussion.

What can I expect?
Concussion typically results in the rapid onset of short-lived impairment that resolves spontaneously over time. You can expect that you will be told to rest until you are fully recovered (that means resting your body and your mind). Then, your doctor will likely advise that you go through a gradual increase in exercise over several days (or longer) before returning to sport.

[www.cjsportmed.com]

FIGURE 13-1 Sports Concussion Assessment Tool (SCAT). Used by sideline medical personnel to streamline and standardize assessment of the player with concussion. Note the multifaceted assessment tools. (From the Summary and Agreement Statement of the Second International Symposium on Concussion in Sport, Prague, 2004.)

seizures, and imbalance.[8] Any athlete presenting with these symptoms must be evaluated by a sideline physician or qualified athletic trainer. Deficits that are persistent or progressive must be referred to the emergency room for further evaluation and diagnostic workup.

On the other hand, postconcussive syndrome is a constellation of somatic, affective, or cognitive symptoms that persist following mild to moderate head trauma. Common postconcussive symptoms include headache, nausea, vomiting, drowsiness, numbness/tingling, balance impairment, vertigo, sleep impairment, light/noise sensitivities, difficulty concentrating/remembering, depression, anxiety, dizziness, irritability, and fatigue.[9,10] The diagnosis of postconcussive syndrome can be difficult, since symptoms are subjective to the athlete's interpretation, and often vary in severity. Often, several sources of information are necessary to make the diagnosis, including input from family members, neuropsychological testing, physical examination, diagnostic imaging, and information from the patient.[10]

Second Impact Syndrome/Diffuse Cerebral Swelling

Concussion syndrome can be further complicated by "second impact syndrome" (SIS). SIS is of concern because it reportedly has a mortality rate of 50% and a morbidity rate of 100%.[11,12] The mechanism of SIS is when an athlete suffers a second head injury, before resolution of symptoms from a prior concussion. The second impact is often less traumatic than the initial episode, but can result in sudden loss of consciousness. At the vascular level, the brain's ability to regulate the cerebral perfusion pressure is disrupted, causing cerebral congestion, an elevation of intracranial pressure, and possible herniation of the brainstem. This results in diffuse cerebral edema, coma, and respiratory failure. SIS remains a controversial topic in sports medicine; McCrory and Johnston reviewed all documented cases and published evidence of second impact syndrome in 2001 and 2002.[12,13] Furthermore, they recommended replacing the term with "diffuse cerebral swelling," which has been documented in traumatic brain injury research. Despite the controversy, many authors agree that athletes with persistent symptoms should not be allowed to play and should follow the recommended guidelines prior to returning to any physical activity.[12,13]

CERVICAL SPINE INJURIES

Cervical spine injuries are common in both contact and noncontact sports, with a 10% to 15% chance of injury in football athletes.[14] Cervical injures in football players are of concern because of the potential risk for permanent disability or paralysis. Injury can involve any of the anatomic structures of the spine including the bony vertebra, ligaments, muscles, and neurovascular elements. Advancements (described later) and research have made football considerably safer in respect to the prevention of catastrophic injuries and the ability for an athlete to return to play following most injuries.

Cervical Strains and Sprains

In football, the majority of cervical spine injuries are self-limiting muscular strains. An excessive loading or stretching of the muscle causes disruption of muscle fibers and localized pain.[14] Cervical sprain is an injury involving the cervical ligaments and facet joint capsules. The mechanism of injury is similar to cervical muscular strains. Both cervical muscular strains and sprains are associated with focal pain, muscle "spasms," and a decrease in both active and passive range of motion. However, only cervical muscular strains have focal muscular tenderness on palpation.

Muscular strains typically do not require diagnostic testing and symptoms generally resolve with time. Muscular strains are treated conservatively with rest, ice, compression, and anti-inflammatory medications. Cervical sprains usually require an x-ray to rule out bony pathology or cervical instability. Uncomplicated cervical sprains can also be treated conservatively with rest, ice, compression, and anti-inflammatory medications. Athletes can return to physical activity when they can demonstrate a painless, full cervical range of motion.

Burner Syndrome

Trauma involving the brachial plexus or cervical nerve roots can result in transient pain and paresthesias in a single limb. Approximately 49% to 65% of college football players have experienced at least one burner episode.[15,16] Controversy exists on whether the symptoms are produced by direct involvement of the brachial plexus or of the cervical nerve roots. A traction injury occurs when the shoulder is forced

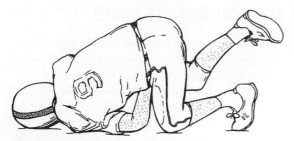

FIGURE 13-2 Traction injury. This is a common mechanism for injury to the brachial plexus, such as with a "burner." (From Anderson MK, Hall SJ. *Fundamentals of Sports Injury Management.* Baltimore: Willams & Wilkins; 1998.)

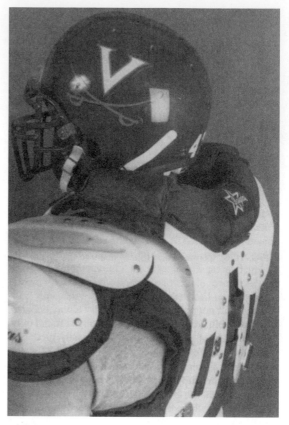

FIGURE 13-3 Cervical neck roll. Note limitations of hyperextension and lateral movements of the cervical spine. (From Perrin DH. *The Injured Athlete.* 3rd ed. Philadelphia: Lippincott-Raven; 1999.)

downward and the cervical spine distracted and rotated away (Fig. 13-2). A compressive injury occurs when the cervical spine is forced into the ipsilateral shoulder.[17]

Following an acute injury the athlete is often seen shaking out the affected limb when returning to the huddle or to the sideline. Acute symptoms often present in the C5-C6 nerve root distribution and include burning, numbness, and tingling of the affected limb. Examination should include a complete neurologic exam including motor, sensory, and reflexive testing. An athlete can return to play if there are no neurologic deficits on examination, a negative Spurling maneuver, and an unrestricted and pain-free range of motion of the cervical spine. Noncomplicated injuries respond to rest, ice, compression, and gentle range of motion of the affected limb. If symptoms persist, the cervical spine should be immobilized and the athlete should be further evaluated to rule out bony or neurovascular injury.

To reduce the potential risk of potential burner events, athletes must practice proper blocking and tackling techniques (described later). Protective equipment includes a properly fitting helmet and shoulder pads as well as a cervical neck roll (Fig. 13-3). The cervical neck roll will limit both hyperextension and lateral flexion of the cervical spine. One study compared the Cowboy Collar, the A Force Neck Collar, and the 5.08-cm foam neck roll. The study concluded that in a controlled setting, the Cowboy Collar was best at reducing hyperextension but that none of the collars significantly reduced passive lateral flexion of the cervical spine.[18]

Cervical Spinal Cord Injury

Injury to the cervical spine can result in bony fracture and/or dislocation of the spinal elements. The disruption of normal spinal anatomy can result in permanent neurologic deficits. A comparison of team sports showed that football, gymnastics, and ice hockey had the highest risk of traumatic spinal cord injury.[19] The proposed mechanism of injury is from axial loading and compression of the cervical spine. A review of 209 cases of football-related tetraplegia showed that axial loading caused 52% of the injuries; hyperflexion (10%) and hyperextension (3%) accounted for only 13% of the injuries.[20] Seventy-three percent of permanent tetraplegia occurred in college defensive backs, and only 52% at the high school level.[20] A review article showed that in high school athletes, special teams (13%) and linebackers (10%) are also at risk for permanent tetraplegia.[21]

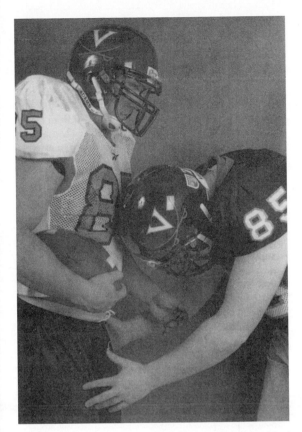

FIGURE 13-4 Head down tackling. Note removal of cervical spine lordosis, which can transmit forces down the spinal column instead of to the surrounding structures. (From Perrin DH. *The Injured Athlete*. 3rd ed. Philadelphia: Lippincott-Raven; 1999.)

Axial loading of the cervical spine is greatest in "head-down" contact (Fig. 13-4). The cervical spine in 30 degrees of flexion removes the natural cervical lordosis and becomes straight, acting like a segmented column. Force is transmitted down the center of the cervical column instead of to the surrounding structures. Traumatic fracture, subluxation, or dislocation occurs when the force generated exceeds the maximum vertical compression threshold. A position statement from the National Athletic Trainers' Association concluded that significant injury can occur with as little as 150 ft-lb of kinetic energy.[22] Since 1976, when rule changes made such "spear tackling" illegal, there has been a reduction in catastrophic spine injuries. Coaching staff and game officials have been essential in implementing and enforcing proper tackling and blocking techniques. The emphasis has been to make the shoulder the initial point of contact, and that

tackling should occur with the head in the up position. The motto "hit what you see" has been emphasized from the professional to the high school level. Despite previous efforts, increased awareness is still necessary; in a recent study nearly one-third of sampled high school athletes were not aware that "spear tackling" was an illegal offense.[23]

Trauma involving the cervical spinal cord can also result in transient sensory and motor deficits. Sensory symptoms include burning pain, numbness, and tingling involving the upper and/or lower extremities. Motor symptoms include weakness or paralysis of two or more extremities, and usually resolve within 10 to 15 minutes, but occasionally last up to 48 hours. Transient tetraparesis occurs commonly in football and other contact sports, with an estimated 1.3 episodes per 10,000 athletes, or an incidence of 6 per 10,000 athletes.[24] Transient tetraparesis can also occur following hyperextension of the cervical spine (Fig. 13-5). Hyperextension results in

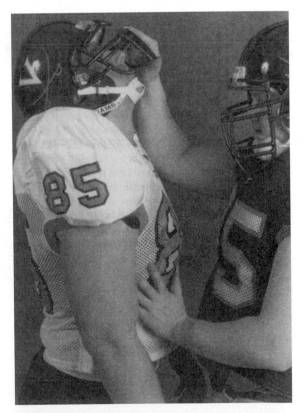

FIGURE 13-5 Neck hyperextension. This may result in transient tetraparesis. (From Perrin DH. *The Injured Athlete*. 3rd ed. Philadelphia: Lippincott-Raven; 1999.)

compression of the spinal cord between the posterior inferior aspect of the superior vertebra and the posterior superior aspect of the inferior vertebra. This "pincer" affects results in a compression/ischemic neuropraxia involving the upper and lower extremities. Involvement of multiple extremities makes a peripheral nerve injury less likely, but cervical neuropraxia is often confused with burner syndrome.

Diagnostic evaluation with magnetic resonance imaging (MRI) is necessary to visualize the spinal cord and the vertebral column. Absolute contraindications to return to play following a neuropraxic event include associated ligamentous instability, persistent neurologic symptoms, or multiple episodes of neuropraxia. Single neurapraxic events with evidence of cervical cord defect or edema are evaluated on a case-by-case basis, but are considered a relative to absolute contraindication for return to play.[25]

SHOULDER

Injuries of the shoulder are the fourth most common musculoskeletal injury involving college football players.[26] The most common injury is acromioclavicular joint separation (41%) followed by anterior shoulder instability (20%), rotator cuff injury (12%), clavicle fracture (4%), and posterior shoulder instability (4%).[26] Defensive players have an increased risk of shoulder instability and rotator cuff injuries, whereas quarterbacks have a higher incidence of acromioclavicular joint sprain, overuse injuries including the rotator cuff, and bicipital tendonitis.[27]

Acromioclavicular Joint Injuries

Acromioclavicular (AC) joint injuries commonly occur in football quarterbacks and offensive players that run and carry the football. Injury commonly occurs after the athlete lands directly onto the lateral aspect of an adducted shoulder. The acromioclavicular ligament is stressed as the shoulder is forced into the opposite direction. Significant force can result in disruption of both the acromioclavicular and the coracoclavicular ligaments.

Athletes with AC joint injuries complain of pain involving the top of the shoulder or focal pain over the AC joint and will have reproducible tenderness with palpation over the affected joint. Range of motion of the shoulder will be limited, and focal pain over the AC joint will be reproduced with the

cross-body adduction test. The O'Brien test (described in Chapter 10) can also be used to differentiate between AC joint and labral pathology of the shoulder. Diagnosis of AC joint injuries can often be made clinically, but x-ray may be necessary to evaluate bony anatomy. AC joint injuries are classified into one of six categories based on the involvement of the acromioclavicular and costoclavicular ligaments and the degree of clavicular displacement (Fig. 13-6). Simple injuries respond well to conservative treatment, but more complex injuries should be surgically evaluated.

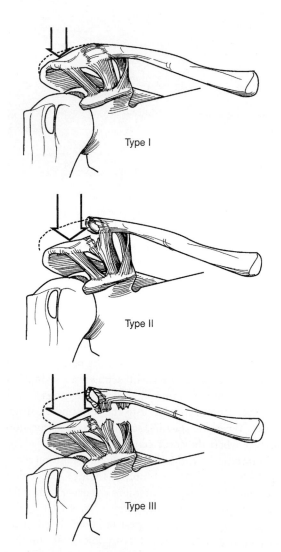

FIGURE 13-6 Classification of acromioclavicular joint injuries. (From Perrin DH. *The Injured Athlete.* 3rd ed. Philadelphia: Lippincott-Raven; 1999.)

Impingement and Rotator Cuff Injury

The rotator cuff is susceptible to impingement caused by repetitive overhead throwing and direct shoulder trauma. Quarterbacks and overhead throwing athletes are at high risk for rotator cuff pathology, though linemen and linebackers are also commonly affected.[27,28] Impingement is the result of a narrow rotator cuff outlet, resulting in impingement of the rotator cuff muscles. The musculotendinous junction of the supraspinatus muscle is most commonly affected.[27] Since the supraspinatus muscle has a poor blood supply, recurrent impingement will eventually result in partial or complete rotator cuff tears. However, a significant acute traumatic event may result in a partial or complete rotator cuff tear without preexisting impingement syndrome.

Impingement symptoms include anterior/lateral shoulder pain, crepitus, and muscle weakness of the involved shoulder. Palpation often produces pain over the bicipital tendon and at the insertion of the superspinatus tendon. Neer, Hawkins, and Yocum impingement tests can be helpful to confirm impingement syndrome, along with the painful arc sign (Fig. 13-7). Athletes with a complete rotator cuff tear will have difficulty with initiating and holding the shoulder in abduction. Provocative tests include the supraspinatus test and the drop arm test. Diagnostic imaging includes x-rays, MRI (gold standard), and arthrogram.

Rotator cuff treatment includes both surgical and nonsurgical options. Nonoperative treatment includes reducing inflammation with anti-inflammatory medications, rest, and modalities such as ultrasound. Glenohumeral joint motion is maintained with a progressive mobilization program starting with passive, then active-assist, and finally active range of motion. Strengthening of the dynamic and static shoulder muscles should progress from isometric to isotonic exercises, and closed kinetic chain to open kinetic chain exercises. A subacromial corticosteroid injection can also be considered in both acute and chronic injuries. Young active athletes should consider having

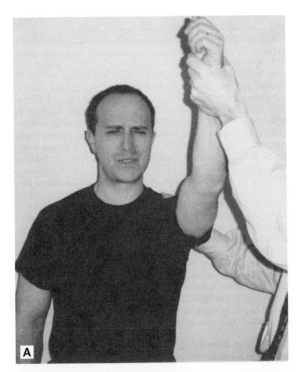
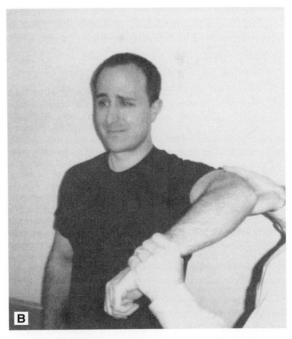

FIGURE 13-7 A. Neer test. The shoulder is passively flexed; reproduction of pain is indicative of rotator cuff impingement. This maneuver can also be performed with the arm in internal rotation. **B.** Hawkin test. The shoulder is abducted 90 degrees and internally rotated; reproduction of pain is indicative of rotator cuff impingement. This maneuver can also be performed in the scapular plane. (From DeLisa JA, Gans BM, Walsh NE, et al. *Physical Medicine & Rehabilitation: Principles and Practice.* 4th ed. Philadelphia: Lippincott Williams & Wilkins; 2005.)

acute complete or partial (> 40% involvement) rotator cuff tears surgically corrected.

ELBOW

The elbow is rapidly extended in throwing athletes, which increases the forces and stress on the muscles, tendons, and ligaments of the joint. A review of elbow injuries in professional football players demonstrated that elbow sprains (76%) were the most common injury, followed by elbow dislocations/subluxations (17%) and fractures (4.4%).[29] Most of the acute elbow sprains were caused by hyperextension of the joint (55.7%); the medial (20%) and lateral (2.9%) collateral ligaments were also susceptible to acute injury.[29]

Tendonitis

Athletes can develop pain involving the muscles that flex and extend the wrist and fingers. The mechanism of injury is typically due to overuse of the muscles or improper biomechanics involving the wrist and elbow. The extensor muscles originate at the lateral epicondyle of the humerus, and the flexor muscles originate from the medial epicondyle of the humerus. The diagnosis of both medial and lateral epicondylitis is often made clinically, without the need for diagnostic imaging. The athlete with lateral epicondylitis will have pain on palpation distal to the origin of the wrist extensors. Resisted extension of the index and middle fingers will reproduce pain over the extensor muscles. Medial epicondylitis is often seen in throwing athletes, including quarterbacks; pain is reproduced with resisted flexion of the wrist and palpation over the common flexor tendon origin.

Treatment includes rest, ice, and anti-inflammatory medications while maintaining range of motion and strength. Also, the main focus must be on identifying the underlying cause and correcting the problem. If symptoms do not resolve with conservation treatment, a corticosteroid injection may be considered. An MRI or diagnostic ultrasound can be ordered to rule out underlying bony or muscular pathology. Surgical intervention may be considered in persistent symptoms that fail standard therapy regimens.

Elbow Collateral Ligament Injuries

The collateral ligaments of the elbow are susceptible to traumatic and overuse injuries. Most commonly the medial collateral ligament is injured following a

traumatic dislocation, repetitive overhead throwing, and a valgus force on a planted hand.[29] The athlete with this condition typically will have palpable pain and tenderness over the medial aspect of the elbow. In more severe cases, laxity of the joint will be demonstrated with a valgus force directed on the elbow. Following an acute injury, treatment should include immobilization, ice, and anti-inflammatory medications. If conservative therapy fails, surgical reconstruction of the medial collateral ligament may be considered.

HAND

Football consists of blocking, tackling, falling, and catching, which leave the wrist and fingers susceptible to injury.

Common Finger Injuries

Shaft fractures involving the fingers are relatively common in all physical activities, including football. Diagnosis is often made without diagnostic imaging, but imaging studies may be necessary to rule out involvement of the interphalangeal joint space. Most simple fractures can be treated conservatively with immobilization of the joint, ice, and anti-inflammatory medications. However, if the fracture involves the joint space or is associated with multiple fragments, the athlete should have a surgical evaluation.

Mallet finger is caused by the rupture of the extensor tendon at its insertion point onto the distal phalanx.[30] The mechanism of injury is passive flexion of the distal phalanx, resulting in loss of extensor tendon continuity with or without avulsion fracture (Fig. 13-8). On examination, the athlete will not be able to extend the distal phalanx. Treatment consists of immobilization of the middle phalanx and distal phalanx in extension for a minimum of 6 to 8 weeks. If x-ray demonstrates an avulsion involving greater than one-third of the joint, surgical evaluation and repair is usually necessary.

"Jersey finger" involves the rupture of the flexor digitorum tendon from its insertion on the distal phalanx. The injury commonly occurs when the athlete's finger gets caught in an opponent's jersey. On examination, the athlete will not be able to flex the distal interphalangeal joint. All athletes presenting with a Jersey finger should be sent for a surgical evaluation.

The ulnar collateral ligament of the thumb can be sprained or torn following a valgus force at the metacarpophalangeal joint. This is often called "gamekeepers"

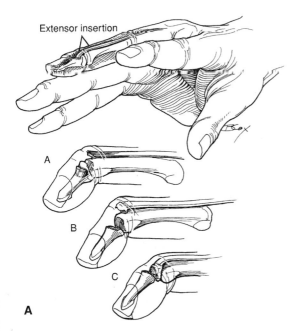

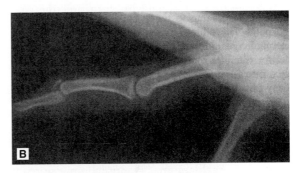

FIGURE 13-8 A. Mallet finger. Note disruption of the extensor tendon at its insertion point on the distal phalanx. **B.** Avulsion fracture associated with mallet finger. (From Perrin DH. *The Injured Athlete*. 3rd ed. Philadelphia: Lippincott-Raven; 1999.)

or "skier's" thumb. On examination, the athlete will have pain with an applied valgus force and either laxity or gapping of the joint space (Fig. 13-9). Diagnostic imaging is not necessary but can help to rule out underlying bony pathology. Treatment consists of conservative management including immobilization for 4 weeks in a thumb spica splint, ice, and anti-inflammatory medications.[31]

HIP

Hip and pelvic injuries account for 5% to 6% of all adult athletic injuries[32] and up to 9% of injuries in high school athletes.[33] The most common conditions involve strains and sprains of the muscles and ligaments in and around the hip joint, as well as contusions due to direct trauma from falling or being tackled. Less common, but still possible, are osseous injuries such as fractures and dislocations.

Contusions

Contusions in the hip region most commonly occur at the anterior thigh or the iliac crest, which is also called a "hip pointer." The presentation of these contusions can include immediate pain, muscle spasm, and even transient loss of muscle function.[34] A

hematoma or ecchymosis may be present. The injured player will have pain when activating the affected musculature.

Management of contusions includes relative rest, ice, compression, and anti-inflammatory medications. Keeping the affected musculature "on stretch"

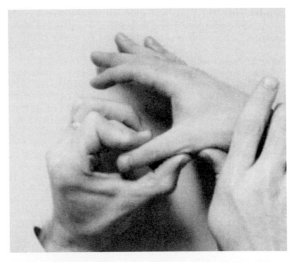

FIGURE 13-9 Skier's thumb evaluation. Note valgus force applied to thumb. (From DeLisa JA, Gans BM, Walsh NE, et al. *Physical Medicine & Rehabilitation: Principles and Practice*. 4th ed. Philadelphia: Lippincott Williams & Wilkins; 2005.)

will help avoid muscle and soft-tissue shortening.[34] Strengthening exercises begin with isometrics with a gradual progression to isotonic and isokinetic exercises, with emphasis on eccentric contractions and should include both open and closed kinetic chain exercises.[34,35] Both agonist and antagonist muscle groups should be strengthened.[33] Return to play is generally allowed when the athlete has achieved full range of motion and strength, without pain. Protective padding should be worn over the contused area.[35]

Hip Labral Tears

The labrum of the hip joint is the fibrocartilage rim around the acetabulum that deepens the "socket" of the hip and provides stability. It can be injured from twisting motions, such as dislocation or subluxation, or from underlying acetabular dysplasia that may stress the lateral labrum.[33] A torn labrum can result in recurrent hip instability or an irreducible dislocation of the hip.[36]

Symptoms of a torn labrum include groin pain, limited motion, an audible click, and/or a painful "catch" with movement.[33,36] Having the patient lay supine and fully flexing, abducting, and laterally rotating the hip assesses the anterior labrum, whereas the posterior labrum is assessed with the hip flexed, adducted, and medially rotated.[37] Reproduction of symptoms with or without a click is considered a positive test.[37] Imaging studies to assess the integrity of the labrum include MRI and arthrography. The use of these two studies in combination has been found to be 90% sensitive and 91% accurate in evaluating labral abnormalities.[36]

Management of these injuries should begin conservatively and follow the process outlined previously. Partial weight bearing is recommended for up to 4 weeks.[33] In addition to conservative treatment, local anesthetic injection may be used and can be both diagnostic and therapeutic.[33] If conservative management fails, surgery is recommended and is performed either arthroscopically, or via open arthrotomy.[33–36]

KNEE

Football-related knee injuries are mostly acute but can be chronic as well. The most common acute conditions are ligamentous and meniscal injuries, whereas chronic conditions are often secondary to overuse or improper biomechanics. The focus of this section will be on acute football-related knee injuries.

Anterior Cruciate Ligament

Injury to the anterior cruciate ligament (ACL) is often the result of a sudden deceleration or pivot with the foot fixed, which places a rotational or hyperextension force on the knee. Often there is no physical contact involved; if, however, there is physical contact, it is most often a posterolateral to anteromedial force and results in an associated medial meniscus tear 50% of the time.[38,39] The O'Donoghue triad, also known as the "terrible" or "unhappy" triad, is a combination of damage to the ACL, medial collateral ligament (MCL), and medial meniscus.[38,40,41] This is a common injury resulting from a valgus force in a flexed and rotated knee.

The athlete will often report hearing or feeling a "pop" with immediate pain and will be unable to continue playing due to pain and instability. An effusion may develop within the first few hours, depending on the severity of the tear. As the effusion continues to grow, the player will have increased pain and decreased range of motion. Examination of a knee with a suspected ACL tear involves comparison to the opposite (asymptomatic) knee. Range of motion may be limited in both flexion and extension due to an effusion and/or pain. The Lachman and anterior drawer tests are the most common tests performed to assess ACL integrity. In addition to clinical examination, diagnostic tests may include plain x-rays and MRI. X-rays are important to rule out a fracture, such as a Segond fracture, which is an avulsion of the tibial plateau.[39] MRI is the best imaging study for visualizing the ACL and has a sensitivity of 95% with a specificity of 98% for detecting ACL tears (Fig. 13-10).[42]

The initial treatment of an acute ACL injury focuses on reducing pain and swelling using the "PRICE" (protection, rest, ice, compression, elevation) approach and anti-inflammatory medications. Joint aspiration can also be helpful by reducing the pressure within the joint and removing some of the inflammatory fluid. The knee can be protected with a hinged knee brace to provide stability and to prevent hyperextension. The positive benefits of bracing may be due to a subjective sense of better stability, which allows better participation in and improved results from the rehabilitation process.[43] Crutches may be used until pain and an antalgic gait are reduced.

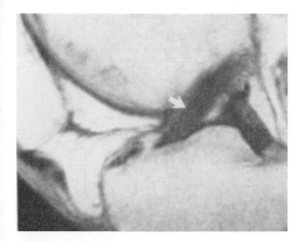

FIGURE 13-10 Oblique sagittal MRI of the knee. *Arrow* points to the anterior cruciate ligament; borders and attachments are clearly visualized. (From DeLisa JA, Gans BM, Walsh NE, et al. *Physical Medicine & Rehabilitation: Principles and Practice*. 4th ed. Philadelphia: Lippincott Williams & Wilkins; 2005.)

Surgery is indicated for younger individuals, especially those involved in high-impact athletics. ACL injuries rarely heal spontaneously,[43–45] and therefore those who are older or do not have an active lifestyle may still require surgery if there is persistent instability. If surgery is not performed in these situations, there is an increased risk of meniscal injury and acceleration of degenerative changes due to continued instability.[35,46] In these cases, rehabilitation should emphasize regaining strength and proprioception. A functional hinged knee brace is often required with a 15- to 20-degree extension stop.[35]

Rehabilitation for ACL tears is similar, whether or not surgery is performed. The step-wise approach discussed earlier should be followed by the rehabilitation of these injuries. The goal should be to achieve full extension by 1 week and gradually increase weight bearing over the first 2 to 3 weeks, with weaning off of the crutches, although a brace may still be worn for several months. Range-of-motion exercises may involve an exercise bike or other closed kinetic chain exercises with progression to an open kinetic chain program. Recent studies have shown that the difference in strain placed on the reconstructed ACL by open and closed kinetic chain exercises is not clinically significant.[47] Both of these types of exercises should be incorporated into the rehabilitation program and have not been shown to have significantly different effects on the healing process of the ACL graft.[47]

After 1 month, functional activities and proprioceptive training should be instituted. Jogging and sport-specific exercises may begin 2 to 3 months after injury.

Meniscal Injuries

Meniscal injuries are common in football as a result of the frequent twisting of the knee as players cut side-to-side while running. The posterior horn of the medial meniscus is most commonly torn and injury typically occurs as a result of rotation of the knee while it is flexed with the foot fixed.[35] On the other hand, lateral meniscus tears tend to occur more with a rotational force while squatting (with the knees fully flexed), such as during heavy weight lifting.[38] Players often feel sudden discomfort at the time of injury. They are usually able to ambulate and may even attempt to return to play the same day. Depending on the severity of the injury, an effusion can develop within a few hours or over the next 24 to 48 hours. The player may complain of knee stiffness and may experience mechanical symptoms such as locking, catching, or popping. These symptoms are often due to a free-floating, torn tissue fragment getting caught in the joint and occur more often in knee flexion.[35]

Examination will often reveal an effusion and joint line tenderness. Special testing includes the McMurray test, which will produce a painful click or thud when positive. When compared to arthroscopy and/or arthrotomy, this test had a sensitivity of 59% and a specificity of over 90%.[48] Diagnostic studies include x-rays to assess for bony injuries and to rule out other diagnoses such as osteochondral injuries. MRI provides excellent visualization of the menisci (Fig. 13-11).

If the knee is stable without mechanical symptoms, surgery is often not necessary. Conservative treatment begins with PRICE and anti-inflammatory medications. It is important to avoid loading the joint with associated rotational forces. Weight bearing should be protected with crutches. If an effusion persists despite conservative treatment, aspiration of the joint followed by a corticosteroid injection can be helpful in reducing inflammation which, when present, can inhibit normal muscle contraction.[35] When strength and range of motion have been regained, advancement to sport-specific agility training can begin. If there are mechanical symptoms or conservative treatment has failed, arthroscopy is the treatment of choice, especially since repair is likely to be required.[35] Damage to the outer one-third can often be repaired as there is vascularization in this region.[49]

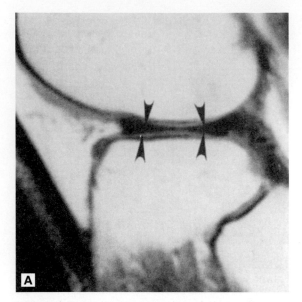
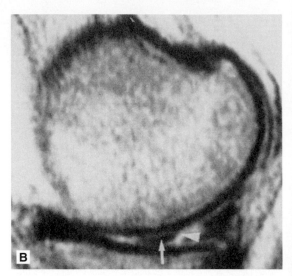

FIGURE 13-11 A. Sagittal MRI of the knee (normal). Note classic "bow-tie" appearance of a normal, lateral meniscus. **B.** T2-weighted knee MRI through the medial meniscus. Note so-called "bucket-handle" tear (*arrowhead*) of the posterior horn of the medial meniscus. *White arrow* is the inner fragment displaced centrally. (From DeLisa JA, Gans BM, Walsh NE, et al. *Physical Medicine & Rehabilitation: Principles and Practice.* 4th ed. Philadelphia: Lippincott Williams & Wilkins; 2005.)

The player should be on protected weight bearing for a longer duration (i.e., until there is pain-free range of motion) and must avoid deep squats for 6 months.[50] If there is injury to the inner two-thirds, the tissue is often resected due to poor ability to heal. Weight bearing usually is allowed as tolerated within 1 to 2 days. Postoperative rehabilitation is similar to that for non-operative care.

ANKLE

Because of the multiple planes of movement possible within the ankle, it is less stable than the knee. Therefore, it is prone to injury and is one of the most commonly injured joints in football players. The stop-and-go and sudden change of direction motions associated with football can put stress on the supporting ligaments that may go beyond their capable range of resistance. As with the knee, most football-related ankle injuries are acute in nature.

Lateral Ankle Sprain

Lateral ankle sprains are also known as inversion sprains due to the mechanism of injury. This is the most common type of ankle sprain, accounting for

85% of all ankle sprains.[9] Injury to the ligaments tends to progress from anterior to posterior depending on the severity. The anterior talofibular (ATF) ligament is generally injured first, followed by the calcaneofibular (CF); (Fig. 13-12) and the posterior talofibular (PTF) ligaments in more severe injuries. In sprains that involve inversion with dorsiflexion, the CF may be the only ligament injured. The PTF is injured in severe sprains or if there is an associated posterior talar displacement.[51]

The injured player will often report a history of "rolling over" the ankle and may or may not have heard a "pop." Depending on the severity, there may be immediate pain, swelling, and/or instability. The more severe the sprain, the more quickly the symptoms will present. On examination, there may be ecchymosis and swelling. Lower-grade sprains may present with only mild swelling and point tenderness over the anterolateral ankle. The most common provocative tests for assessing the integrity of the lateral ligaments are the anterior drawer and talar tilt tests (Fig. 13-13). The anterior drawer test is considered the gold standard for testing the ATF.[37] The talar tilt test mainly assesses the CF integrity.[37] Separation of the talus from the tibia with this test suggests a CF tear. Comparisons should always be made to the unaffected ankle.

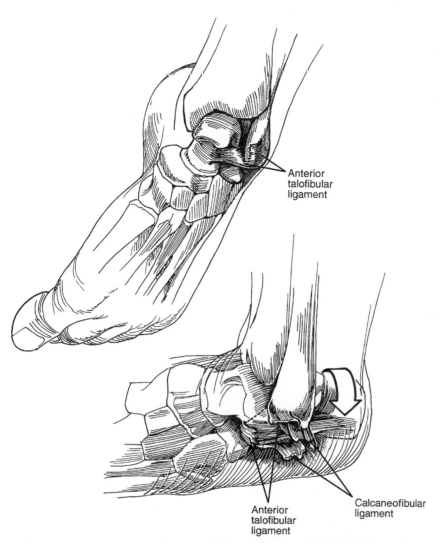

FIGURE 13-12 Lateral ankle ligament sprains. Note single-ligament sprain with plantarflexion, and double-ligament sprain with inversion *(arrow)*. (From Perrin DH. *The Injured Athlete*. 3rd ed. Philadelphia: Lippincott-Raven; 1999.)

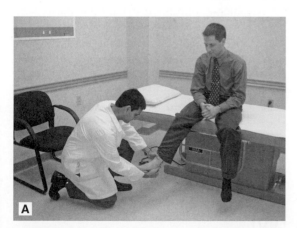

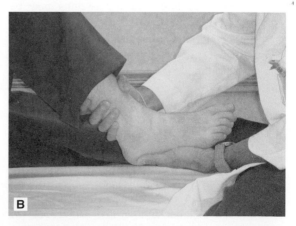

FIGURE 13-13 A. Anterior drawer test of the ankle. Note anterior force directed at the heel to subluxate the talus from the tibia. The examiner notes degree of displacement, degree of pain, and whether or not a firm end-point is reached. **B.** Talar tilt test. Inversion force applied to the ankle to test the calcaneofibular ligament. A positive test is indicated by laxity and/or pain.

Inversion sprains are usually graded I to III. A grade I sprain is mild and presents with minimal swelling and local anterolateral tenderness without instability. There may be a partial tear of the ATF but the CF and PTF remain intact.[37] The anterior drawer and talar tilt tests are usually negative.[37] A grade II sprain presents with more diffuse swelling and some ecchymosis. Often there is instability on exam with difficulty in toe walking. In this case, the ATF is completely torn with a positive anterior drawer test. The CF may be partially torn but the talar tilt test is often negative.[35] A grade III inversion sprain is considered a complete tear of the lateral ligament complex. The player may have significant swelling, ecchymosis, and diffuse lateral ankle pain. Range of motion and weight-bearing tolerance will be limited due to pain and swelling. There may also be marked instability. The anterior drawer and talar tilt tests are usually positive.[35]

If x-rays are necessary, they should include AP, lateral, and mortise views. The mortise view is taken with the lower leg in 20 degrees of internal rotation of the foot and ankle. This allows full assessment of the talar dome and distal tibia and fibula. The medial tibia-talus and lateral fibula-talus distances should be equal.[51] Stress views can also be done with the anterior draw and talar tilt tests to further assess for laxity as well as to look for an avulsion fracture.

Early weight bearing as tolerated is allowed with the use of a brace and crutches for support. Casting should be avoided, even in grade III sprains, as it may slow recovery.[52,53] Initially, pain and swelling should be treated with PRICE and anti-inflammatory medications. After 48 hours, further swelling may be reduced with contrast baths or other modalities such as ice and electrical stimulation. Rehabilitation should then begin with range-of-motion exercises (e.g., writing the alphabet with the foot and ankle) and stretching of the gastrocnemius. After the pain and swelling have been managed, weight-bearing allowance should be increased and strengthening of the inverters, everters, dorsiflexors, and plantar-flexors should begin. Once full range of motion and strength have been regained, special attention should be given to proprioception retraining. Regaining proprioception has been found to be a critical component to the rehabilitation of ankle injuries and can reduce the recurrence of ankle sprains.[54,55] The entire rehabilitation process may take between 2 to 8 weeks depending on the severity.[39] Players who have sustained a more severe sprain should continue to wear a brace while playing. According to one study, 95% of grade III sprains with a talar tilt >9 degrees and anterior translation >10 mm were mechanically stable after functional rehabilitation.[56] A surgical consult is indicated if there is instability noticed on imaging, if a fracture is present, or if conservative treatment has failed.

Syndesmosis Injury

Injury to the syndesmosis is also known as a high ankle sprain. The mechanism of injury may be hyperdorsiflexion with eversion, forced external rotation, or some rotational force added to the injury mechanisms listed above for inversion and eversion sprains. Upon examination, there is often swelling and tenderness to deep palpation along the anterior aspect of the ankle. One complication associated with this type of sprain is a Maisonneuve fracture.[35] This is a fracture of the proximal fibula due to high forces that rupture the anterior tibiofibular ligament and are then transmitted throughout the interosseous membrane.[35]

Special tests to assess the integrity of syndesmosis ligaments include the squeeze test and external rotation test (Fig. 13-14).[37–39] Because of the potential for instability associated with this injury, imaging studies are often warranted and should include AP, lateral, and mortise views. Harper and Keller reported that the most reliable method of detecting syndesmotic widening is the width of the space between the tibia and fibula on the AP and mortise views.[57] Weight bearing x-rays should be performed and are positive for syndesmotic disruption if the tibiofibular space is >6 mm on the AP and mortise views and there is <6 mm overlap of the fibula and tibia on the AP view with <1 mm of tibiofibular overlap on the mortise view.[57] The integrity of the ligaments is better assessed with MRI. The initial treatment and rehabilitation for syndesmosis sprains is similar to that for inversion and eversion sprains, but the recovery time is often longer.[35] Surgical consultation is indicated if there is widening on x-rays, associated fracture, or failed conservative treatment (Fig. 13-15).

FOOT

The foot is composed of many small bones and moves in multiple planes. The strong and repetitive forces associated with football place the foot at high

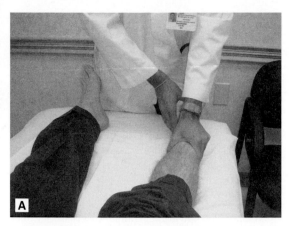
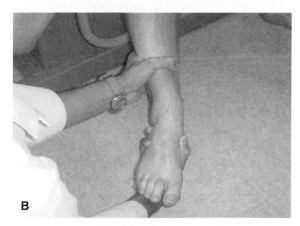

FIGURE 13-14 A. Ankle squeeze test. The squeeze test involves gently squeezing the tibia and fibula together around the distal one-third of the leg. A positive test will elicit severe pain in the distal tibiofibular junction. **B.** Ankle external rotation test. The external rotation test is done with the patient seated and knee bent 90 degrees. If the patient has distal tibiofibular junction pain with passive external rotation of the ankle/foot, the test is positive.

risk for injury. There are several possible injuries that may occur within the foot but the most common is turf toe.

Turf Toe

Turf toe refers to a sprain of the metatarsophalangeal (MTP) joint. This most common occurs at the first toe. The mechanism of injury is hyperextension of the joint. This phenomenon was given its name due to the increased incidence in players who participate on artificial turf.[39] This condition more commonly occurs on artificial turf because it is a stiff and unforgiving surface.[35] Although this appears to be a minor injury, some studies have shown that it results in a greater loss of playing time than other sprains.[39]

Findings on examination include localized swelling and tenderness, usually on the plantar surface. Range of motion of the first MTP joint may be limited with increased pain with passive dorsiflexion

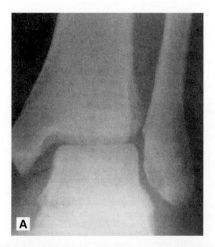
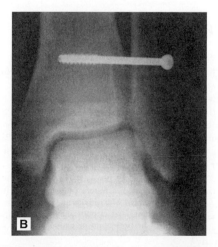

FIGURE 13-15 A. Ankle mortise x-ray view. Note decreased tibia/fibula overlap, which indicates syndesmosis injury. **B.** Ankle mortise x-ray view (postfixation). Note correction of syndemosis injury and normal anatomic alignment in this joint. (From Perrin DH. *The Injured Athlete.* 3rd ed. Philadelphia: Lippincott-Raven; 1999.)

and especially during push-off when running. This injury is graded I to III. A grade I represents only a stretch of the capsule with mild symptoms and the player can return to play, whereas a grade III is a complete tear and even simple walking will be difficult.[39] X-rays may be taken, depending on the severity, to assess for associated bony pathology such as an avulsion fracture.

Treatment for this condition is usually conservative with PRICE and nonsteroidal anti-inflammatory drugs (NSAIDs). Severe injuries may require immobilization with taping, a rocker bottom shoe, or orthotics that protect the joint from dorsiflexion. This should be continued for 1 to 2 weeks with a restriction on athletic participation for up to 6 weeks.[39] If pain and inflammation are severe enough to limit rehabilitation participation, a corticosteroid injection can be considered.[35]

CONCLUSION

Football is a dynamic sport, with dramatic plays and high physical activity. Furthermore, it is a collision sport and the risk for potential injuries always exists. As elucidated above, these injuries can involve virtually any part of the body, ranging from minor sprains to more severe traumatic brain and spinal cord injury leading to long-term sequelae. In order to ensure the safest athletic environment, continued research, education, and stricter safety regulations must be pursued.

REFERENCES

1. American Football History. Available at: http://www.essortment.com/americanfootbal_rwff.htm. Accessed November 4, 2007.
2. Cahill BR. American football and the evolution of modern sports medicine. *J Orthop Surg.* 2003;11:107–109.
3. Rimel RW, Giordani B, Barth JT, et al. Disability caused by minor head injury. *Neurosurgery.* 1981;9:221–228.
4. Yarnell PR, Lynch S. Retrograde memory immediately after concussion. *Lancet.* 1970;1:863–864.
5. Macciocchi S, Barth JT, Alves W, et al. Neuropsychological functioning and recovery after mild head injury in collegiate athletes. *Neurosurgery.* 1996;39:510–514.
6. Matser EJ, Kessels AG, Lezak MD, et al. Neuropsychological impairment in amateur soccer players. *JAMA.* 1999;282:971–973.
7. Pellman, EJ, Powell JW, Viano, et al. Concussion in professional football: epidemiological features of game injuries and review of the literature—part 3. *Neurosurgery.* 2004;54:81–96.
8. McCrory PR, Johnston KM. Acute clinical symptoms of concussion. *Physician Sports Med.* 2002;30:43–47.
9. Kushner D. Concussion in sports: minimizing the risks of complications. *Am Fam Physician.* 2001;64:1007–1014.
10. Chen SH, Kareken DA, Fastenau PS, et al. A study of persistent post-concussion symptoms in mild head trauma using positron emission tomography. *J Neurol Neurosurg Psychiatry.* 2003;74:326–332.
11. Cantu RC. Neurologic athletic head and neck injuries. *Clin Sports Med.* 1998;17:37–44.
12. McMrory PR, Berkovic SF. Second impact syndrome. *Neurology.* 1998;50:677–683.
13. McCrory P. Does second impact syndrome exist? *Clin J Sports Med.* 2001;11:144–149.
14. Malanga GA, Kim D. Cervical spine sprain/strain injuries. *eMedicine* 2005. Available at: http://www.emedicine.com/sports/TOPIC24.HTM. Accessed November 4, 2007.
15. Sallis RE, Jones K, Knopp W. Burners: offensive strategy for an underreported injury. *Phys Sportsmed.* 1992;20:47–55.
16. Clancy WG Jr, Brand RL, Bergfeld JA. Upper trunk brachial plexus injury in contact sports. *Am J Sports Med.* 1975;5:209–216.
17. Nissen S, Laskowski E, Rizzo T Jr. Burner syndrome: recognition and rehabilitation. *Phys Sportsmed.* 1996;24:57–64.
18. Gorden JA, Straub SJ, Swanik CB, et al. Effects of football collars on cervical hyperextension and lateral flexion. *J Athl Train.* 2003;38:209–215.
19. Cantu RC, Mueller FO. Catastrophic spine injuries in football (1977–1989). *J Spinal Disord.* 1990;3:227–231.
20. Torg JS: *Athletic Injuries to the Head, Neck, and Face.* 2nd ed. St. Louis: Mosby-Year Book; 1991.
21. Torg JS, Quedenfeld TC, Burstein A. National football head and neck injury registry: report on cervical quadriplegia, 1971 to 1975. *Am J Sports Med.* 1979;7:127–132.
22. Heck JF, Clarke KS, Peterson TR, et al. National Athletic Trainers' Association position statement: head-down contact and spearing in tackle football. *J Athl Train.* 2004;39:101–111.
23. Lawrence DS, Stewart GW, Christy DM. High school football-related cervical spinal cord injuries in Louisiana: the athlete's perspective. Available at: http://www.injuryprevention.org/states/la/football/football.htm. Accessed July 15, 2007.
24. Torg, JS, Pavlov H, Genuario, SE. Neurapraxia of the cervical spinal cord with transient quadriplegia. *J Bone Joint Surg.* 1986;68:1354–1370.
25. Torg JS, Ramsey-Emrhein JA. Suggested management guidelines for participation in collision activities with congenital, developmental, or postinjury lesions involving the cervical spine. *Med Sci Sports Exerc.* 1997;29:256–272.
26. Kaplan LD, Flanigan DC, Norwig J, et al. Prevalence and variance of shoulder injuries in elite collegiate football players. *Am J Sports Med.* 2005;33:1142–1146.
27. Kelly BT, Barnes RP, Powell JW, et al. Shoulder injuries to quarterbacks in the National Football League. *Am J Sports Med.* 2004;32:328–331.
28. Foulk DA, Darmelio MP, Rettig AC, et al. Full-thickness rotator-cuff tears in professional football players. *Am J Orthop.* 2002;31: 622–624.
29. Kenter K, Behr CT, Warren RF. Acute elbow injuries in the National Football League. *J Shoulder Elbow Surg.* 2000;9:1–5.

30. Bendre AA, Hartigan BJ, Kalainov DM. Mallet finger. *J Am Acad Orthop Surg*. 2005;13:336–344.

31. Heim D. The skier's thumb. *Acta Orthopaedica Belgica*. 1999;65:440–446.

32. Boyd KT, Peirce NS, Batt ME. Common hip injuries in sport. *Sports Med*. 1997;24:273–288.

33. Anderson K, Strickland S, Warren R. Hip and groin injuries in athletes. *Am J Sports Med*. 2001;29:521–533.

34. Arnheim DD, Prentice WE. *Principles of Athletic Training*. 9th ed. Madison, WI: Brown & Benchmark; 1997.

35. Malanga GA, Nadler SF, Bowen JE, et al. Sports Medicine. In: Delisa JA, ed. *Physical Medicine and Rehabilitation: Principles and Practice*. 4th ed. Philadelphia: Lippincott Williams & Wilkins; 2005:557–575.

36. Scopp JM, Moorman CT III. Acute athletic trauma to the hip and pelvis. *Orthop Clin North Am*. 2002;33:555–563.

37. Magee DJ. *Orthopedic Physical Assessment*. 4th ed. Philadelphia: Saunders; 2002.

38. Baker BE, Peckham AC, Pupparo F, et al. Review of meniscal injury and associated sports. *Am J Sports Med*. 1985;13:1–4.

39. Greene WB, ed. *Essentials of Musculoskeletal Care*. Rosemont, IL: American Academy of Orthopaedic Surgeons; 2001.

40. Drake DF, Nadler SF, Chou LH. Sports and performing arts medicine. 4. Traumatic injuries in sports. *Arch Phys Med Rehabil*. 2004;85:S67–S71.

41. O'Donoghue DH. Surgical treatment of fresh injuries to the major ligaments of the knee. *J Bone Joint Surg*. 1950; 32:721.

42. Ha TP, Li KCP, Beaulieu CF, et al. Anterior cruciate ligament injury: fast spin-echo MR imaging with arthroscopic correlation in 217 examinations. *Am J Roentgenol*. 1998; 170:1215–1219.

43. Swirtun LR, Jansson A, Renstrom P. The effects of a functional knee brace during early treatment of patients with a nonoperated acute anterior cruciate ligament tear. *Clin J Sport Med*. 2005;15:299–304.

44. Fujimoto E, Sumen Y, Ikuta Y. Spontaneous healing of acute anterior cruciate ligament (ACL) injuries: conservative treatment using an extension block soft brace without anterior stabilization. *Arch Orthop Trauma Surg*. 2002;122: 212–216.

45. Malanga GA, Giradi J, Nadler SF. The spontaneous healing of a torn anterior cruciate ligament. *Clin J Sport Med*. 2001;11:118–120.

46. Fithian DC, Paxton EW, Stone ML. Prospective trial of a treatment algorithm for the management of the anterior cruciate ligament-injured knee. *Am J Sports Med*. 2005;33: 335–346.

47. Fleming BC, Oksendahl H, Beynnon BD. Open- or closed-kinetic chain exercises after anterior cruciate ligament reconstruction? *Exerc Sport Sci Rev*. 2005;33:134–140.

48. Corea JR, Moussa M, al Othman A. McMurray's test tested. *Knee Surg Sports Traumatol Arthrosc*. 1994;2:70–72.

49. Ellen MI, Young JL, Sarni JL. Musculoskeletal rehabilitation and sports medicine. 3. Knee and lower extremity injuries. *Arch Phys Med Rehabil*. 1999;80:S59–S67.

50. Fu FH, Baratz M. Meniscal injuries. In: Delee JC, Drez D Jr, eds. *Orthopaedic Sports Medicine*. Philadelphia: Saunders; 1994:1146–1248.

51. Renstrom PA, Kannus P. Injuries of the foot and ankle. In: Delee JC, Drez D Jr, eds. *Orthopedic Sports Medicine*. Philadelphia: Saunders; 1994:1705–1767.

52. Buschbacher R. The use and abuse of ankle supports in sports injuries. *J Back Musculoskeletal Rehabil*. 1993;3:57–68.

53. Kannus P, Renstrom P. Treatment for acute tears of the lateral ligaments of the ankle. *J Bone Joint Surg Am*. 1991;73: 305–312.

54. Osborne MD, Rizzo TD Jr. Prevention and treatment of ankle sprain in athletes. *Sports Med*. 2003;33:1145–1150.

55. Verhagen E, van der Beek A, Twisk J. The effect of a proprioceptive balance board training program for the prevention of ankle sprains: a prospective controlled trial. *Am J Sports Med*. 2004;32:1385–1393.

56. Konradsen L, Holmer P, Sondergaard L. Early mobilizing treatment for grade III ankle ligament injuries. *Foot Ankle*. 1991;12:69–73.

57. Harper MC, Keller TS. A radiographic evaluation of the tibiofibular syndesmosis. *Foot Ankle*. 1989;10:156–160.

CHAPTER 14

Elizabeth A. Grossart and Johnny G. Owens

Soccer Injuries

Concerning football [soccer] playing, I protest to you it may rather be called a friendly kind of fighting, rather than recreation.

—Author Unknown

Soccer, known as football in most of the world, has roots in the Far East as well as Europe. Once played as a form of military training for Roman soldiers, previous versions of the game were brutal contests with few rules and unlimited players contending for the ball across entire villages. Injuries from these violent, disorganized competitions were undoubtedly unpredictable and severe, which led to laws banning soccer in many European cities. This changed in 1863 when the Football Association of England was established to define the sport and set basic rules that forbade tripping of opponents and carrying the ball.

Modern soccer remains a contact sport in which 11 players (10 field players and 1 goalkeeper) on each side attempt to direct the ball into the opponent's goal using any part of the body excluding the arms and hands. Soccer has tremendous global appeal, attracting players of all national, cultural, religious, and socioeconomic backgrounds. Participation continues to increase in the United States, with approximately 18 million people playing organized soccer. Worldwide, soccer participation is estimated at over 240 million. The Fédération Internationale de Football Association (FIFA) serves as the international governing body of soccer, as well as its sister sports, futsal and beach soccer.[1]

Because of its wide appeal, soccer players vary widely in age, size, fitness, and ability level. However, all soccer athletes are susceptible to some common injuries. Effective, sport-specific injury prevention and rehabilitation interventions are critical because of the physical demands of soccer; the average adult player covers 10 km during a 90-minute game, running approximately 75% the time.[2] Our goal is to discuss soccer equipment and skills, epidemiology of soccer injuries, factors that may contribute to injury, some common soccer injuries (from the foot up), and their evaluation, treatment, and soccer-specific rehabilitation, and finally, equipment and exercise programs designed to prevent soccer injuries.

EQUIPMENT AND SKILLS

Equipment

Shoes

The first soccer boots were constructed with a high ankle support, similar to basketball shoes. However, as the game evolved, external ankle stability was sacrificed for increased foot and ankle motion. Modern boots typically have a flexible upper support composed of leather or synthetic leather and a thin but rigid outsole to which molded studs are attached. Shoes specific for indoor or turf use small short studs or a court-type outsole. Cushion and arch support are minimal owing to the absence of a midsole in most boots. The soccer boot's ergonomic function is described as protecting the foot and enabling it to perform necessary motions in the context of the game.[3]

Shin Guards

Shin guards are worn over the anterior surface of the tibia and are the only protective padding routinely worn by soccer players. In theory, shin guards act to dissipate impact over a larger surface area and may reduce soft-tissue injury. An analysis of tibia and fibula fractures in soccer players, in which 90% of players were wearing shin guards when they sustained fractures, suggested that while shin guards protect the shank from minor injuries to skin and soft tissue, they are not likely to be preventive beyond a certain critical force.[4]

Ball

The soccer ball is characterized by its mass, diameter, internal pressure, surface texture, and composition. Modern soccer balls are constructed of an outer layer of synthetic panels stitched together over a rubber bladder. Balls are available in various sizes. Although size 5 (circumference 27–28 in, weight 14–16 oz, pressure 8.5–15.6 pounds per square inch [psi] at sea level) is used in regulation play by adults and adolescents >14 years of age; size 4 (circumference 25–26 in, weight 12–13 oz); and size 3 (circumference 23–24 in, weight 11–12 oz) balls may be more appropriate for children, especially for decreasing the risk of head and neck injury.[5]

Goal Posts

FIFA mandates that goal posts and crossbars must be made of wood, metal, or other approved material and be square, rectangular, round, half-round, or elliptical in shape. The width and depth of the crossbar must not exceed 5 inches (12 cm). The common dimensions of a full-size goal are approximately 24 feet in width by 8 feet in height and 6 feet in depth.[6] Collisions with goal posts and falling goal posts have been associated with severe injuries, including death. Padded goal posts have been proposed as a means to prevent such injuries. A study of force characteristics of padded goal posts and injuries resulting from player/padded goal post collisions showed that no injuries resulted from the collisions during a 3-year period. A survey of players and coaches revealed that neither felt that padded goal posts negatively impacted game play.[7]

Surface

Soccer can be played on natural or artificial turf surfaces. The quality of natural turf is affected by grass species, weather conditions, and wear, making it theoretically less desirable. Artificial surfaces have greater peak decelerations for high-energy impacts; this suggests an increased likelihood of injury from falls.[3] Formal studies of indoor (artificial turf) versus outdoor (natural turf) soccer injuries reveal similar rates of injury on both surfaces.[8] FIFA rules specify that competitive international matches be played on natural turf.

Skills

A variety of physical skills are necessary for participation in soccer. Of the most commonly used skills (passing, trapping [receiving and controlling the ball], tackling [challenging the opponent to steal the ball], jumping, running, sprinting, starting and stopping, changing direction, and falling), kicking has been the subject of the most biomechanical studies. The basic kick in soccer involves an approach of one or more strides followed by contact with the ball at the instep, while the opposite foot remains planted to the side and slightly behind the ball. The kick is initiated by bringing the kicking leg backward with the knee flexed. The thigh of the kicking leg is subsequently brought forward by pelvic rotation around the supporting leg. Knee flexion initially increases and then extends vigorously as the thigh decelerates to near-stationary upon contact with the ball. During follow-through, the hip and knee flex, and the foot may reach above the level of the hip. Optimal approach angle is 30 to 45 degrees. Plant foot placement in elite players has been noted to be 38 cm behind the ball center and 37 cm to the side of the ball center. Players generate higher ball speeds using a five- to eight-stride approach than kicking from a stationary position. Passing involves striking the ball with the medial aspect of the foot, which allows more accurate placement of the ball.[3] Punting and drop-kicking are skills used by goalkeepers and are not discussed here.

The throw-in is utilized to restart the game after the ball has been played out-of-bounds across one of the sidelines. It is the only time the hands can be used by a field player, and thus is impacted by injuries to the upper extremities. A throw-in can be performed from the standing or running positions as long as both feet are in contact with the ground when the ball is released. A run-up approach allows the thrower to achieve a greater distance. In this technique, the legs and abdominal musculature are involved, in addition to the shoulders, arms, and hands.[3]

"Heading," or using the forehead to direct the ball, is a skill unique to soccer. When executed with the proper technique, there is little risk of injury. The head should contact the ball at or just below the hairline. At contact, the neck musculature is isometrically contracted and the trunk is flexed forward to provide a counterforce; thus the upper body, neck, and head become a single unit whose mass is relatively larger than the ball or the head alone.[9] Specific heading techniques that can be instructed by coaches include centering the ball on the forehead, correct timing, and strengthening of neck muscles.[8]

EPIDEMIOLOGY

Sports injury research is often hampered by differences in methodology that prevent comparing or combining incidences. However, a recent review of soccer injuries and their prevention estimates that elite male players sustain at least one performance-limiting injury annually.[10] Limited data are available on the incidence of injuries in elite female players, although an increased frequency of anterior cruciate ligament (ACL) injuries in women has been established.[11,12] Injuries occur during match play at a rate of four to six times greater than during practice sessions.[10] Traumatic (acute) injuries (80%) outnumber overuse (chronic) injuries (20%). Many acute injuries are reaggravations of previous injuries.[13] Most injuries sustained are minor injuries such as contusions, sprains, and strains to the lower legs and thighs.[10] Injury patterns in children vary by age, with upper extremity injuries and fractures being relatively more common in the 5- to 9-year-old age group.[14] Physical contact with another player or the ground is the most common mechanism resulting in injury.[15] However, more severe injures, including ACL tears, often occur in noncontact settings. Types of injuries appear to be similar in indoor and outdoor soccer.[16]

Few studies have been conducted with the aim of identifying specific risk factors for injury. In youth soccer, a previous history of injury increases the risk of subsequent injury.[17] In elite male players, a previous injury and increasing age have been identified as risk factors.[18] Among elite female players, defenders (usually players in the fullback position, defending the goal) and strikers (forward players whose role is to score) have a higher risk of injury than midfielders and goalkeepers; more injuries occur to the dominant leg, and the risk of sustaining an ACL injury is higher in players who have had a previous ACL injury.[19] Likewise, previously sprained ankles have significantly higher risk of reinjury of the same type.[20] Muscle tightness and poor flexibility are likely risk factors for thigh muscle strains and tendonitis in soccer players.[21] Muscle imbalance, particularly alteration in the quadriceps to hamstring strength ratio,

also is a probable risk factor for hamstring strain.[22] Other important risk factors for soccer injuries are low skill level and foul play.[13]

ANKLE INJURIES

Ankle sprains are extremely common among both elite and amateur soccer players, accounting for 20% of injuries to male players and 21% of injuries sustained by female players. This can be attributed to the close proximity of the foot and ankle to the ball, as most foot and ankle injuries are the result of contact between players during tackling.[23] Ankle sprains are more likely to occur when the injured ankle is weight-bearing and neutral or pronated in the sagittal plane; foot and ankle injuries have been associated with foul play as well as tackles from the side.[24]

Sprains involving the lateral ligaments, principally the anterior talofibular ligament (ATFL), are far more common than syndesmosis or medial ligament sprains in soccer, as in other sports involving cutting and jumping.[25,26] The mechanism of injury in lateral ligament sprain is inversion, usually while the ankle is plantar flexed. Examination reveals edema and/or ecchymosis over the lateral ankle and foot, with tenderness to palpation over the ATFL and occasionally the calcaneofibular ligament. Imaging is usually unnecessary unless there is exquisite bony tenderness or crepitus.

Initial treatment of the soccer athlete's ankle sprain includes nonsteroidal anti-inflammatory drugs (NSAIDs), rest/protected weight-bearing, ice, and compression with the goal of reducing pain and inflammation at the injury site. During this period, the athlete can engage in core stabilization exercises. Side planks, prone planks, and bridging are effective ways to strengthen the core with minimal stress to the injured ankle (Figs. 14-1 and 14-2). Initial rehabilitation includes passive and gentle active range of motion, with an emphasis on dorsiflexion. Because the anterior talus is wider than the posterior talus, the ankle gains stability in dorsiflexion with less stress than the anterior talofibular ligament, which is lax in this position.[27] Full, stable dorsiflexion is also critical for passing and tackling. Strengthening of the ankle evertors provides optimum support to the plantar-flexed, inverted ankle during ball strike.[28]

Once the athlete is able to bear weight on the injured side without pain, functional rehabilitation and proprioceptive training should take precedence

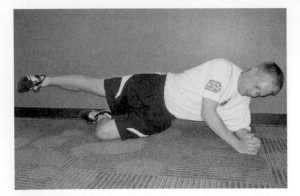

FIGURE 14-1 "Side planks" allow the athlete to strengthen the core musculature with minimal stress to the injured ankle.

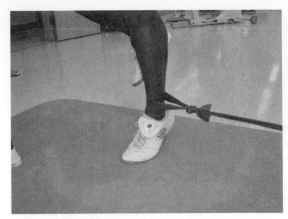

FIGURE 14-3 Functional rehabilitation of the ankle. Strengthening and proprioceptive work are introduced after the athlete can bear weight without pain.

(Figs. 14-3 to 14-5). A soccer-specific functional progression might consist of running, jumping, and kicking exercises. There is no consensus on the best criteria for return to play. In the authors' clinic, the athlete may return to play once he or she passes a unilateral jump test with a side-to-side difference <15% and is able to cut, land, and tackle without pain or instability. Prescription of an ankle stirrup orthosis (Fig. 14-6) may be warranted during initial return to play and for prevention of reinjury. Players should be permitted to participate only in training sessions on level surfaces at first. Functional testing for return to play is optimally conducted at the conclusion of a training session, as fatigue is a factor in ankle sprains.[29]

Potential complications of improper or incomplete rehabilitation include recurrent sprain, chronic instability, impingement ("footballer's ankle"), and arthritis.

KNEE INJURIES

Anterior Cruciate Ligament Injuries

Perhaps the most devastating injury for both amateur and elite soccer players is traumatic rupture of the anterior cruciate ligament (ACL). The ACL is the primary restraint to anterior displacement of the tibia relative to the femur and also acts to restrain internal–external rotation.[30] While ACL injuries occur in soccer

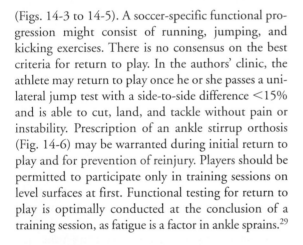

FIGURE 14-2 "Prone planks" allow core strengthening without stressing the ankle.

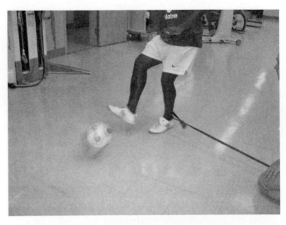

FIGURE 14-4 Advanced ankle rehabilitation. Soccer skills are incorporated into the rehabilitation program.

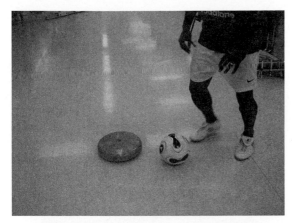

FIGURE 14-5 Ankle rehabilitation. Stepovers onto unstable surfaces are one component of an advanced rehabilitation program.

players of both genders, epidemiologic studies indicate that they are two to five times more common in female players.[12,31] Risk factors for ACL injuries in women include greater anteroposterior knee joint laxity, a smaller intracondylar notch and ligament, and possibly decreased proprioception compared to men. Other factors that contribute to ACL injuries in soccer players are abnormal quadriceps and hamstring interactions, altered neuromuscular control, shoe to surface interface, playing surface, and the athlete's

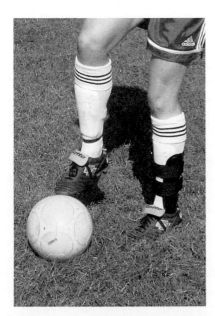

FIGURE 14-6 An ankle stirrup orthosis is shown on the left ankle.

playing style. It has been suggested that the extensor mechanism may play a role in ACL injuries, pulling the tibia anteriorly during a strong closed-chain eccentric contraction of the quadriceps, as may occur during a deceleration or changing direction.[32] Position played does not seem to impact the incidence of ACL tears, although some studies suggest that strikers and defenders are more likely to sustain injuries than midfielders and goalkeepers.[19]

The majority of ACL injuries occur to the dominant leg during noncontact incidents. The mechanisms of injury have not been elucidated, but common elements are sudden deceleration, abrupt change in direction, and a fixed foot. At the time of injury, the knee is often near full extension with the tibia internally rotated relative to the body. The athlete may report a popping sound at the time of injury. Most patients are unable to resume playing.[32] Massive effusion secondary to hemarthrosis ensues within hours of the injury. NSAIDs, ice, compression, elevation, and protected weight-bearing until the gait normalizes are components of initial management. Radiographs are particularly useful in adolescents, in whom it is important to exclude avulsion fracture. The diagnosis is usually established clinically via the Lachman test, which demonstrates increased tibial translation =5 mm compared to the contralateral side when positive. The pivot shift test will elicit a posterolateral shift of the tibia as the knee is gradually flexed with a valgus stress.[33] Magnetic resonance imaging (MRI) is utilized to evaluate for concomitant meniscal and chondral injuries as well as bone bruising prior to surgical reconstruction of the ACL. Surgical intervention is necessary for most soccer players who wish to return to playing soccer or an active lifestyle.[30]

Postoperative ACL Rehabilitation

Optimal postoperative rehabilitation varies by surgeon and technique. It appears that early range of motion and early weight-bearing help to decrease morbidity associated with immobilization and anterior knee joint pain (associated with harvest of the middle one-third of the patellar tendon). Early motion has not been associated with increased joint laxity at follow-up.[34] The two most common types of reconstruction—bone-patellar tendon-bone graft and multistrand hamstring graft—both have advantages and disadvantages. Patellar tendon grafts are associated with increased anterior knee pain and crepitus and decreased knee extension strength compared with the noninjured side. Hamstring grafts are sometimes associated with prolonged weakness of the knee flexors.[30] Rehabilitative and functional knee orthoses do not alter long-term outcomes or risk of reinjury.[35]

Soccer-specific rehabilitation after ACL reconstruction must consider cutting, turning, running, and landing in addition to dribbling, passing, and kicking the ball. Cutting tasks need to be rehabilitated in positions that protect the healing graft, and then advanced to more soccer-specific positions. Foot strike for cutting maneuvers typically occurs at 22 degrees of knee flexion, which is an anatomically vulnerable position for the ACL.[36] Also, the low angle of knee flexion decreases the mechanical advantage of the hamstrings and can result in decreased stabilization due to hamstring activity. Precutting exercises should work to establish cocontraction of the quadriceps and hamstrings at differing knee flexion angles. As good control is established, deeper knee flexion angles are started for dynamic activities with emphasis on control and maintenance of form. Valgus moments at the knee are also a concern. Female players in particular are at risk for reinjury secondary to increased adductor moments, smaller peak knee flexor moments, and increased quadriceps activity during deceleration and cutting tasks.[37] Athletes should incorporate jump training with emphasis on decreasing valgus posture and increasing knee flexion upon landing to decrease strain on the ACL and recruit the hamstrings, respectively.[38,39] The athlete can be trained initially in proper landing techniques, and then advanced from double- to single-leg jumping tasks.

Kicking, passing, and dribbling should also be incorporated into the rehabilitation program. Knee extensors and hip flexors are agonists in the kicking leg and are optimally trained concentrically (Figs. 14-7

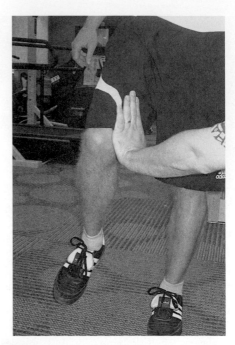

FIGURE 14-8 Dynamic knee-strengthening exercises, with resistance.

and 14-8).[40] Stretch-shortening activities (plyometrics) such as bounding and squat jumps can facilitate this. Likewise, the hamstrings and gluteus maximus act eccentrically throughout the majority of the kicking motion and should be strengthened accordingly. The Russian hamstring exercise (Fig. 14-9) is a useful eccentric exercise for the posterior thigh.

The angle of approach to kick the ball must also be considered. Angles between 45 and 60 degrees allow the player to take advantage of significant translational and rotational forces from the plant leg.[40] Adequate hip abduction and core strength help to stabilize the support leg at increasing angles of kicking.[41] If the plant leg is the leg being rehabilitated, then an interval kicking program is used to moderate increasing stresses to the leg. The program we use starts with the least stress on the plant leg and slowly increases the stress as the player demonstrates mastery of each phase. The first phase is a straight approach pass. The next phase is an instep kick using a straight approach. During this phase, the player is taught to quickly transfer forces from the plant leg through the kicking leg by quickly coming off of the plant leg at ball strike and landing on the kick leg after the follow-through. This decreases stress on the plant leg and increases

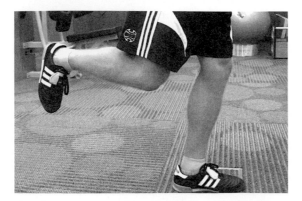

FIGURE 14-7 Dynamic knee-strengthening exercises.

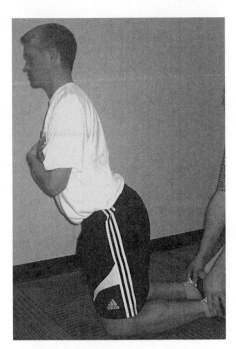

FIGURE 14-9 The Russian hamstring exercise.

power through the ball.[40] The next phase incorporates increasing the angle of approach to the ball with passing. Last, an angled approach with an instep kick is practiced, again with the player landing on the shooting leg after the follow-through.

Return to play is allowed once the athlete passes functional jump tests and demonstrates proficiency in passing, dribbling, shooting, and cutting tasks. Isokinetic testing can aid in assessing for deficits of the injured side versus the contralateral side in hamstring-to-quadriceps ratio and adequate peak torque to body weight. Return-to-play testing is ideally performed at the completion of a therapy or training session, as fatigue is a known risk factor for noncontact ACL injury.[42]

Other Knee Injuries

Soccer players are also susceptible to other, less serious knee injuries. Frequent starting and stopping, cutting, and jumping predispose athletes to anterior knee pain from patellar tendonitis. This typically responds to ice massage, rest, and NSAIDs. Iliotibial band syndrome can also temporarily sideline soccer players. No sport-specific intervention is required for these minor knee pain syndromes.

THIGH INJURIES

Because of the roles of the hamstrings and quadriceps in the movements of soccer, the thigh is susceptible to strains and contusions. Injuries to the thigh account for 25% of soccer-related injuries.[43] Muscle strains in the first few minutes of the game are usually secondary to inadequate warm-up and stretching. Those occurring in the latter half of the game are usually secondary to fatigue.[22] Hamstring strains are particularly common in soccer athletes and can be recurrent, with reinjury rates ranging from 12% to 30%.[44] The musculotendinous junction of the hamstring is strained during an eccentric contraction as the athlete attempts to accelerate, decelerate, or stretch for the ball.[45] He or she may report a pop or tearing sensation along with acute pain. Edema and ecchymosis are uncommon but may be present in the distal posterior thigh. Avulsion of the proximal hamstring insertion is rare in soccer but requires surgical consultation. The rehabilitation of uncomplicated hamstring strains should address recovery as well as the risk factors associated with hamstring injuries. Eccentric training for the hamstrings and hip extensors is emphasized in the sport-specific phase of recovery. The quadriceps can also be strained in soccer, most commonly as the result of a blocked kick or tackle. A direct blow from a collision or misplaced kick can lead to myositis ossificans or calcification of contused or damaged muscle tissue.[45] Muscle contusions resolve quickly and do not usually require additional treatment beyond icing, compression, and possibly padding for future competitions.[22]

HIP, GROIN, AND PELVIS INJURIES

Injuries to the hip and pelvis are particularly common in soccer. In contrast to other sports where the incidence of hip/pelvis injuries is 5% to 6%, such injuries may account for up to 13% of soccer injuries.[46] Adductor strain is likely to occur in sports that involve kicking or pivoting actions, especially with the hip externally rotated as in trapping or passing a soccer ball or engaging in a tackle that results in forced abduction. The adductor longus is frequently injured near the musculotendinous junction; the insertion site is relatively small with poor regional blood supply, which may contribute to injury of this muscle. The athlete with an acute injury and a history consistent with adductor strain should be managed with rest, ice, compression, protected weight-bearing, and NSAIDs, as indicated. Because most adductor strains are incomplete injuries, nonoperative treatment is warranted. Initial rehabilitation involves gentle passive and active assisted motion within limits of pain. Transverse friction massage at the pubic tubercle is occasionally helpful. Once range of motion (ROM) is pain free, the athlete can begin isometric strengthening, progressing to isokinetic strengthening, while gradually increasing weight. Proprioception and agility training followed by introduction of soccer-specific movements can begin once the athlete has reached 70% of normal strength and has pain-free ROM. In particular, a dual focus on flexibility and stabilization for landing and cutting, as well as concentric strengthening for kicking, may benefit the soccer athlete.[47] If rehabilitation is inadequate or incomplete, the athlete may go on to experience chronic groin pain.[48]

Chronic Groin Pain

Osteitis Pubis

Recurrent or chronic groin pain in soccer players has most commonly been attributed to osteitis pubis, but the differential diagnosis includes several other conditions, including abdominal and urologic diseases and other musculoskeletal problems, such as acetabular labral tears and other intra-articular hip pathology.[49,50] Athletes with osteitis pubis usually complain of gradual onset of unilateral groin pain that is worse with soccer activity or running. Physical exam reveals tenderness to palpation over the pubic symphysis. Plain radiographs may show symmetric bone resorbtion, widening of the symphysis pubis, or sclerosis along the pubic rami.[48] Nuclear medicine bone scan (technetium[99] scintigraphy) may assist with the diagnosis; increased uptake at the pubic symphysis on delayed views suggests osteitis pubis, while increased uptake at the pubic tubercle suggests adductor insertion strain.[51] The pain has been attributed to abnormally increased motion at the symphysis pubis, and rest from activities that produce pain is the recommended treatment. Injection may hasten resolution of symptoms and enhance participation in rehabilitation, including hip ROM, adductor stretching, and strengthening.[48] A recent study comparing magnetic resonance imaging of soccer players with chronic symphysis pain revealed microtears of the adductor enthesis in 48% of subjects, isolated osteitis pubis in 9%, and a combination of both findings in 42%. The athletes with adductor microtears with or without osteitis pubis were treated with symphyseal injections of bupivicaine and corticosteroids with good

relief, which suggests that injection may be a reasonable approach in either diagnosis.[52]

Sports Hernia

Another possible cause of chronic groin pain in the soccer athlete is sports hernia. The etiology of pain and/or dysfunction in this entity, also called athletic hernia, athletic pubalgia, incipient hernia, and "Gilmore's groin," is somewhat controversial. However, the different terms generally describe a weakening or deficiency in the innermost portion of the inguinal canal (transversalis fascia) associated with chronic activity-related groin pain. Participation in kicking sports and sports that involve rapid changes are probable predisposing factors.[49] One possible cause of shearing and/or tears of the transversalis fascia is an imbalance between the hip adductors and the lower abdominal musculature.[53]

Athletes typically report insidious onset of dull groin pain, which they may initially attribute to repeated adductor strain. In 30% of cases, there is history of an acute injury such as a blocked kick resulting in sudden deceleration of the lower limb.[51,54] Pain is worse with athletic activity and may be particularly aggravated by sit-ups or resisted hip flexion.[55] Specific findings on physical exam (conducted by inserting the small finger through an inverted scrotum into the external inguinal canal) are tenderness and dilation of the superficial inguinal ring.[48] A bone scan or MRI may help to exclude femoral or pubic ramus stress fractures and intra-articular hip pathology. Injection of the pubic symphysis under fluoroscopy may also aid in the diagnosis. Herniography is diagnostic for sports hernia only 12% to 36% of the time.[49]

Because many soccer athletes with this diagnosis are unable to play due to pain and tend to have symptoms for several months before the diagnosis is made, they will likely have exhausted conservative treatments. Surgery is indicated in patients who fail to respond to rehabilitation.[51] Restoring the normal anatomy can be accomplished via the open technique and layered suture repair or laparoscopically with mesh. Bilateral repair is often necessary to achieve resolution of symptoms. After open repair, 90% of athletes return to play.[48] Early comparison studies indicate that the laparoscopic approach is similarly efficacious in reducing symptoms and will probably permit faster return to sport.[49,54] One recommended rehabilitation program for soccer athletes after open sports herniography is conducted over a 4-week period and concludes with return to play. During week 1, the athlete is instructed to walk four times per day. In week 2, the athlete begins straight-line jogging and adductor exercises. Running and progression of adductor strengthening occur in week 3. During week 4, the athlete may sprint, resume kicking, and return to competition.[51]

HEAD INJURIES

While the vast majority of severe injuries in soccer occur to the lower limbs, the risk for head injury is becoming more recognized in soccer players due to potential neurocognitive sequelae.[56] Because the head is intentionally used to advance or control the ball in soccer, there is concern over whether repeated head–ball contact over the course of a career can result in neuropsychological impairment. Head and facial injuries reportedly account for 4% to 20% of all soccer injuries.[57] The incidence of concussion in college soccer players over two seasons of play was found to be 59% in male players and 41% in female players; none of the concussions resulted from heading the ball.[58] Data collected from emergency departments over a 10-year period in the United States revealed approximately 28,000 severe head injuries (skull fracture, cerebral contusion, intracranial hemorrhage, subdural or epidural hematoma), which translated to 1 to 2 injuries per 10,000 players per year. Goalkeepers are particularly at risk for head injuries due to collisions with other players and potentially the goal posts.[59] The most likely sites of getting a head injury on the field are within the penalty area and at midfield, where players are challenging for balls in the air.[57]

Cognitive Effects

Studies of retired Norwegian soccer players, active Dutch professional soccer players, and amateur soccer players demonstrated abnormalities on neuropsychological testing that were surmised to have resulted from repetitive heading and chronic traumatic brain injury. Deficits noted were in domains of attention, concentration, memory, judgment, planning, and visuoperceptual tasks; these were significant when compared with a control group of swimmers and track athletes.[60–62] On the other hand, a study of active U.S. National Soccer Team players revealed no difference in MRI findings compared with track athletes; symptoms correlated with history of concussion.[63] Also, no acute neuropsychological effects were seen in college soccer athletes who were tested before and after a training

session involving heading and compared to controls who did no heading.[64] National Collegiate Athletic Association Division I soccer players, when compared to nonsoccer athletes and nonathletes, demonstrated no impairment in cognitive function or scholastic aptitude, nor was there a significant relationship between history of soccer-related concussion and neurocognitive performance.[65] Thus, controversy remains regarding the presence and origin of cognitive deficits in soccer athletes.

While neuropsychological impairment was initially attributed to cumulative subconcussive impacts sustained during purposeful heading, confounding factors like alcohol abuse, prior head injury, and existence of learning disabilities may have biased the results of those studies. Many authors suggest that neurocognitive deficits are more likely due to the cumulative effect of concussions sustained by soccer athletes during their careers. The odds of a male, high-level amateur soccer player sustaining at least one concussion during a 10-year career are estimated to be near 50%.[57] However, the definition and reporting of concussions have not been consistent and are subject to recall bias, as well as the notion that loss of consciousness is required for the diagnosis.[57] Formal studies demonstrate that forces occurring upon contact of the head with the ball are well below the tolerance thresholds established for head injuries identified in boxing.[57] More research is needed to determine whether a long-term risk of neurocognitive impairment exists for soccer players. Preventive headgear has been developed, but its efficacy is uncertain at this time (see below). There are no soccer-specific interventions for diagnosis, treatment, and rehabilitation of mild traumatic brain injury in soccer players. A concise, thorough discussion of the definition, evaluation, and management of concussion in athletes can be found in the American College of Sports Medicine Team Physician Consensus Statement.[66]

PREVENTION

Prevention of soccer-related injuries obviously promotes the success of high-level club and professional teams, to the financial gain of both players and team owners. At this level and less competitive levels, decreasing the number of injuries to the ankle, knee, and head may help to prevent disability later in life. Arthritis of the knee and ankle are known sequelae of trauma and instability in those joints, which may ensue from soccer injuries.[8] Neurocognitive impairment may also be mitigated with equipment or other preventive strategies.

Nonspecific Interventions

The first prevention studies evaluated multiple interventions and followed the incidence of all injuries in the study group. Interventions included correction of training, provision of shin guards and special winter-training shoes, prophylactic ankle taping in players with clinical instability or history of sprain, supervised rehabilitation, exclusion of players with gross knee instability, information about the importance of disciplined play and the increased risk of injury at training camps, and correction and supervision of team physicians and physical therapists. Over the 6-month follow-up period, those in the trained group sustained 75% fewer injuries than those in the control group.[68] A 7-week preseason conditioning program with emphasis on sport-specific cardiovascular conditioning, plyometrics, strength training, and flexibility resulted in a 14% incidence of injury in adolescent females versus 34% in the control group.[69] An educational intervention for coaches and male youth players decreased the incidence of injury by 21%, with mild, overuse, and training injuries reduced the most.[10]

Ankle

Specific interventions to reduce the risk of ankle sprain have also been studied. Proprioceptive training using ankle discs and use of a semirigid or air stirrup ankle orthosis (Fig. 14-6) are beneficial for secondary prevention of ankle sprains in high-risk sports such as soccer.[70–72]

Knee

Healthy female athletes can compensate for an inherently greater laxity by increasing recruitment of the lateral hamstring and increasing knee flexion to control anterior tibial translation forces at the knee produced when landing or changing direction on a single leg.[73] This biomechanical observation, as well as other neuromuscular control deficits, can be targeted during prevention and rehabilitation programs. Several studies have been conducted to evaluate neuromuscular coordination training's efficacy in preventing ACL injuries in female athletes. The evidence thus far suggests that structured proprioceptive and neuromuscular training

programs decrease severe knee injuries. Specifically, the Prevent Injury and Enhance Performance (PEP) program demonstrated an 88% and 74% decrease in the incidence of ACL injuries in two trained groups followed for 1 year, respectively.[38] Unsupervised balance board training did not change the incidence of traumatic injuries to the lower limb.[74]

Head

Based upon studies showing neuropsychiatric abnormalities in amateur and elite soccer players, several manufacturers have endeavored to develop protective headgear in order to diminish forces of acceleration experienced by the head during intentional contact with the ball. Concussions are frequently caused by rotational accelerations resulting in contracoup injuries—not the actual force of the impact. Padded headgear designed to decrease impact is not likely to reduce the prevalence of these types of concussions. Evaluation of four different types of soccer headgear demonstrated a decrease in peak acceleration at the highest ball speeds and pressures; however, there was no significant difference at lower speeds, suggesting that soccer headgear does not reduce the acceleration experienced during routine, intentional heading.[75] Three headbands were evaluated for their ability to attenuate peak force and impulse, and all were effective at reducing peak impact force for speeds at which a soccer ball is purposefully headed.[76] Mouth guards should be worn by soccer players to decrease the risk of oral and dental injuries; there is no definitive evidence that mouth guards are protective against concussions.

FIFA Medical and Research Centre—"The 11"

A prevention program, "The 11," was developed by FIFA's medical research center (F-MARC) and other international experts. "The 11" is a prevention program that comprises 10 evidence-based or best practice exercises and the promotion of fair play. The exercises focus on core stabilization, eccentric training of quadriceps and hamstrings, proprioceptive training, dynamic stabilization, and plyometrics with attention to proper technique. Because it can be completed in less than 15 minutes, "The 11" can be integrated into every training session following warm-up and stretching. An abbreviated version can be utilized prior to matches as part of warm-up. The benefits of the program include improved performance and also injury prevention.[77]

CONCLUSION

Soccer is a unique contact sport with worldwide popularity and growing participation in the United States. Various factors have been identified as contributing to the risk of injury in soccer. The vast majority of soccer injuries affect the lower limbs, necessitating a sport-specific approach to rehabilitation. Interventions and equipment designed to prevent injuries can play a key role in keeping players in the game and avoiding future disability.

REFERENCES

1. Classic football: the history of football. Available at: http://www.fifa.com/classicfootball/history/game/historygame1.html. Accessed April 13, 2007.
2. Kirkendall DT. Physiology of soccer. In: Garrett WE, Kirkendall DT, eds. *Exercise and Sport Science.* Philadelphia: Lippincott Williams & Wilkins; 2000:857–884.
3. Lees A, Nolan L. The biomechanics of soccer: a review. *J Sports Sci.* 1998;16:211–234.
4. Boden BP, Lohnes JH, Nunley JA, et al. Tibia and fibula fractures in soccer players. *Knee Surg Sports Traumatol Arthrosc.* 1999;7:262–266.
5. Queen RM, Weinhold PS, Kirkendall DT, et al. Theoretical study of the effect of ball properties on impact force in soccer heading. *Med Sci Sports Exerc.* 2003;35:2069–2076.
6. Consumer Product Safety Commission. Guidelines for movable soccer goal safety: CPSC document #326. Available at: http://www.cpsc.gov/cpscpub/pubs/326.html. Accessed April 15, 2007.
7. Janda DH, Bir C, Wild B, et al. Goal post injuries in soccer: a laboratory and field testing analysis of a preventive intervention. *Am J Sports Med.* 1995;23:340–344.
8. Giza E, Micheli LJ. Soccer injuries. In: Maffulli N, Caine DJ, eds. *Epidemiology of Pediatric Sports Injuries: Team Sports.* Basel: Karger; 2005:140–169.
9. Kirkendall DT, Jordan SE, Garrett WE. Heading and head injuries in soccer. *Sports Med.* 2001;31:369–386.
10. Junge A, Dvorak J. Soccer injuries: a review on incidence and prevention. *Sports Med.* 2004;34:929–938.
11. Arendt E, Dick R. Knee injury patterns among men and women in collegiate basketball and soccer: NCAA data and review of literature. *Am J Sports Med.* 1995;23:694–701.
12. Bjordal JM, Arnoy F, Hannestad G, et al. Epidemiology of anterior cruciate ligament injuries in soccer. *Am J Sports Med.* 1997;25:341–345.
13. Inklaar H. Soccer injuries II: aetiology and prevention. *Sports Med.* 1994;18:81–93.
14. Adams AL, Schiff MA. Childhood soccer injuries treated in U.S. emergency departments. *Acad Emerg Med.* 2006;13:571–574.
15. Neilson A, Yde J. Epidemiology and traumatology of injuries in soccer. *Am J Sports Med.* 1989;17:803–807.
16. Putukian M, Knowles WK, Swere S, et al. Injuries in indoor soccer: the Lake Place Dawn to Dark soccer tournament. *Am J Sports Med.* 1996;24:317–322.
17. Kucero KL, Marshall SW, Kirkendall DT, et al. Injury history and a risk factor for incident injury in youth soccer. *Br J Sports Med.* 2005;39:462–466.
18. Arnason A, Sigurdsson SB, Gudmundsson A, et al. Risk factors for injury in football. *Am J Sports Med.* 2004; 32(suppl): S5–S16.
19. Faude O, Junge A, Kindermann W, et al. Risk factors for injuries in elite female soccer players. *Br J Sports Med.* 2006;40:785–790.
20. Ekstrand J, Gillquist J. Soccer injuries and their mechanisms: a prospective study. *Med Sci Sports Exerc.* 1983;15:267–270.
21. Ekstrand J, Gillquist J. The avoidability of soccer injuries. *Int J Sports Med.* 1983;4:124–128.
22. Fried T, Lloyd GJ. An overview of common soccer injuries: management and prevention. *Sports Med.* 1992;14:269–275.
23. Wong P, Hong Y. Soccer injury in the lower extremities. *Br J Sports Med.* 2005;39:473–482.
24. Giza E, Fuller C, Junge A, et al. Mechanisms of foot and ankle injuries in soccer. *Am J Sports Med.* 2003;31: 550–554.
25. Lewin G. The incidence of injury in an English professional soccer club during one competitive season. *Physiotherapy.* 1989;75:601–605.
26. Woods C, Hawkins R, Hulse M, et al. The football association medical research programme: an audit of injuries in professional football: an analysis of ankle sprains. *Br J Sports Med.* 2003;37:233–238.
27. Casilla M. Ligament injuries of the foot and ankle. In: DeLee JC, Drez D, Miller MD, eds. *DeLee and Drez's Orthopaedic Sports Medicine: Principles and Practice.* 2nd ed. Philadelphia: Saunders/Elsevier; 2002.
28. Zoch C, Fialka-Moser V, Quittan M. Rehabilitation of ligamentous ankle injuries: a review of recent studies. *Br J Sports Med.* 2003;37:291–295.
29. Garrick JG. The epidemiology of foot and ankle injuries in sports. *Clin Podiatr Med Surg.* 1989;12:653–665.
30. Beynnon BD, Johnson RJ, Abate JA, et al. Treatment of anterior cruciate ligament injuries, part 1. *Am J Sports Med.* 2005;33:1579–1602.
31. Rozzi S, Lephart S, Gear W, et al. Knee joint laxity and neuromuscular characteristics of male and female soccer and basketball platers. *Am J Sports Med.* 1999;37:312–319.
32. Kirkendall DT, Garrett WE Jr. The anterior cruciate ligament enigma. *Clin Orthop Relat Res.* 2000;372:64–66.
33. Gerbino P, Nielson J. Knee injuries. In: Frontera WR, Herring SA, Micheli LJ, et al., eds. *Clinical Sports Medicine Medical Management and Rehabilitation.* Philadelphia: Saunders; 2007:421–439.
34. Beynnon BD, Johnson RJ, Abate JA, et al. Treatment of anterior cruciate ligament injuries, part 2. *Am J Sports Med.* 2005;33:1751–1767.
35. Wright RW, Fetzer GB. Bracing after ACL reconstruction: a systematic review. *Clin Orthop Relat Res.* 2007;455:162–168.
36. Scott C, Anthony F, Bing Y, et al. Electromyographic and kinematic analysis of cutting maneuvers. *Am J Sports Med.* 2000;28:234–240.

37. Sigward S, Powers C. The influence of gender on knee kinematics, kinetics and muscle activation patterns during side-step cutting. *Clin Biomech.* 2006;21:41–48.

38. Mandelbaum BR, Silvers HJ, Watanabe DS, et al. Effectiveness of a neuromuscular and proprioceptive training program in preventing anterior cruciate ligament injuries in female athletes: 2-year follow-up. *Am J Sports Med.* 2005;33:1003–1010.

39. Hewett T, Lindenfeld T, Riccobene J, et al. The effect of neuromuscular training on the incidence of knee injury in female athletes. *Am J Sports Med.* 1999;27:699–706.

40. Barfield W. Biomechanics of kicking. In: Garrett W, Kirkendall D, eds. *Exercise and Sport Science.* Philadelphia: Lippincott Williams & Wilkins; 2000:551–562.

41. Masuda K, Demura K, Yamanaka K. Relationship between muscle strength in various isokinetic movements and kick performance among soccer players. *J Sports Med Phys Fitness.* 2005;45:44–52.

42. Chappell J, Herman D, Knight B, et al. Effect of fatigue on knee kinetics and kinematics in stop-jump tasks. *Am J Sports Med.* 2005;37:1022–1029.

43. Hawkins RD, Hulse MA, Wilkinson C, et al. The association football medical research programme: an audit of injuries in professional football. *Br J Sports Med.* 2001;35: 43–47.

44. Woods C, Hawkins R, Maltby S, et al. The football association medical research programme: an audit of injuries in professional football. Analysis of hamstring injuries. *Br J Sports Med.* 2004;38:36–41.

45. Reilly T, Howe T, Hanchard N. Injury prevention and rehabilitation. In: Reilly T, Williams AM, eds. *Science and Soccer.* 2nd ed. London: Routledge; 2003:136–147.

46. Scopp JM, Moorman CT III. Acute athletic trauma to the hip and pelvis. *Orthop Clin North Am.* 2002;33:555–563.

47. Sizer P. The hip: physical therapy management utilizing current evidence. *Current Concepts of Orthopaedic Physical Therapy.* 2nd ed. (APTA independent study monograph.) 2006, p. 22.

48. Lynch SA, Renström P. Groin injuries in sport: treatment strategies. *Sports Med.* 1999;28:137–144.

49. Swan KG Jr, Wolcott M. The athletic hernia: a systematic review. *Clin Orthop Relat Res.* 2006;455:78–87.

50. Saw T, Villar R. Footballer's hip: a report of six cases. *J Bone Joint Surg Br.* 2004;86B:655–658.

51. Gilmore J. Groin pain in the soccer athlete: fact, fiction, and treatment. *Clin Sports Med.* 1998;17:787–793.

52. Cunningham PM, Brennan D, O'Connell M, et al. Patterns of bone and soft-tissue injury at the symphysis pubis in soccer players: observations at MRI. *AJR.* 2007;188: W291–W296.

53. Anderson K, Strickland SM, Warren R. Hip and groin injuries in athletes *Am J Sports Med.* 2001;29:521–533.

54. Ingoldby CJH. Laparoscopic and conventional repair of groin disruption in sportsmen. *Br J Surg.* 1997;84:213–215.

55. Myers WC, Foley DP, Garrett WE, et al. Management of severe lower abdominal or inguinal pain in high-performance athletes. *Am J Sports Med.* 2000;28:2–8.

56. Goga I, Gongal P. Severe soccer injuries in amateurs. *Br J Sports Med.* 2003;37:498–501.

57. Kirkendall DT, Jordan SE, Garrett WE. Heading and head injuries in soccer. *Sports Med.* 2001;31:369–386.

58. Boden B, Kirkendall D, Garrett W. Concussion incidence in elite college soccer players. *Am J Sports Med.* 1998; 26:238–241.

59. Al-Kashmiri A, Delaney J. Head and neck injuries in football (soccer). *Trauma.* 2006;8:189–195.

60. Tysvaer AT, Løchen EA. Soccer injuries to the brain: a neuropsychologic study of former soccer players. *Am J Sports Med.* 1991;19:56–60.

61. Matser JT, Kessels AGH, Jordan BD, et al. Chronic traumatic brain injury in professional soccer players. *Neurology.* 1998;51:791–796.

62. Matser E, Kessels A, Lezak M, et al. Neuropsychological impairment in amateur soccer players. *JAMA.* 1999;282: 971–973.

63. Jordan SE, Green GA, Galanty HL, et al. Acute and chronic brain injury in U.S. national team soccer players. *Am J Sports Med.* 1996;24:205–210.

64. Putukian M, Echemendia RJ, Mackin S. The acute neuropsychological effects of heading in soccer: a pilot study. *Clin J Sport Med.* 2000;10:104–109.

65. Guskiewicz KM, Marshall SW, Broglio SP, et al. No evidence of impaired neurocognitive performance in collegiate soccer players. *Am J Sports Med.* 2002;30:157–162.

66. American College of Sports Medicine. Concussion (mild traumatic brain injury) and the team physician: a consensus statement. *Med Sci Sports Exerc.* 2006;38:395–399.

67. Lohmander LS, Östenberg A, Englund M, et al. High prevalence of knee osteoarthritis, pain, and functional limitations in female soccer players twelve years after anterior cruciate ligament injury. *Arthritis Rheum.* 2004;50:3145–3152.

68. Ekstrand J, Gillquist J, Liljedahl SO. Prevention of soccer injuries: supervision by doctor and physiotherapist. *Am J Sports Med.* 1983;11:116–120.

69. Heidt RS, Sweeterman LM, Carlonas RL, et al. Avoidance of soccer injuries with preseason conditioning. *Am J Sports Med.* 2000;28:659–662.

70. Tropp H, Askling C, Gillquist J. Prevention of ankle sprains. *Am J Sports Med.* 1985;13:259–262.

71. Surve O, Schwellnus MP, Noakes T, et al. A fivefold reduction in the incidence of recurrent ankle sprains in soccer players using the sport-stirrup orthosis. *Am J Sports Med.* 1994;22:601–606.

72. Thacker SB, Stroup DF, Branche CM, et al. The prevention of ankle sprains in sports: a systematic review of the literature. *Am J Sports Med.* 1999;27:753–759.

73. Robinson P, White L. The biomechanics and imaging of soccer injuries. *Semin Musculoskel Radiol.* 2005;9:397–420.

74. Soderman K, Werner S, Pietila T, et al. Balance board training: prevention of traumatic injuries of the lower extremities in female soccer players? A prospective randomized intervention study. *Knee Surg Sports Traumatol Arthrosc.* 2000;8:356–363.

75. Naunheim RS, Ryden A, Standeven J, et al. Does soccer headgear attenuate the impact when heading a soccer ball? *Acad Emerg Med.* 2003;10:85–90.

76. Broglio SP, Ju Y, Broglio MD, et al. The efficacy of soccer headgear. *J Athl Train.* 2003;38:220–224.

77. Federation Internationale de Football Association (FIFA). "The 11": The Prevention Programme. Available at: http://www.fifa.com/aboutfifa/developing/medical/the11/index.html. Accessed May 13, 2007.

Running Injuries

R unning continues to be one of the most popular forms of aerobic exercise despite increasing trends and advancement in the development of stationary equipment (elliptical machines, low-impact treadmills, etc.) and aerobics classes. Nearly 30 million Americans participate in running on a regular basis.[1-4] Running appears to be an attractive form of exercise as it requires no equipment beyond footwear, can be done anywhere, is inexpensive, can be done alone, and requires a minimal amount of skill. However, errors of training, biomechanical flaws, and poor equipment selection can lead to musculoskeletal injury.[1,2,5-10] This chapter is intended to provide an overview for the clinical evaluation and rehabilitation of an athlete who has sustained a running injury.

PATHOGENESIS/EPIDEMIOLOGY

The overall incidence of running injuries has been reported to be approximately 37% to 56% per year.[11] The incidence of all running injuries per 1,000 hours of running ranges from 3.6 to 5.5 for recreational runners and from 2.5 to 5.8 for competitive athletes.[11] Nevertheless, certain factors seem to be rather consistently implicated in increasing the risk of injury. The factors contributing to the etiology of running injuries can be divided into extrinsic and intrinsic factors.

Extrinsic factors include training errors (which are most common), running terrain, running surfaces, and running shoes. Training errors that may make the runner more susceptible to injury are persistently sustained high-intensity training without rest periods, abrupt increases in intensity and mileage, repetitive hill training, and competitive training sessions (i.e., marathons or other long-distance events). Frequent

up- or downhill running also contributes to the development of injury. Downhill running causes increased knee flexion, net extensor moment, increased patellofemoral forces, and increased power absorption of the knee extensors. Patellofemoral pain and iliotibial band friction syndrome result from excessive downhill running. Uphill running results in Achilles tendinitis and plantar fasciitis. Frequent running on hard surfaces results in mechanical shock, with joint and tendon overload, increasing the susceptibility to injury.

Intrinsic factors are divided into basic, primary, and secondary categories. Basic factors include age, gender, growth, weight, and height. Primary factors consist of bone alignment, structural variation, muscle conditioning (strength, flexibility, neuromuscular coordination, and ligamentous laxity). Secondary (acquired) dysfunction includes mechanical factors, muscle asymmetry (imbalances, localized weakness, localized inflexibility), and previous recurrent injuries.

Most authors agree that training errors account for the majority of injuries,[1,2,7,8] and one study reported that less than 20% of injuries were related to identified anatomic problems.[7] Common errors include changing to a harder running surface,[1] abruptly increasing mileage by more than 10% per week,[1,6,8,12,13] a sudden increase in running intensity,[1,2] hill running,[6] running on crowded roads, inadequate rest, and previous injury.[14]

The most common site of injury is the knee,[1,2,15] which is estimated to account for 30% to 50% of all injuries.[1,2,16,17] Typical problems include patellofemoral tracking disorders[16,18,19] and hamstring strains.[20] The lower leg, ankle, and foot are also problematic areas. Plantar fasciitis may alter training programs severely.[6,21,22] Up to 50% of runners report having sprained an ankle at one time or another in their running careers.[2] Stress fractures have been reported as the cause of up to 10% of all injuries presenting to a running clinic.[23] Achilles tendinitis is one of the most frequently identified diagnoses for which running orthotics are prescribed.[5] The hip, pelvis, and back collectively, which make up close to 20% of all injuries,[1] are frequent sites of overuse injuries as well as muscular tightness and strength imbalance.

THE ACTION OF RUNNING

Management of the injured runner requires a basic understanding of the biomechanical events that occur during running. The gait cycle begins when one foot contacts the ground—the beginning of the stance phase—and ends when the same foot makes initial contact with the ground again. Stance phase ends when the foot is no longer in contact with the ground. Toe-off marks the beginning of swing phase of the gait cycle.[3] The transition from walking to running occurs when periods of double limb support during the stance phase of gait (both feet in contact with the ground at the same time) give way to two periods of double float at the beginning and the end of the swing phase of gait (i.e., neither foot is in contact with the ground). As speed increases, initial contact changes from being on the hindfoot to the forefoot (i.e., the change from running to sprinting).[3] Stance phase during walking occupies >50% of the

gait cycle. There are two periods of double-limb support; running toe-off occurs before 50% of the gait cycle is complete, and there are no periods with both feet in contact with the ground (Fig. 15-1). Sprinters virtually always exhibit a total forefoot strike pattern.

Runners typically strike the ground with their feet 800 to 2,000 times/mile. The ground reaction forces at the time of initial contact are usually two to four times body weight. Electromyograph (EMG) evaluation of muscle activity during running demonstrates that the muscles of the lower extremity are most active in anticipation and just following initial contact.[3] Both the rectus femoris and the quadriceps are important in preparing the limb for contact with the ground, for shock absorption, and for energy transfer between segments (from knee to the hip); they contract from late swing to the midstance phase of the gait cycle.[3]

Pelvic motion is minimized to conserve energy and to maximize efficiency. The pelvis tilts and the trunk leans forward in order to lower the body's center of mass and to produce a horizontal force that maximizes forward acceleration and propulsion.[3] The body's center of mass (position and acceleration) determines the magnitude and direction of the ground reaction force. Kinematics of the hip demonstrate maximum extension just before toe-off and maximum hip flexion during mid to terminal swing. With an increase in velocity, maximum hip flexion also increases, resulting in a longer step length. During running, the knee flexes to approximately 45 degrees

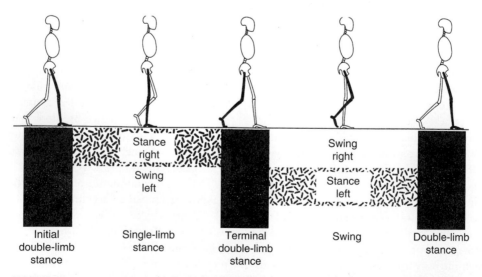

FIGURE 15-1 Normal gait cycle. (Reprinted from Perry J. *Gait Analysis: Normal and Pathological Function.* Thorofare, NJ: Slack; 1992: Fig. 1.2, p. 5. With permission.)

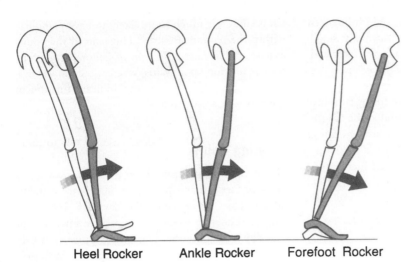

FIGURE 15-2 Three ankle rockers. (Reprinted from Perry J. *Gait Analysis: Normal and Pathological Function.* Thorofare, NJ: Slack; 1992: Fig. 3.19, p. 33. With permission.)

Heel Rocker   Ankle Rocker   Forefoot Rocker

during the absorption phase of stance, followed by approximately 25 degrees of knee extension during the propulsion phase.[3] Maximum knee flexion during the swing phase is approximately 90 degrees, with increasing knee flexion as running speed increases. During running, greater ankle dorsiflexion is required to allow initial heel contact. The ankle dorsiflexes as body weight is transferred to the stance leg in the absorption phase of running.[3]

Perry[24] described the biomechanics of the foot during gait with the three "ankle rockers" during stance phase (Fig. 15-2). The first rocker occurs during the loading response phase of the gait cycle; starting the gait cycle at heel strike (0%), the ankle joint undergoes rapid plantar flexion, which is at a maximum at 7% of the cycle, concluding with the foot flat on the floor (first rocker or initial double-limb support). Next, the ankle progressively dorsiflexes until roughly 40% of the gait cycle (second rocker or single-limb support), then plantar flexion starts, reaching maximum at toe-off or 60% of the gait cycle (third rocker or double-limb support). The second rocker occurs during the midstance phase of the gait cycle, and the third rocker occurs during the terminal stance phase of the gait cycle. During the third phase of the gait cycle the foot acts as a rigid lever for toe-off. Acting through the windlass mechanism, dorsiflexion of the toes helps to stabilize the plantar arch of the foot by shortening the plantar aponeurosis, which in turn results in elevation of the arch, passive inversion of the heel, and increased stability. This action also converts the normally flexible foot into a rigid lever which is used for push-off. When the foot is fixed to the ground, ankle dorsiflexion results in tibial internal

rotation and foot pronation (pronation/supination of the foot relative to the tibia occurs through the subtalar joint). The hindfoot is inverted during initial contact, which is followed by pronation as the limb is loaded during the absorption phase of stance. Pronation results in "unlocking" of the transverse tarsal joints, which increases the flexibility of the foot, allowing more effective shock absorption. Maximal pronation occurs at approximately 40% of the stance phase. With progression of stance the foot supinates, resulting in a "locked"/rigid transverse tarsal joint, providing a more effective lever arm for push-off.

The ankle and foot remain relatively supinated through the airborne phase, and forward swing of the leg and is mildly supinated when the foot is just about to strike the ground again.[1,8] Problems with the sequencing and control of ankle–foot motion can lead to foot/ankle pathology or affect any of the links in the biomechanical chain. For example, excessive pronation and midfoot collapse with sustained internal rotation of the tibia place an increased load on the medial aspect of the knee due to valgus stress.

Knee flexion at initial contact facilitates shock absorption when the foot impacts the ground. As the lower extremity progresses through the gait cycle, the center of gravity shifts from behind the knee (at initial contact) to in front of the knee, and thereby develops an extension moment. During midstance, the knee is flexed approximately 30 to 40 degrees and progresses to nearly full extension at toe-off. Rotation of the tibia at the knee is highly influenced by the amount of pronation (internal rotation of the tibia) or supination (external rotation of the tibia) at the subtalar joint. The femur rotates in the same direction as the tibia, and the femoral neck angle influences knee angle and foot position. The normally small amount of tibia varum at heel strike may be increased in runners (especially women) who cross over the midline of the body with the feet.[1,8,25]

The amount of energy expended during running is quite variable, and a runner's natural stride length typically produces the most economical running style.[26] An increase in stride length beyond the natural limit is accompanied by an observed increase in energy expenditure for a given running speed, thus reducing efficiency.[26]

THE RUNNER'S HISTORY

It is important for the clinician to perform a detailed and thorough history of the runner in order to accurately diagnose both the mechanism and type of injury. Analysis of the entire running program, including changes in mileage and training conditions, is essential. Several key aspects of the runner's history must be evaluated to accurately assess the athlete. These include chronology of injury, nature of the pain, age, running habits, equipment, terrain, previous injuries, review of symptoms, goals, and ability to cope with an injury.

Chronology of the Injury

How long has the runner had the pain, and when did the pain first appear? Was the onset of pain sudden or gradual? Unless a race is at stake or a major injury is involved, runners rarely show up at a physician's office when injury or symptoms first occur. They tend to seek help when running performance and/or their training regimens are threatened.

Nature of the Pain

Is the pain constant or intermittent? What makes it more tolerable, and what exacerbates it? Is the pain associated with weight-bearing, and how soon does it appear after beginning activity? Is the pain associated with inflammation?

Age Considerations

The differential diagnosis of distal Achilles tendon pain in the skeletally immature runner must include calcaneal apophysitis (Sever disease), whereas the adult runner is much more likely to have pathology within the tendon itself.[27,28] Hip pain in the young athlete should raise suspicion of femoral stress fracture or traction apophysitis, whereas the same symptoms in the adult runner can indicate fracture or symptomatic spinal stenosis.[27,28]

Running Habits

How long has the runner been training? How many miles per session and per week? What pace is maintained? Does the runner take days off? Has there been a sudden increase in frequency, intensity, or duration of workouts? Does the runner routinely stretch before and/or after exercising? Which muscle groups are stretched? Does the runner train alone or with others, and who determines the running pace? Is the patient a competitive runner who regularly enters races, or a recreational jogger? These questions are important in identifying potential errors of training that can cause breakdown.

Equipment

What type of shoes does the runner use? How often are new pairs purchased and old pairs discarded? Has the runner recently started wearing a new style of shoe? Does the runner wear orthotics? When were the orthotics originally constructed and for what purpose? These questions help to provide insight into potential errors of training and biomechanical imbalances.

Terrain

Where does the athlete typically run? Does the runner train on a level dirt path, on a banked concrete surface, on a treadmill at a health club, or a flat circular track? Does the runner hill train? Have any of these factors changed recently? Poor selection of running course may create imbalances at the level of the foot and ankle that are transmitted up the biomechanical chain to the more proximal structures. For example, running on a banked surface causes uphill foot pronation, which stresses the medial ankle, and creates a knee valgus force, hip abduction, and elevation of the ipsilateral hemipelvis; whereas "downhill" foot supination stresses the lateral ankle and creates a knee varus force, hip adduction, and lowering of the ipsilateral hemipelvis.[1,25]

Number of Previous Injuries

How many other injuries have been sustained? What were the locations? Were they managed nonsurgically or surgically? These questions help to identify patterns of overtraining and provide a sense of how much the athlete is willing to endure to continue running on a regular basis.

Symptoms

Does the runner get chest pain or palpitations during exercise? Is it harder to do the same amount of work? Has the runner started experiencing wheezing or shortness of breath during or after runs? Does the runner experience constant fatigue and difficulty in getting rid of colds or infections? Has weight loss occurred, and was it on purpose? Has a female athlete runner stopped menstruating, and is there a reason to suspect osteoporosis? What medications are being used? Are anabolic steroids being taken? Although the major focus of this chapter is musculoskeletal problems, one must not fail to identify other factors that may heavily influence the runner's overall health.

Goals

Why does the patient run? For fun and fitness, or in preparation for competition? As part of a program for weight control, stress management, or health maintenance? Is the running a substitute for something that is missing in the patient's life or a reflection of a problem in the larger psychosocial context? An overweight middle-aged man who has just started running as part of a generic fitness program may be amenable to trying a new form of exercise if running causes knee pain. On the other hand, a gaunt young woman who presents with pelvic stress fractures and amenorrhea, yet whose primary concern is fear of gaining weight, raises the possibility of disordered body image and/or other emotional issues. Such issues may require the input of a psychologist or psychiatrist, so that running rehabilitation can occur.

Coping Skills

How does the loss of running affect the person's life? Can the athlete tolerate relative or complete rest? What will he or she do if running is no longer an option for an undetermined amount of time? A more holistic approach to the injured athlete, with input from a sports psychologist or psychiatrist, may be essential to successful rehabilitation.

PHYSICAL EXAMINATION

A thorough physical examination is critical in developing a diagnosis-specific rehabilitation and/or treatment program. The runner's entire back and lower limbs should be evaluated while standing, sitting, lying while prone and while supine, as well as during walking and running. It is critical to adhere to the concept of the kinetic chain and to recognize that biomechanical dysfunction in one body region may cause injury at a distance. Consequently, examination of the low back, hip, knee, and ankle regions should be routine in virtually all injured runners. The basic components of a runner's physical examination are reviewed below.

Observation

The entire lower extremity must be evaluated for asymmetry of static and dynamic alignment and function. The patient is first examined while standing. This allows attention to any gross abnormalities of the spine and lower limbs, including the pelvis down to the toes. Common anatomic structural abnormalities may include genu varum or valgum, tibia vera, tibial torsion, hindfoot varus or valgus, patellar malalignment (medial/lateral, alta/baja), and pes planus or cavus foot.[29] Frequently, knee pain in runners may be caused by lower limb malalignment ("miserable malalignment"), which consists of a broad pelvis, femoral neck anteversion, genu valgum, excessive Q-angle, hypermobile patella, external tibial torsion, and foot pronation.[29] The examination at rest helps to identify such entities as limb-length discrepancy, scoliosis, excessive lordosis, pelvic asymmetry, genu varum/valgum, tibial torsion, side-to-side differences in muscle bulk, static ankle–foot deformities, blisters and clauses, and visible evidence of inflammation.

The walking examination may reveal signs of foot pronation or supination, early heel rise from a tight gastroc-soleus complex, increased knee valgus/varus, and hip abductor weakness (Trendelenburg sign).

The greatest insight is achieved with direct visualization of running itself. Treadmill evaluations provide an excellent opportunity in this regard. Analysis of video recordings of the runner at varying speeds, with and without shoes and with and without orthotics, is recommended. This strategy enables the clinician to identify more subtle biomechanical imbalances as well as flaws in running style. Video recordings are not only a useful diagnostic aid but also a vehicle for patient education. The recording/projecting system should be capable of high resolution when played at normal, fast-forward, or slow-motion speeds.

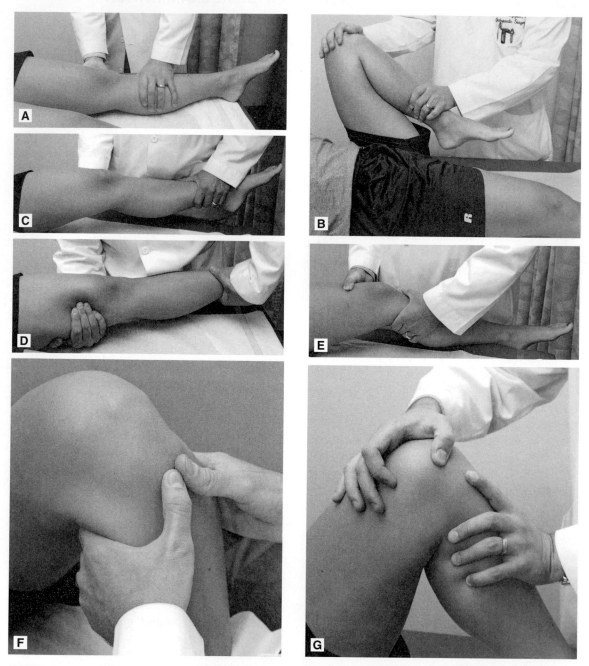

FIGURE 15-3 A. Full knee extension. **B.** Full knee flexion. **C.** Valgus stress on the left knee. **D.** Varus stress on the left knee. **E.** Lachman test. **F.** Anterior drawer test. **G.** Posterior drawer test (exam is done by placing thumb/or finger on both the medial femoral condyle and the medial tibial plateau and noting whether the tibia is placed more anterior to the femur).

Foot and Ankle

The examiner must first look for any blisters, calluses, forefoot (hallux valgus, metatarsus adductus, dorsal bunion), or hindfoot (subtalar varus or valgus) deformities. Common foot abnormalities that may result in runner's injuries include the hyperpronated foot, cavus foot, and Morton foot. Foot hyperpronation is characterized by a very flexible foot with excessive subtalar motion. The cavus foot is described as rigid with a high arch. This foot type adapts poorly to running surfaces and does not adequately absorb shock, frequently resulting in Achilles tendinitis and plantar fasciitis. The foot with an extremely mobile first ray and elongated second metatarsal has been described as the Morton foot.

In examination of the ankle and foot, the following maneuvers are considered to be the minimum: palpation of the Achilles tendon along with the origin and insertion of the plantar fascia; intrinsic ankle motion as well as range of motion of the talar, subtalar, and midtarsal joints; and evaluation of laxity in the lateral and medial ligaments of the ankle. It is also important to assess the flexibility of the gastrocsoleus complex by dorsiflexing and plantar-flexing the ankle with the knee fully extended. Evaluation of the forefoot for presence of varus/valgus malalignment also aids in detecting areas of tightness that need stretching, or regions of connective-tissue laxity in need of orthotic devices for protection, stability, and support.[10]

Knee

Assessment of range of motion in the knee is followed by evaluation of patellar position, mobility, tracking, and retropatellar pain. Range of motion of the knee allows assessment of flexion and extension (i.e., flexion contractures or muscle tightness/imbalances), as well as instability. Instability of the knee is assessed with examination (Fig. 15-3). The Q-angle is measured from the angle formed between straight lines drawn from the anterior superior iliac spine (ASIS) to the distal femur and from the tibial tuberosity through the middle of the patella (Fig. 15-4). The Q-angle is considered to be abnormal if it measures over 20 degrees.[1,16,30,31] The combination of hypermobility of the patella, external tibial torsion, increased Q-angle, femoral neck anteversion, a broad pelvis, and pes planus with pronation defines malalignment syndrome, which is associated with

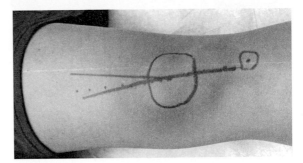

FIGURE 15-4 Q-angle measurement. A line is drawn from the ASIS to the distal femur and from the tibial tuberosity to the center of the patella. The angle that is created is the Q-angle. Normal Q-angle is approximately 15 degrees.

medial knee pain.[16,30,32] The Ober test (Fig. 15-5) is used to evaluate tightness of the tensor fascia lata.[33]

In cases of anterior knee pain, the examination focuses on patellar orientation (internal/external rotation, presence of patella baja or alta, abnormal patellar tilt), defects in the medial or lateral retinacula, apprehension, increased laxity or pain with patellar mobilization (Fig. 15-6), evidence of poor patellar tracking within the trochlea, retropatellar crepitus, and atrophy of the vastus medialis obliquus.

Hip and Pelvis

The hip should be evaluated with the patient supine. The hip and groin region should be palpated for any soft-tissue abnormalities, starting at the least painful

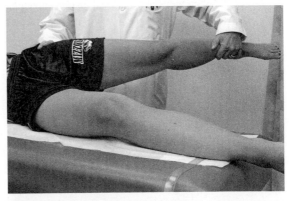

FIGURE 15-5 Ober test, performed by abducting and extending the affected hip, and then allowing the thigh to adduct passively toward midline. A positive test is indicated when the thigh does not return to at least a neutral position or lateral hip pain is produced.

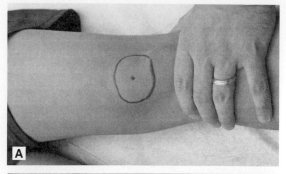

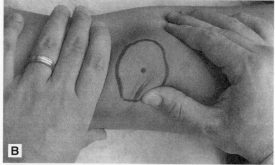

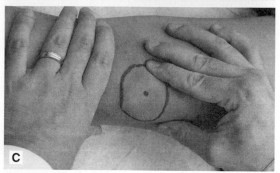

FIGURE 15-6 A. Patellar mobility assessment: neutral. **B.** Patellar mobility assessment: medial displacement (left knee). **C.** Patellar mobility assessment: lateral displacement (left knee).

areas. Although the hip joint itself is too deep to directly palpate, this examination may give clues as to areas of pathology. An understanding of the anatomy of the muscular attachments around the hip and palpation of these bony landmarks is useful for evaluation of bursitis, avulsion fractures, and/or apophysitis. The iliac crest is the attachment site for the abdominal oblique, transverses, and gluteus medius muscles, which can be irritated at the bone tendon interface by accentuated arm motion while running. The sartorius muscle originates at the ASIS and is frequently injured during sprinting or hurdling.[33] The rectus femoris muscle originates on the

anterior inferior iliac spine. The medial and lateral hamstrings originate on the ischial tuberosity. Avulsion of the ischial tuberosity occurs from eccentric hamstring contraction with the hip in a flexed position and the knee extended. The greater trochanter is the insertion site for the gluteus medius and minimus, as well as the hip external rotators. The iliopsoas tendon inserts on the lesser trochanter. These insertion sites are more commonly involved in insertional muscle strain as opposed to avulsion-type injuries. It is important to assess hip range of motion (both active and passive) in both flexion and extension as well as internal and external rotation. Limitations in hip range of motion may be a result of tight hip flexors, extensors, and adductors and may be a factor in the development of the runner's injury.[2,15]

Stabilizing the pelvis with one hand while attempting a straight leg raise with the other gives a sense of hamstring tightness, as retro-tilting of the pelvis begins to occur when maximal length is approached. The patient brings both knees up to the chest and then tries to let one leg descend to a flat lying position on the examination table (Thomas test; Fig. 15-7). If hip flexor tightness is present, the patient cannot place the leg flat on the table. Tightness of the piriformis and external hip rotators can be checked with knee flexion and internal hip rotation with the patient lying prone. Placing the hip in end-range flexion plus abduction and external rotation (FABER) stresses the hip joint itself (Fig. 15-8). The Gaenslen maneuver may be used to stress the sacroiliac joint.

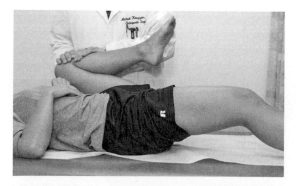

FIGURE 15-7 Thomas test. The patient has both knees flexed up to the chest and then attempts to move one leg to a flat lying position on the table.

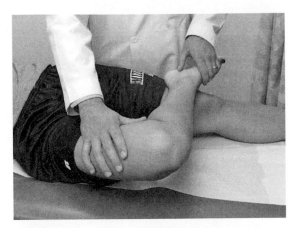

FIGURE 15-8 FABER test. The hip is *F*lexed, *AB*ducted, and *E*xternally *R*otated.

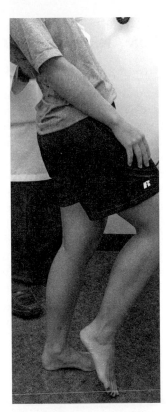

FIGURE 15-9 One-legged hyperextension test. The patient is asked to extend the spine while standing on one leg. If this elicits pain, it may be an indication of active posterior element irritation and/or symptomatic spondylolysis.

The patient also needs to be checked for symmetry in the evaluation of the sacroiliac joint. In addition, the ASIS is a fixed landmark typically used in limb-length measurement, down to the medial malleolus. Limb-length inequalities have been estimated to have three times as much an effect on the runner as on the walker.[8]

Spine

An evaluation of the back takes into account all of the observations from the lower body segments; again, the concept of the kinetic chain must not be overlooked. Lumbosacral spine motion is intimately related to motion at the level of the hip and pelvis. Tightness of the lower-extremity muscles attaching to the pelvis can interfere with the normal smooth combination of spine flexion-pelvic rotation and spine extension-pelvic derotation (lumbopelvic rhythm), observed during trunk flexion and extension.[34] During spine flexion and extension, it is essential to identify the major motion segments—80% to 90% of the motion in the lumbosacral spine should be at L4-L5 and L5-S1.[34] Migration of the motion upward toward the thoracolumbar junction, altered tone of the paraspinal muscles, and lack of a springing sensation in the lower spine during anterior glides (placement and release of pressure along the spine while the patient is relaxed in the prone position) suggest spinal segment dysfunction. Weakness of abdominal muscle and thoracolumbar fascia further indicate that the spine is in need of conditioning.[35] Many individuals who appear to be otherwise highly fit from constant aerobic exercise fail to perform regular exercise that conditions the supportive musculature of the spine. In the young runner with back pain, provocative tests such as extending the spine while standing on one leg (one-legged hyperextension test; Fig. 15-9) help identify active posterior element irritation and/or symptomatic spondylolysis.

Miscellaneous Components of the Examination

Finally, the running shoes should be inspected for signs of breakdown and correct fit for the runner's foot. In general, pronation is controlled better with a straight board-lasted shoe with good rear-foot control, whereas the supinator does better with a flexible and curve-lasted shoe.[1,5,8]

SPECIFIC RUNNING INJURY EVALUATION AND REHABILITATION

Muscle Strains and Tendinitis (Hip)

The most common site of injury involving the muscles around the hip is at the proximal myotendonous junction of the biceps femoris (hamstrings); however, the iliopsoas, rectus femoris, and adductor muscle groups may all be affected.[25,33,36] These type of injuries can account for 33% of all sports injuries and are some of the most common causes of "hip" pain in runners. Muscle strains typically occur during eccentric loading. They are a result of sudden acceleration/deceleration, sudden direction change, or eccentric contraction, coupled with a muscle's failure to withstand the applied force. Risk factors for this type of injury include poor flexibility, improper technique, fatigue, regional muscle weakness/imbalances, prior injury, inadequate warm-up, and increased age.[20,25,33,37,38]

A history of localized pain, weakness, stiffness, swelling, and/or bruising is common among runners presenting with muscle strain and/or tendinitis. On physical examination, one may find a limited range of motion, tenderness to palpation of regional muscle groups, edema, ecchymosis, crepitation, and muscle group weakness. Muscle strains can be classified as grade 1 (minimal fiber disruption), grade 2 (partial tear without muscle retraction), and grade 3 (complete rupture of the myotendinous unit).[33]

Initial treatment should begin with rest, ice, and protected weight-bearing. Nonsteroidal anti-inflammatory drugs (NSAIDs) can be used for pain relief. Heat, gentle range-of-motion (ROM) activity, and isometric strengthening can be initiated after several days. Stretching significantly enhances the rehabilitation program for muscle strain injuries and can facilitate earlier return to sporting activities.[33] Isometric strengthening is introduced when the athlete is pain free. For full stretching of the hamstrings, the athlete must be able to maintain knee extension with the hip flexed to 90 degrees and the ankle dorsiflexed (Fig. 15-10). This is done most safely with the patient starting from a supine position.

There have been several approaches to prepare the athlete to return to running. One may begin with slow running for one-third the usual distance, alternating with a day of rest. This should only be started once all symptoms have resolved, full hip ROM has been restored, and at least 90% of strength has been

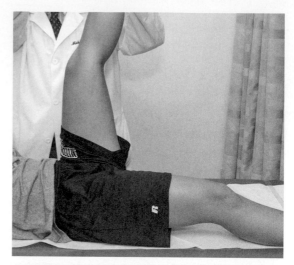

FIGURE 15-10 Hamstring stretch. For full stretching of the hamstrings, the athlete must be able to maintain knee extension with the hip flexed to 90 degrees and the ankle dorsiflexed.

regained compared to the uninjured leg. There should be equalization of the quadriceps:hamstring strength ratios.[20,25,37] If the athlete continues to remain pain free, then mileage, speed, and intensity may be slowly increased. It is crucial that rest days are maintained for at least 4 to 6 weeks, and cross-training should be incorporated.[33] As the athlete begins to return to running, technique errors and extrinsic factors must be addressed to prevent reinjury.[20,25,33,37,38]

Iliotibial Band Friction Syndrome

Iliotibial band syndrome (ITBS) is the most common cause of lateral knee pain in runners, but may also result in lateral hip pain.[29,32,33,39] The iliotibial band originates at the iliac crest and inserts on the lateral tibia at the Gerdy tubercle, the fibular head, and the lateral patellar retinaculum. It is the continuation of the tensor fascia lata and gluteus maximus muscles. Excessive and/or sudden increase in running distance or frequency, leg length discrepancy, genu varum, pes cavus, muscle weakness (especially weak hip abductors), inexperience, running on banked surfaces, inappropriate footwear, and hip inflexibility may all result in irritation of the ITB.[6,9,29,32,33,39] Patients with ITBS typically will present with sharp or burning pain along the lateral hip, thigh, or knee that is worsened with activity and subsides with rest.

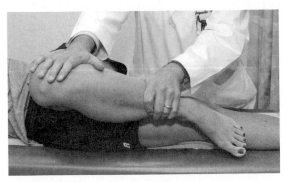

FIGURE 15-11 Noble compression test. This examination is performed by placing the patient on their side, with the affected knee flexed 90 degrees. As pressure is placed over the ITB at the level of the lateral femoral condyle, the knee is extended. Pain is a positive finding (this typically occurs as the knee approaches 30 degrees of flexion, which is the position in which the tensed ITB rubs directly on the lateral femoral condyle).

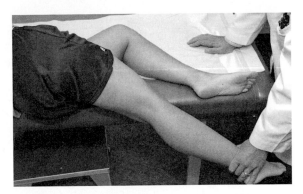

FIGURE 15-12 IT band stretching.

On physical examination patients typically will have local tenderness over the distal ITB (2–3 cm proximal to the joint line of the knee where the ITB moves over the lateral femoral condyle). They may also present with crepitation, snapping, and edema at the area. The Noble compression test (Fig. 15-11) may also elicit pain.[39]

Initial management of athletes with ITBS should begin with activity modification and with attempts to reduce inflammation. NSAIDs, ice massage, phonophoresis, and iontophoresis are all useful modalities to break the inflammatory cascade. Occasionally, local corticosteroid injection may be helpful in reducing inflammation and pain. Once acute inflammation has subsided, stretching exercises may be initiated (Fig. 15-12). Contraction–relaxation exercises of the ITB/tensor fascia lata are helpful to lengthen tight muscles. This exercise should be performed in three sets of 7-second submaximal contractions followed by 15-second stretches.[39] Standing ITB stretch has been shown in biomechanical studies to be effective.[39] These may be performed with the arms at the side, arms extended overhead, and arms reaching diagonally downward.[39,40] Once ROM has been fully recovered, strengthening exercises, especially of the hip adductors, may be initiated. The adductors counter the pull of the tight ITB (gluteus maximus and TFL) and must be strengthened to avoid overuse.[37] Patients may return to running once

strength has been regained. As with muscle strain rehabilitation, running should progress slowly with alternate day rest periods and a gradual increase in distance and frequency.

Anterior Knee Pain

Patellofemoral pain syndrome, causing anterior knee pain, is one of the most common knee problems in runners.[11,19,32] It is essential in the examination of any athlete with anterior knee pain to thoroughly evaluate the extensor mechanism, including quadriceps development; muscle contractures; position of the vastus medialis; patellar position, tracking, and stability; pain during knee ROM; Q-angle; fat pad tenderness; crepitation; and quadriceps and/or patellar tenderness.[19,30,32] Reaction forces of the patellofemoral joint are increased markedly during the single-leg support phase of running because the quadriceps contracts vigorously while the knee is in flexion.[19,30]

Runners with patellar tilt—excessive lateral pressure syndrome—present with diffuse anterior knee pain that may localize to the patella as the major site of discomfort. Physical examination is often unremarkable, with the exception of the lateral retinaculum, which may be tight or tender to palpation. A tight lateral retinaculum prevents the patella from being brought to the horizontal plane when the knee is fully extended and the quadriceps relaxed. The examiner may also test the degree of patellar mobility by stabilizing the medial patella and pulling up on the lateral patella. Additionally, the examiner must be aware of any crepitus or tenderness along the lateral border of the patella, which may be an indication of degenerative changes of the articular cartilage. Radiographic evaluation of the patella is important to assess if it is correctly positioned within the sulcus of the distal femur. This is best seen on an axial view such as the Merchant or Laurin view.[32]

Patellar instability is characterized by episodes of patellar subluxation or even dislocation. Again, because of the patellar maltracking there are increased compressive forces within the patellofemoral joint, resulting in pain and possible articular cartilage damage. Laxity in the medial retinaculum, high Q-angle, weak vastus medialis, shallow sulcus, patella alta, genu valgum, femoral neck anteversion, and compensatory pronation all can contribute to, or be associated with, patellar instability. Observation of patellar tracking during active flexion and extension is necessary. Lateral movement at terminal displacement (J sign) is highly suggestive of maltracking. Lateral pressure on the patella with the knee flexed at 30 degrees can demonstrate lateral instability; the patella should normally be stable in the sulcus with the knee in this position. If the Q-angle is greater than 20 degrees, there is a tendency for abnormal lateral displacement of the patella by the quadriceps.

Patellar tracking and subluxation can be managed initially with quadriceps rehabilitation and closed-chain exercises. Athletes should not return to running until they are pain free.[32,37] RICE (rest, ice, compression, elevation) and anti-inflammatory medications are initiated. Problems with the malalignment syndrome must be corrected. Consideration is given to fitting the runner with orthotics only if biomechanical deficits persist after achieving full flexibility of the gastrocsoleus complex, hamstrings, and iliotibial band and after full-strength training of the vastus medialis obliques (VMO). Taping of the patella to simulate proper alignment, accompanied by neuromuscular reeducation of the knee musculature (McConnell technique), may also be beneficial.[41] Patellar stabilizing braces may be considered but should not be the first plan of attack. Strengthening of the VMO is facilitated via short arc ($<$30 degrees of flexion to full extension) quadriceps exercises.[30] Adductor squeezes and short-arc knee extensions with a closed kinetic chain also help with VMO training.

Achilles Tendinitis and Tendinosis

Injury to the Achilles tendon often starts as inflammation of the peritendinous structures and bursa, which progresses to involvement of the entire tendon (tendinosis). During the peritendinous stage, the tendon itself is not involved. With progression and involvement of the tendon itself, damage occurs in the form of tears, necrosis, or calcification. Achilles tendinitis can either be of the insertional or the noninsertional type. Insertional tendinitis involves pathology at the bone-tendon junction. Commonly, there is an associated Haglund deformity (excessive posterosuperior spurring/prominence of the calcaneal tuberosity). This results in inflammation of the superficial and retrocalcaneal bursa, causing tendinitis. There is often a palpable bony prominence posteriorly as well as a tight heel cord. Noninsertional Achilles tendinitis is characterized by pain and tenderness 2 to 6 cm proximal to the Achilles tendon insertion and is worsened with dorsiflexion.[37,42] Repeated episodes of microtrauma result in microtearing of the tendon in the region of the least vascularity, approximately 2 to 6 cm above the tendon insertion.[11,37,42,43] Excessive pronation, tight heel cords, and rear-foot or forefoot varus can induce this problem, along with overtraining, a single excessively strenuous workout, and hill running.[37,42] Aside from the location of pain, symptoms are similar to those experienced with insertional tendinitis. It is important to recognize that although the majority of patients feel that they have an acute inflammatory problem (tendinitis), in fact, they probably have a chronic problem (tendinosis), in which asymptomatic intratendinous degeneration has occurred over time.[11,44]

Treatment consists of anti-inflammatories, rest, ice message, and Achilles stretching (Fig. 15-13). A heel lift should be used in all shoes, including running shoes, during the rehabilitation phase of recovery. Although heel lifts often provide some pain relief in early rehabilitation, they should not be used indefinitely, because they promote shortening of the heel cord. Ultrasound may be useful in chronic cases in which old, scarred connective tissue must be loosened and stretching is difficult.[37] Reduction in weight-bearing activity is mandatory. These patients are good candidates for aquatic-based conditioning. As pain is reduced, the patients should go through a gradual program of first concentric and ultimately eccentric strengthening of the plantar flexors. If pain continues despite all the above measures, magnetic resonance imaging (MRI) of the Achilles tendon may reveal previously unidentified partial tendon tears, musculotendonous tears, retrocalcaneal bursitis, or stress fractures.[11,37,44]

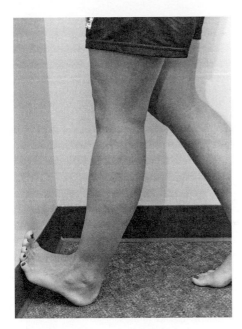

FIGURE 15-13 Achilles tendon stretching.

Posterior Tibial Tendinitis

Patients who present with posterior tibial tendinitis typically have pain at the medial aspect of the ankle behind or slightly distal to the medial malleolus; less commonly, this is present at the navicular bone. Treatment consists of anti-inflammatory medications, ice massage, and shoe modifications (medial heel and sole wedge, especially for hyperpronators).[42] Pain relief may be obtained by injection of long-acting anesthetic (such as bupivicaine), which may help disrupt adhesions within the tendon sheath. Athletes with persistent cases may require casting for 4 to 6 weeks to allow the inflammation to subside.

Plantar Fasciitis

Plantar fasciitis is one of the most common causes of heel pain in runners.[29] Patients typically experience pain during the first few steps taken in the morning upon arising from bed—the "dreaded first step of the morning." Pain also develops at the beginning of a run, diminishing with time and recurring when the run is complete. Physical examination elicits tenderness to palpation at the attachment of the plantar fascia to the heel. The pathologic process of plantar fasciitis involves an inflammatory reaction and traction-induced microtears of the plantar fascia and associated

structures at the insertion on the calcaneus.[22,29,45] The runner's foot may have biomechanical abnormalities related to cavus or pronation, with increased eversion of the heel and forefoot varus. Ordinarily, the fascia tightens passively with toe extension, resulting in an arch elevation (windlass effect). Limited ankle dorsiflexion, a tight gastroc-soleus complex, and excessive pronation decrease the foot's ability to achieve the rigidity needed to push off the ground, and make the development of plantar fasciitis more likely. Other support structures, such as the medial portion of the plantar fascia, are then subject to greater tensile forces. Patients will typically adapt by increasing the amount of time on the forefoot during running as well as developing a "choppy" stride.[22,37]

Treatment consists of rest, ice, anti-inflammatory medications; consideration can be made for injection of corticosteroids into the calcaneal attachment, although many clinicians do not recommend this. Orthotic devices may also be helpful, including arch supports, counterforce taping, felt heel pads, horseshoe-shaped pads, or flexible laminated devices.[21,22,29,37] Stretching of the plantar fascia, gastroc-soleus complex, hamstrings, and intrinsic strengthening of the foot are quite important.[22,29] This injury can take 3 to 4 months to resolve in chronic cases; alternative aerobic conditioning programs (i.e., rowing, swimming, aqua running, and occasionally cycling) should be considered.

It is also important to keep in mind the other possible causes of heel pain, including entrapment of the medial calcaneal branch of the tibial nerve (medial-sided heel pain) and tarsal tunnel syndrome (entrapment of the tibial nerve with medial heel and ankle pain).

Stress Fractures

A stress fracture is defined as a skeletal defect resulting from repeated application of a stress that is less than that required to fracture a bone with a single load, but greater than the bone's ability to fully recover.[16,23,46] Runners at risk are those who have asymmetric limb lengths, pronate excessively, or run on rigid surfaces.[23,47] The tibia is the most common site (34%), followed by the fibula (24%), metatarsals (20%), and femur (14%).[23] Distance runners and track athletes have been shown to be prone to developing stress fractures.[46] Pain that is relatively well localized is a major clinical feature.[23] Pain produced over the suspected fracture site with application of a vibrating tuning fork to the affected area or with percussion of the bone away from the affected site may also suggest stress fracture.[25,37] Because they frequently do not produce a full cortical defect, stress fractures are difficult to detect by routine radiography early in their course. Bone scans or MRI are recommended in cases of increased clinical suspicion when plain film study is negative.[46]

Treatment consists of rest, and if needed, nonweight-bearing and immobilization until the stress fracture is healed and symptoms resolve. A supervised, graduated physical therapy program is important to outline the duration, frequency, and intensity of activities as the athlete progresses from rest back to training and eventually competition. The first step in the rehabilitation of athletes with a stress fracture is to stay below the level of activity that induces symptoms. Running on dry land is prohibited until an adequate amount of time for healing has passed—approximately 3 weeks for the fibula, 4 to 8 weeks for the tibia (although considerably longer if the tibial plateau has been affected), and 3 months (with limited weight-bearing) for the neck of the femur.[23,37] In the past, athletes with stress fractures were primarily restricted to alternative forms of aerobic exercises, such as swimming and bicycling, which were of general conditioning value but were not particularly specific to running. Aqua running is also an acceptable alternate mode of training. Women with the female athlete triad and stress fractures should be monitored for adequate caloric intake to support energy output and fracture healing.

CONCLUSION

The runner can present with a multitude of symptoms and injuries. It is critical that the physician has a thorough understanding of the basic biomechanics of running as well as the pathology that can result from imbalance. It is also important to understand that the athlete will develop compensatory changes in stride and running technique, which can further induce injury and prolong recovery. These factors must be addressed and rehabilitated in a concise, organized fashion with a team approach. For successful rehabilitation, it is critical that the athlete, physician, and physical therapist have an open line of communication and knowledge of both the treatment and rehabilitation plan.

REFERENCES

1. Brody DM. Running injuries. Prevention and management. *Clin Symp.* 1987;39:1–36.
2. O'Toole ML. Prevention and treatment of injuries to runners. *Med Sci Sports Exerc.* 1992;24:S360–S363.
3. Novacheck TF. The biomechanics of running. *Gait Posture.* 1998;7:77–95.
4. Novacheck TF. Running injuries: a biomechanical approach. *Instr Course Lect.* 1998;47:397–406.
5. Gross ML, Davlin LB, Evanski PM. Effectiveness of orthotic shoe inserts in the long-distance runner. *Am J Sports Med.* 1991;19:409–412.
6. Messier SP, Pittala KA. Etiologic factors associated with selected running injuries. *Med Sci Sports Exerc.* 1988;20:501–505.
7. Paty JG Jr. Diagnosis and treatment of musculoskeletal running injuries. *Semin Arthritis Rheum.* 1988;18:48–60.
8. Subotnick SI. The biomechanics of running. Implications for the prevention of foot injuries. *Sports Med.* 1985;2:144–153.
9. Sutker AN, Barber FA, Jackson DW, et al. Iliotibial band syndrome in distance runners. *Sports Med.* 1985;2:447–451.
10. Newell SG. Functional neutral orthoses and shoe modifications. *Phys Med Rehab Clin North Am.* 1992;3:193–222.
11. Renstrom AF. Mechanism, diagnosis, and treatment of running injuries. *Instr Course Lect.* 1993;42:225–234.
12. Noble CA. Iliotibial band friction syndrome in runners. *Am J Sports Med.* 1980;8:232–234.
13. O'Neill DB, Micheli LJ. Overuse injuries in the young athlete. *Clin Sports Med.* 1988;7:591–610.
14. Hoeberigs JH. Factors related to the incidence of running injuries. A review. *Sports Med.* 1992;13:408–422.
15. van Mechelen W, Hlobil H, Zijlstra WP, et al. Is range of motion of the hip and ankle joint related to running injuries? A case control study. *Int J Sports Med.* 1992;13:605–610.
16. Lutter LD. The knee and running. *Clin Sports Med.* 1985;4:685–698.
17. Newell SG, Bramwell ST. Overuse injuries to the knee in runners. *Physician Sports Med.* 1984;12:81–92.
18. Cox JS. Patellofemoral problems in runners. *Clin Sports Med.* 1985;4:699–715.
19. Putnam CA, Kozey JW. *Biomechanics of Sport.* Boca Raton, FL: CRC Press; 1989.
20. Young JL, Laskowski ER, Rock MG. Thigh injuries in athletes. *Mayo Clin Proc.* 1993;68:1099–1106.
21. Kibler WB, Chandler TJ, Stracener ES. Musculoskeletal adaptations and injuries due to overtraining. *Exerc Sport Sci Rev.* 1992;20:99–126.
22. Kibler WB, Goldberg C, Chandler TJ. Functional biomechanical deficits in running athletes with plantar fasciitis. *Am J Sports Med.* 1991;19:66–71.
23. McBryde AM Jr. Stress fractures in runners. *Clin Sports Med.* 1985;4:737–752.
24. Perry J. *Gait Analysis: Normal and Pathological Function.* Thorofare, NJ: Slack; 1992.
25. Roy S, Irvin R. *Sports Medicine: Prevention, Evaluation, Management, and Rehabilitation.* Englewood Cliffs, NJ: Prentice-Hall; 1983.
26. Astrand PO, Rodahl K. *Textbook of Work Physiology.* New York: McGraw-Hill; 1986.

27. Apple DF Jr. Adolescent runners. *Clin Sports Med.* 1985;4:641–655.
28. Apple DF Jr. End stage running problems. *Clin Sports Med.* 1985;4:657–670.
29. Brody DM. Running injuries. *Clin Symp.* 1980;32:1–36.
30. Bourne MH, Hazel WA Jr, Scott SG, et al. Anterior knee pain. *Mayo Clin Proc.* 1988;63:482–491.
31. Kuland DN. *The Injuried Athlete.* 2nd ed. Philadelphia: Lippincott; 1988.
32. James SL. Running injuries of the knee. *Instr Course Lect.* 1998;47:407–417.
33. Paluska SA. An overview of hip injuries in running. *Sports Med.* 2005;35:991–1014.
34. Cailliet R. *Low Back Pain Syndrome.* 5th ed. Philadelphia: Davis; 1995.
35. Saal JA. Rehabilitation of sports related lumbar spine injuries. *Phys Med Rehabil State Art Rev.* 1987;1:613–638.
36. Smith AM, Scott SG, Wiese DM. The psychological effects of sports injuries. *Sports Med.* 1990;9:352–369.
37. Guten GN. Running Injuries. Philadelphia: W.B. Saunders Co; 1997.
38. Agre JC. Hamstring injuries. Proposed aetiological factors, prevention, and treatment. *Sports Med.* 1985;2:21–33.
39. Fredericson M, Wolf C. Iliotibial band syndrome in runners: innovations in treatment. *Sports Med.* 2005;35:451–459.
40. Fredericson M, White JJ, Macmahon JM, et al. Quantitative analysis of the relative effectiveness of 3 iliotibial band stretches. *Arch Phys Med Rehabil.* 2002;83:589–592.
41. McConnell J. The management of chondomalacia patellae: a long-term solution. *Aust J Phys.* 1986;32:215–219.
42. Baxter DE, Zingas C. The foot in running. *J Am Acad Orthop Surg.* 1995;3:136–145.
43. Kibler WB, Chandler TJ, Pace BK. Principles of rehabilitation after chronic tendon injuries. *Clin Sports Med.* 1992;11:661–671.
44. Leadbetter WB. Cell-matrix response in tendon injury. *Clin Sports Med.* 1992;11:533–578.
45. Kwong PK, Kay D, Voner RT, et al. Plantar fasciitis. Mechanics and pathomechanics of treatment. *Clin Sports Med.* 1988;7:119–126.
46. Feingold D, Hame SL. Female athlete triad and stress fractures. *Orthop Clin North Am.* 2006;37:575–583.
47. Daffner RH, Pavlov H. Stress fractures: current concepts. *AJR Am J Roentgenol.* 1992;159:245–252.

Skiing and Snowboarding Injuries

S kiing and snowboarding are two of the most popular winter sports worldwide, with over 58 million estimated participants annually in the United States alone. Although the two sports are quite distinct, with differing techniques, equipment, and even terminology, the participants coexist side by side, accessing the same terrain and facilities. Due to the nature and season of these sports, many people are inadequately prepared physically, before hitting the slopes, and may be more prone to injury, particularly if they are only able to ski or snowboard a few days a year. This chapter will review the common injury patterns seen in these two sports, including demographics, epidemiology, injury prevention, and rehabilitation.

Skiing has a long history, dating back 5,000 years to when hunters traversed the snow using animal tusks, but did not gain popularity in the United States until after the 1932 Lake Placid Winter Olympics. Snowboarding did not develop into a mainstream winter sport until the 1970s, but has grown exponentially over the past two decades, with an estimated 6 million snowboarders on U.S. ski hills in recent years. Both sports encompass a wide range of styles, including downhill, telemark, and cross-country in the case of skiing, with a number of competitive classes and different types of equipment specific to each style.

DOWNHILL (ALPINE) SKIING

Downhill skiing involves thrusting oneself down a snowy slope on two small planks, ideally in a controlled fashion, making turns to regulate speed and direction of descent. In the United States, the slopes are classified according to degree of difficulty, with no official standard across the country. Green circles,

or "bunny slopes," are the easiest and are relatively flat and smooth. Blue squares are medium in difficulty, whereas black diamonds are more difficult with steep slopes and may include rough terrain, such as moguls. Double black diamonds are reserved for experts only, and are natural slopes without the man-made influence of grooming. The competitive classes of alpine skiing include downhill, slalom, giant slalom, and super-G. There are also freestyle events that can include jumps, moguls, and trick skiing. Moguls are steep slopes that are ungroomed to the point where piles of snow, or moguls, create severe bumps and troughs that the skier must negotiate using abrupt pivoting turns. Due to the quick turning maneuvers, mogul slopes are usually only used by skiers, and not snowboarders.

Alpine boots are typically hard shell, and may be front entry, rear entry, or hybrid. Boots are secured to the ski by the binding, and it is here, at the boot-binding interface, where continuous improvements in technology have translated into fewer injuries. The binding must be adjusted to the individual skier to maximize safety and to release during a fall without allowing premature release during normal skiing.

Telemark Skiing

Telemark skiing, also known as "free-heel skiing" or "pinning," is the oldest form of alpine or downhill skiing, with the free-heel binding dating back to the mid-1800s when it was developed by Sondre Norheim, the father of modern day skiing, in Telemark, Norway. In telemark skiing the skier's foot is only attached to the ski at the toe, with boots that flex at the forefoot, allowing the skier to perform the lunge turn typical of this sport (Fig. 16-1). Many telemark skiers, particularly at the advanced level, currently favor reinforced plastic boots for improved

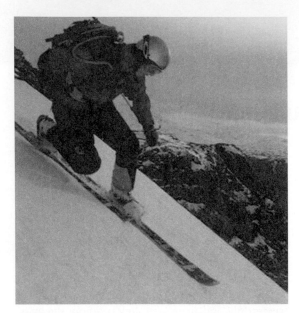

FIGURE 16-1 A telemark skier performing the typical lunge turn unique to this style, which is made possible by the free heel binding system. (Photo reproduced courtesy of Vail Resorts Inc.)

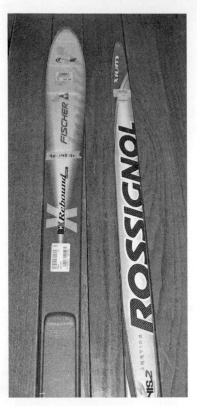

FIGURE 16-2 Two different styles of cross-country skis: the wider style is used for back-country ski touring, while the lighter, narrower style is used on well-groomed trails (wide smooth trails for skate skiing and narrower trails with two ruts to guide the skis for the classical style).

control and performance. However, the use of such boots has been associated with higher rates of knee injuries as compared to leather boots,[1] while the increased height of the plastic boots has been credited with decreasing foot and ankle injuries.[2] Despite the availability of releasable bindings, most telemark skiers still prefer to use nonreleasable bindings.[3]

CROSS-COUNTRY SKIING

Cross-country (XC) skiing originated in Scandinavia out of necessity to travel across the snow, and was first included as an Olympic Winter Games sport in 1924. Now, XC skiing has two distinct styles, classic and skating, with the latter gaining popularity within the last 20 years. In the classic style, the skis remain parallel in a traditional gliding walking motion, which is typically recommended for beginners. The skating style is much like in-line skating, performed at a faster pace and requiring more athleticism than classical XC skiing. The equipment should fit the style of XC skiing and type of terrain; for well-groomed trails, skis are typically lighter and narrower (Fig. 16-2). Skis were originally sized according to the skier's height, but with advancements in technology,

skis are now fitted to account for stiffness and flexibility based upon the individual's weight, strength, and skill level. Boots are also selected based upon terrain and style of XC skiing; classic boots are less stiff than the skating style. Correct pole selection is important, as poles that are too long can place excessive strain on the shoulder, and poles that are too short can result in back pain.

DISABLED SKIING

There is also a large population of disabled skiers who can participate with the use of specially adapted equipment. Disabled skiers who are able to stand can use adaptive equipment such as outriggers (modified Canadian crutches with a small ski on the end), ski bras (clips attaching the tips of the skis together), tethers (rope held by coaches to control speed and turns), or

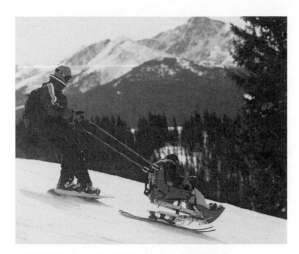

FIGURE 16-3 An instructor guiding a disabled skier, using a specially adapted monoski system. Many such skiers are able to navigate the ski runs independently, without the aid of an instructor. (Photo reproduced courtesy of Vail Resorts Inc.)

adaptive ski schools with both professional instructors and volunteers available to train and assist disabled skiers.

SNOWBOARDING

There are several different styles of snowboarding (free ride and carving are the most popular), as well as different classes of competition including freestyle, slalom, and giant slalom, which are comparable to the similarly named alpine ski events. There is also a newer discipline, boarder cross, in which a group of snowboarders race together down varied terrain including jumps and designated gates. Different boards, boots, and bindings are available for the various different styles of snowboarding (Fig. 16-4). Boots can be soft and flexible, hard and stiff (similar to a ski boot), or hybrid with a rigid base but soft upper. Soft boots generally allow for better flexibility and superior board control, which is important in freestyle or free ride riding styles (where riders perform various tricks or maneuvers); whereas stiff boots perform better during racing or alpine snowboarding. A variety of bindings are available to secure the rider to the board, including a strap-in binding used with soft boots, and step-in or plate bindings, with which the rider clips in using a mechanism similar to clipless bike pedals (Fig. 16-4). All bindings are nonreleasable.

a walker with attached modified skis. If a skier is unable to stand, due to paralysis or lack of neuromuscular control of the lower limbs, other types of skis have been developed, in which the individual sits on the ski and uses outriggers as balance aids. The upper bucket assembly connects through a binding to either a monoski or a bi-ski, with an associated shock absorber to smooth out rough terrain (Fig. 16-3). Many ski areas in the United States have

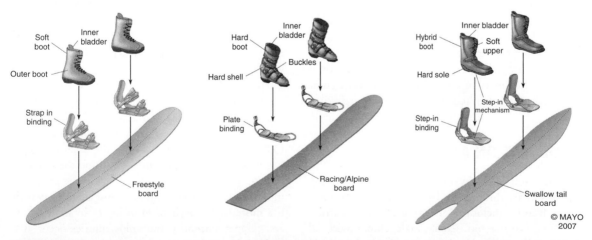

FIGURE 16-4 The three main types of snowboard boots with their respective binding mechanisms are depicted. Variations on boot/binding combinations can be made. Freestyle and swallow tail boards are available in split style (dotted line), allowing the board to be split and used with climbing skis for backcountry ascent.

TABLE 16-1	Examples of More Common Snowboarding Terminology

Bail/biff/bust/crater/eat snow/face plant/pack/spill—All terms used to describe a crash or fall (e.g., "he packed into that snowbank and broke his leg"). Variations include "scorpion," which is to face plant with the low back and hips extending so as to resemble a scorpion; and "yard sale," which is to biff so hard one loses his or her equipment.

Bone—Extending one or both legs during an aerial maneuver.

Bonk—Intentionally hitting a no-snow object with the snowboard (e.g., a tail bonk could be hitting a picnic table with the tail of the snowboard).

Boost—Catching air off a jump (e.g., "he boosted ten feet out of the halfpipe").

Fakie—A term for riding backward, also known as switchstance or switch.

Flying squirrel air—Bending at the knees and grabbing the heel edge of the snowboard with both hands, the front hand near the front foot, and the rear hand near the rear foot.

Goofy footed—Riding the board with the right foot in the forward position.

Huck—To throw oneself at or off any form of snow ramp (e.g., a kicker, pipe, cliff, etc.).

Jib—The act of riding on something other than snow (e.g., rails, trees, garbage cans, logs).

McTwist—An inverted aerial where the rider performs a 540-degree backside rotation in combination with a front flip, landing facing forward.

Rail slide—To slide the rails of the snowboard onto almost anything, other than a flat slope (e.g., fallen tree branches, logs, the coping of a halfpipe, a picnic table).

Railing—A term used to describe making fast and hard turns.

Stalefish air—The rear hand grabs the heel edge behind the rear leg and in between the bindings while the rear leg is boned.

Switch—To ride with the tail of the board forward.

As a physician treating these athletes, it is helpful to have a basic understanding of the sport, including equipment and terminology, not only to avoid making the mistake of confusing a "stale fish" with a "flying squirrel" (Table 16-1) but also to help identify the mechanism of injury and assist with accurate diagnosis. For example, when a boarder reports injuring his knee while attempting a "crippler air but then cratering out into the wall of the halfpipe," this would translate to an attempt at a forward-facing 180-degree rotation combined with a flip, but rather than landing as intended in a forward-facing position, colliding with the wall of the halfpipe. The terminology is almost a language of its own, but a number of the more common terms are listed in Table 16-1.

A POPULATION AT RISK

Accurate injury rates in the skiing and snowboarding population are difficult to determine, due to a number of factors, including the wide range of participants (e.g., young, old, female, male, elite, novice, all of whom have differing injury profiles)[4]; the widely varying exposure rates of each participant (with some skiers completing as few as three or four runs in a day while others clock thousands of feet of altitude); and

the widely varying terrain, which changes from run to run even on the same hill, and from day to day depending on weather conditions. Individual factors relevant to injury risk include fitness level, fatigue, technique, and equipment. Determining injury rates is further complicated by the fact that many alpine athletes do not seek medical attention at all[5] or self-triage to medical facilities remote from the ski area where they were injured.[6] Rates of injury for snowboarders have been estimated at 13.5 injuries per 100,000 km traveled or about 4 injuries per 1,000 snowboarder days.[7] Alpine skiers have 2 to 3 injuries per 1,000 skier days, which has decreased from 5 to 8 injuries in the 1970s, likely due to advancements in equipment.[8]

Studies show a clear difference in injury patterns between snowboarding and skiing. Overall, the most common injuries that occur in skiing are to the knee (30%), the head (12% to 20%), the ulnar collateral ligament (UCL) of the thumb (8%), and the shoulder (4% to 11%).[3] Torsional injuries are more common in skiers, as opposed to impact against the slope, which is a more likely mechanism of injury in snowboarders.[9] Upper extremity and ankle injuries occur at a higher rate in snowboarders and tend to be more severe, with a greater proportion of dislocations and fractures[6,7,9–14]; while lower extremity injuries are more common in skiers.[15] Head and abdominal injuries account for the majority of severe injuries in snowboarding and skiing,[16] with fatalities most often resulting from collisions, usually with trees.[17–19] Death by immersion is a risk more associated with snowboarding, and usually occurs in deep powder conditions when riders lose control and fall head first; without the assistance of ski poles, they may be unable to extricate themselves and can quickly suffocate.

The vast majority of the skiing literature pertains to alpine or downhill skiing, with only a handful of articles evaluating injury profiles in the other disciplines within the sport. In cross-country skiing the two most common injuries are sprains of the medial collateral ligament of the knee (MCL) and sprains of the UCL.[20] Telemark skiers injure the foot and ankle most frequently (28%), with about one-third of those being fractures, followed by the knee (20%) and head and neck (17%); beginners tend to injure the foot and ankle whereas advanced telemark skiers are more likely to injure the knee.[2] The binding system, with the heel being free (Fig. 16-5), has been implicated as a causative factor in the high number of foot and ankle injuries, as opposed to downhill skiing where the boot is more rigid, relaying force to the knee. The vast majority of telemark ski injuries result from falls, followed by collisions and jumps.[2] Injury patterns in disabled skiers have not been evaluated in depth; however, incidence and types of injuries seem to be fairly comparable in able-bodied and disabled downhill and XC skiers, although injuries tend to be less severe in disabled skiers.[21,22]

It is helpful to understand the biomechanics of snowboarding to properly evaluate the injured snowboarder. Snowboarders stand affixed to their snowboard, typically with the rear foot at 90 degrees to the long axis and the front foot (or lead leg) at 45 to 90 degrees to the long axis. The mechanisms of turning and stopping incorporate leaning in toward the downhill slope by shifting the center of gravity either toward the front or toward the back (Fig. 16-6), which predisposes to forward falls on the outstretched hands or backward falls on the hands, buttocks, or head. Aerial maneuvers can be performed by launching off an upward incline (either the wall of a halfpipe, a built-up jump, or a natural rise in the terrain), with various combinations of inversion and rotations performed while in the air (Fig. 16-7).

Turning and regular snowboarding maneuvers account for over half of injuries, whereas jumping accounts for about 11%. However, with advancing skill and confidence, snowboarders attempt new tricks

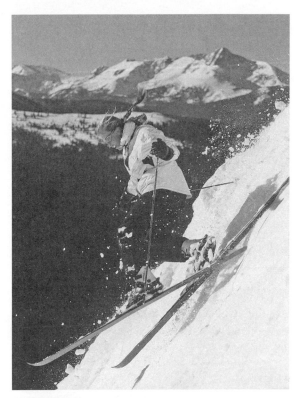

FIGURE 16-5 The binding system, with the free heel, has been implicated as a causative factor in the high number of foot and ankle injuries in telemark skiing, as opposed to downhill skiing where the boot is more rigid, transferring force to the knee. (Photo reproduced courtesy of Vail Resorts Inc.)

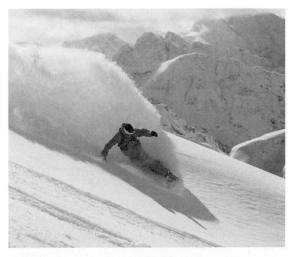

FIGURE 16-6 Snowboarder shown carving with the center of gravity focused on the frontside edge of the board. (©2007 Burton Snowboards.)

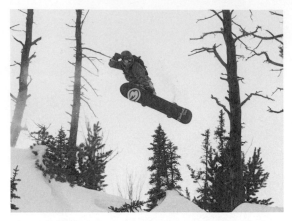

FIGURE 16-7 Snowboarder performing aerial frontside grab. (©2007 Burton Snowboards.)

and ride increasingly difficult terrain (Fig. 16-8), resulting in alteration in injury patterns among competitive snowboarders. The elite snowboarder has a higher incidence of shoulder, clavicular, back, and knee injuries, and a lower incidence of hand and wrist injuries.[11,23]

UPPER EXTREMITY INJURIES

One-half to two-thirds of all snowboarding injuries involve the upper extremities, and almost half of these injuries are fractures.[5,6,24] Wrist injuries account for 22% of all snowboarding injuries and are the most common site of upper extremity involvement (18% to 20%), followed by the shoulder (16% to 7%)

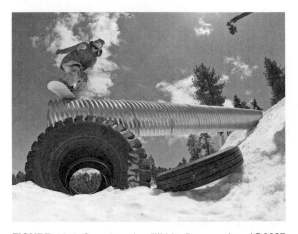

FIGURE 16-8 Snowboarder "jibbing" on a pipe. (©2007 Burton Snowboards.)

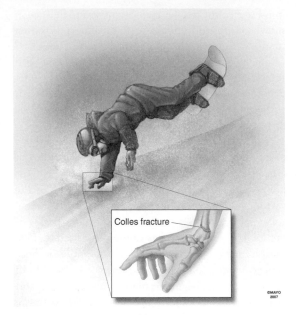

FIGURE 16-9 A forward fall on the outstretched hand is a common mechanism for wrist injury in snowboarding. The snowboarder's feet are fixed to the board and the force of landing on the slope is placed on the hand and transmitted proximally.

and elbow (7.9%)[24]; snowboarders are 10 times more likely to sustain wrist injuries than their skiing counterparts. Ninety-six percent of wrist injuries are caused by falls, and distal radius fractures are twice as likely to occur with a backward fall (Fig. 16-9).[5,11] While sprains, dislocations, and scaphoid fractures are commonly observed, up to 66% of wrist injuries are fractures. Fractures are more common in beginners, women, and younger participants, but intermediate to advanced riders are more likely to sustain more severe fractures, scaphoid fractures, or other hand, shoulder, and elbow injuries.[5]

Nearly one-third of snowboarding injuries involve the shoulder, typically sustained during a forward fall on an outstretched hand or directly on the shoulder. Of these injuries, acromioclavicular separations are the most common (32%), followed by anterior dislocations of the glenohumeral joint.[5] In skiing, shoulder injuries are less frequently encountered, at a rate of 4% to 11% of all skiing injuries, and are usually rotator cuff tears, glenohumeral dislocations or subluxations, or sprains of the acromioclavicular joint.

Elbow injuries, like shoulder and hand injuries, are more likely to occur in the intermediate to advanced snowboarder, usually in association with a fall on an outstretched hand with the elbow in extension. The transmission of longitudinal thrust force through the radial head, ulna, and distal humerus can result in a variety of fracture and dislocation patterns. Although the rate of elbow injuries is low (4% to 8%), snowboarders are three times more likely than skiers to sustain elbow injuries.[5,25]

Injury to the UCL, although originally known as gamekeeper's thumb (related to injuries seen in Scottish rabbit keepers), is now referred to as "skier's thumb." In alpine skiing, the typical mechanism for injury is a fall in powder snow while grasping ski poles. While the open hand is forced downward through the snow by the body's momentum, the pole remains relatively stationary atop the snow's surface, thereby exerting an abduction moment at the first metacarpophalangeal joint (Fig. 16-10).

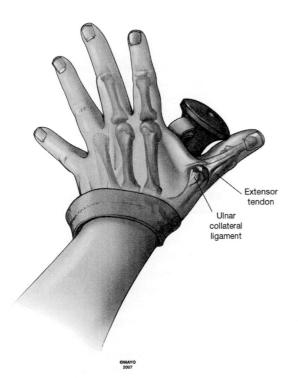

FIGURE 16-10 "Skier's thumb" typically occurs when a skier falls in powder while grasping the ski pole: as the open hand is forced downward through the snow by the body's momentum, the pole remains relatively stationary atop the snow's surface, thereby exerting an abduction moment at the first metacarpophalangeal joint.

Skier's thumb accounts for 8% of all injuries that occur in alpine skiing and is the most common injury seen in adolescents.[3] Typically, a skier will present with a history of falling with pole in hand and noticeable swelling and pain at the base of the thumb. There is exquisite tenderness along the UCL, and ligamentous stress testing reveals pain or valgus laxity with complete tears. A Stener lesion can be seen, with complete disruption of the UCL, when the distal attachment is avulsed and becomes entrapped under the adductor aponeurosis, thereby preventing proper healing and leading to chronic instability of the joint. Due to the risk of long-term disability secondary to pain and associated early degenerative arthritis with complete ruptures of the UCL, surgical repair is recommended. Otherwise, simple sprains to the UCL can be treated conservatively with immobilization for 3 weeks. In contrast to the high incidence of UCL and other hand injuries sustained while skiing, injuries to the hand are relatively infrequent during snowboarding. Advanced-level riders are more likely to sustain hand injuries, and of those, fractures are the most common, followed by sprains and dislocations.[5]

LOWER EXTREMITY INJURIES

Lower extremity injuries occur with less frequency and are typically less severe in snowboarders than in alpine skiers.[6,10,11] When compared with skiers, snowboarders are probably less susceptible to ligamentous injuries of the knee, as the snowboard is fixed to both feet and is unable to act as a lever transmitting rotational forces through the joint.[6] Nearly three-quarters of all lower extremity snowboarding injuries occur in the forward or front leg.[9,11] Equipment selection may also contribute to injury patterns, as most snowboarders prefer a soft boot, which provides minimal ankle support. And while hard-shelled boots reduce the risk of ankle injury, they increase the risk of knee injury.[9–11]

An injury unique to snowboarding and sinister in presentation is a fracture of the lateral process of the talus (LPT), otherwise known as "snowboarder's ankle" (Fig. 16-11). Until snowboarding became mainstream, fractures of the LPT were considered a rarity.[26] Nearly half of snowboarding ankle injuries are fractures, and LPT fractures account for nearly one-third of these, typically after a high-impact fall or landing a jump with a twisting aerial maneuver.[27–30]

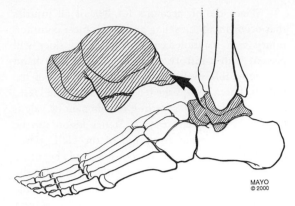

FIGURE 16-11 Lateral perspective of the hindfoot, showing *in situ* anatomy of the lateral process of the talus, with its two articular surfaces: the trochlea, which articulates with the proximal fibula, and the talocalcaneal joint.

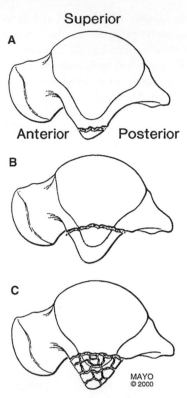

FIGURE 16-12 LPT fractures are classified based on the presence of comminution and involvement of the talofibular and talocalcaneal articular surfaces of the subtalar joint. **A.** Type I: small chip fracture off the anterior and inferior portion of the articular process without involvement of the articular surfaces. **B.** Type 2: simple fracture that involves the articular surface and may or may not be displaced. **C.** Type 3: comminuted fracture, involving the entire lateral process and articular surfaces.

LPT fractures often masquerade as an inversion ankle sprain, with the snowboarder presenting with anterolateral ankle pain and swelling, difficulty weight-bearing, and possible discontinuation of riding for the day (which should always raise suspicion of a severe injury in a snowboarder). Physical examination is often limited by the amount of local swelling and soft-tissue pain, but with LPT fracture there will be point tenderness just inferior to the tip of the lateral malleolus, as opposed to a lateral collateral ligament sprain, which should be more tender anterior and inferior to the lateral malleolus.

One should also have a heightened index of suspicion for LPT fractures when treating a snowboarder with a presumed ankle sprain who has failed conservative therapy or has persistent pain. In this setting it is imperative to search for a definitive diagnosis with imaging studies, as failure to diagnose these fractures promptly may result in sequelae such as avascular necrosis, secondary arthritis, and loose body formation, all of which may lead to significant disability.[6,26,29] Due to the complexity of the ankle joint and the precise degree of internal rotation (10–20 degrees) required to image the LPT, conventional x-rays miss nearly half of LPT fractures and often underestimate the extent of the fracture and degree of displacement of the fracture fragments. For this reason, computed tomography (CT) or magnetic resonance imaging (MRI) is recommended to classify injury and thereby determine treatment.[26]

Management of LPT fractures is based on the fracture type (Fig. 16-12). Surgical intervention is generally warranted for type II and III injuries; Valderrabano et al. demonstrated improved outcomes with open reduction internal fixation (ORIF) of type II fractures after a 3½-year period.[30] Patients treated surgically in this study showed fewer degenerative changes and a higher rate of return to pre-injury activity levels than those treated nonoperatively. Restoration of surface anatomy may not be possible in severely comminuted fractures, in which case debridement is performed, often with drilling of the chondral surface, in an attempt to salvage the joint. In short, LPT fractures are fairly unique to snowboarders and are frequently missed. As the complication rate is high and surgical intervention may be necessary, it is crucial to be aware of LPT fractures in the snowboarding population.

Knee injuries are by far the most common injury seen in skiing, accounting for 30% of all injuries.[3] Ligamentous injuries, especially involving the MCL and anterior cruciate ligament (ACL), dominate, with sprains of the MCL accounting for 18% of all skiing injuries alone. The MCL is typically injured through a rotational or valgus stress placed upon the knee. Isolated MCL injuries can usually be treated nonoperatively, but may be surgically repaired when combined with an ACL rupture.[31]

Isolated ACL injuries in skiing account for 49% of all knee injuries.[32] Common mechanisms of injury to the ACL include the following:

1. Valgus external rotation, when the skier catches the tip of the ski on the snow or a gate.
2. Boot-induced anterior drawer, which usually occurs as a skier lands from a jump or mogul and falls backward—with the knee in a flexed position, pressure from the boot top against the calf produces an anterior drawer, compounded by contraction of the quadriceps as the skier tries to recover.
3. A combination of internal rotation and extension, usually due to the skier crossing the tips of the skis.
4. What is often referred to in the literature as a "phantom-foot" or "phantom-fall" injury.[33,34] The phantom fall mechanism is seen when the skier gets off balance to the rear, with the hips below the knees, while the ski continues to internally rotate, resulting in ACL rupture (Fig.16-13).[33] This can occur when the skier attempts to get up while still moving after a fall, attempts to sit down after losing control, or tries to recover from an off-balance position.

Isolated posterior cruciate ligament tears are rare, accounting for fewer than 1% of knee injuries.[31]

Although multidirectional ski boot-binding release mechanisms have decreased lower extremity fractures by 90%,[35] "boot top" fractures involving the tibia and fibula still occur when the boot-binding mechanism fails to release, resulting in torque forces applied to the tibia and fibula just proximal to the boot. These fractures need immediate medical attention because of the obvious instability of the leg, but also because tibial fractures tend to heal slowly due to poor blood supply necessitating ORIF.

Other tibial bony injuries include tibial plateau fractures, distal tibial plafond fractures, and avulsion fractures of the tibial spine or eminence. The latter can occur with the same mechanism of injury seen in ACL ruptures, but avulsion of the distal attachment

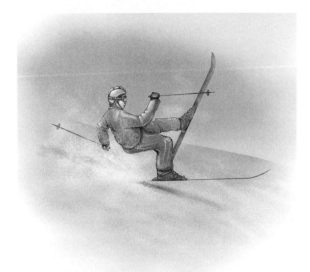

FIGURE 16-13 A "phantom fall" often occurs in beginners, when a skier loses his or her balance backward, with the hips below the flexed knees, the uphill arm dragging behind, the uphill ski unweighted, and weight on the inside edge of the downhill ski tail, while the ski continues to internally rotate, resulting in an ACL rupture.

of the ACL causes a fracture that extends through the epiphysis of the tibia. Although the presentation is very similar to ACL injuries, tibial eminence fractures are typically more painful. The avulsed fragment will be evident on plain radiographs, but further imaging with CT or MRI is warranted, to determine whether conservative management or ORIF is necessary, depending on the degree of displacement and comminution of the fragment. Isolated fibular fractures were commonplace when high ski boots were initially used, but now are relatively rare.

SPINE INJURIES

Spine injuries account for about 3% of snowboarding injuries, and if simple contusions are included, the total goes up to 8%.[10,36] Snowboarders often approach the ski hill with the intent to perform jumps and other aerial maneuvers. Whether hucking a cliff, riding the halfpipe, or jibbing on a rail (Fig. 16-14), they spend more time in the air and are at significantly higher risk for spine injuries compared to skiers.[36,37] A large Japanese study showed that the majority of spine injuries sustained

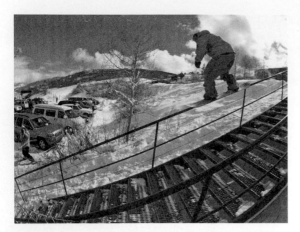

FIGURE 16-14 Snowboarder performing a railslide on a stair rail. (©2007 Burton Snowboards.)

while snowboarding are anterior compression fractures (45%) and transverse process fractures (40%) and occur most frequently in the lumbar spine.[36] Most traumatic spinal cord injuries suffered while snowboarding are a result of backward falls after a poorly controlled intentional jump and are typically of the flexion-distraction type.[36,38,39] Skiers are more at risk of sustaining spine injuries from falling, and although collisions account for only approximately 5% of spine injuries in both populations, they tend to result in the most severe spinal injuries.[40]

HEAD INJURIES

Head injuries are more common in snowboarders than in skiers, with concussions and closed head injuries accounting for 2% to 10% of snowboarding injuries.[10,41] Head injuries occur most frequently in young, male, beginner snowboarders, and typical mechanisms include backward falls and falls during jumping.[41] Most head injuries are mild, with initial Glasgow coma scores of 13 to 15.[42] Tree collisions in both skiers and snowboarders are the most common cause of more severe head injuries with higher mortality rates.[42]

SPLENIC INJURIES

Overall, snowboarders are 6 times more likely to sustain splenic injuries than skiers, likely due to the fact that the majority of boarders ride with the left side of their body forward; the risk for males is 20 times that

for females.[43] The majority of splenic injuries are caused by falls (69.7%) and jumping (25.6%), with less than 5% caused by collisions.[43] In skiers, splenic injuries occur in two patterns: in association with low-energy falls on moguls with delayed presentation, or in high-energy collisions necessitating emergent medical care with other associated abdominal injuries.[44] The textbook complaint after a splenic injury is left upper quadrant pain radiating to the left shoulder (Kehr sign), but symptoms may be more vague. The onset of symptoms can be insidious and range from nausea and vague abdominal discomfort to more classic left upper quadrant or chest pain. Peritoneal signs and left upper quadrant tenderness may be evident on examination. Whether the patient is hemodynamically stable or not, he or she should be urgently evaluated by a surgeon if a splenic injury is suspected.

INJURY PREVENTION

The approach to injury prevention in skiers and snowboarders is multifaceted. Both intrinsic and extrinsic factors should be addressed in preparation for hitting the slopes. Intrinsic factors include physical conditioning, sport-specific training, education, and mental preparedness. Proper equipment selection and care, use of protective equipment, and attention to environmental factors are keys to safe participation in both skiing and snowboarding.[45] Injuries are more common in novice alpine participants, particularly those who have not taken lessons.[10,36,39] Formal on-hill lessons are desirable, but even educational videos have been shown to reduce injury risk in skiing by 30%.[46]

Skiing and snowboarding place high demands on the body. It is important for participants to establish optimal sport-specific strength and power as well as aerobic capacity, as deficits in any of these areas may lead to fatigue and predispose to injury. Baseline fitness should be maintained throughout the winter season as well as during the off-season with an appropriate cross-training program. No specific strengthening programs have been shown to reduce injury rates in skiing or snowboarding; however, recognizing and addressing individual strength deficits can decrease the risk of injury.

Equipment selection and care are critical in injury prevention. Most skiers use a hard boot, but snowboarders have the choice of soft, hard, or hybrid boots. While a more supportive boot may help prevent ankle injuries, there is an increased rate of knee injuries.[9–11] Ski boots with a rearward cuff release have been shown to decrease stress on the ACL during boot-induced anterior drawer-type stress.[47] Ski length and width are also important to consider, as a longer ski is more difficult to turn and can translate torque to the knee. Releasable bindings have dramatically reduced the number of lower extremity injuries, but they may be ineffective if not properly cared for or adjusted for the appropriate skill level.[46,48] The rate of injuries sustained on rental equipment is twice that of injuries on personal equipment.[45] This may in part be due to people overestimating their ability at the time of renting, with lack of equipment adjustment appropriate for skill level.

Beginner snowboarders are particularly at risk for wrist injuries,[5,6,24] and despite the fact that cadaveric studies show little efficacy of wrist guards, clinical studies show a reduced fracture risk of 50% to 100%.[5,49–53] There has been concern that wrist guards may translate force to the elbow, thereby increasing elbow injuries; however, this has not been observed.[5,53] Wrist guards are readily available and should be encouraged.

The role of functional knee bracing after ACL injury is somewhat controversial, although the consensus at this time is that athletes returning to the slopes with an ACL-deficient knee should use a low-profile, lightweight, functional knee stabilizer brace. Biomechanical studies have documented decreased anterior tibial translation, at least under low loads, and most subjects report significant benefit, with increased subjective knee stability.[54] Use of functional bracing in the stable, post-ACL reconstructed knee remains controversial, as the majority of studies to date have not demonstrated improved range of motion, decreased pain, improved graft stability, or decreased reinjury rate,[55] so the overall consensus at this time is that bracing is not indicated.

Given that the rates of injury to the head and cervical spine of skiers and snowboarders can approach 20% of all injuries, the effect of helmet use has been investigated. There has been discussion of helmets obstructing peripheral vision and decreasing auditory acuity, thereby causing more collisions and falls. However, Macnab et al. found no increase in collision rates among children using helmets,[56] and in that same study, the decrease in head injuries did not correlate with an increased risk of cervical spine injury. Overall, the use of a helmet has been found to decrease the risk of head injury among skiers and

snowboarders by 30% to 60%.[56,57] Beginning snowboarders should be educated early as to the risk of head injury and the importance of regular helmet use.

REHABILITATION AFTER INJURY

In the rehabilitation of injured skiers or snowboarders, where the overall goal is to allow the athlete to return to his or her prior level of function as quickly as possible, the rehabilitation principles utilized are relatively standard and can be applied to any injury site. These include pain control, regaining flexibility, strengthening, proprioceptive re-education, and sport-specific training including power, speed, and coordination. One must also take into account any specific factors or deficits that may have contributed to the initial injury when prescribing an individualized program. In addition to the use of physical agents and modalities, therapeutic exercise, and manual medicine techniques, a host of psychological factors may influence recovery, and these should also be addressed, particularly in the elite athlete.[58,59]

In the acute phase of recovery, pain control is achieved through cryotherapy, elevation, and compression,[60] in conjunction with relative rest and splinting as clinically indicated. In any situations where prolonged immobilization is necessary, such as after a fracture, recovery can be optimized with the use of gentle stretching[61] and by eccentric training of the contralateral limb.[62]

Stretching

Throughout the healing process, stretching should be employed to regain full range of motion, with the end goal of achieving symmetric range of motion between limbs and decreasing injury occurrence or recurrence.[63,64] It is important that the athlete understand not only the goal of stretching, but also the correct technique and duration that should be employed. In general, alpine skiing and snowboarding stretches should include the ankle plantar flexors, the hamstrings and quadriceps, the hip groups, the lumbar spine, and the shoulder groups.

Strengthening

As the athlete regains pain-free range of motion with adequate flexibility, a strengthening program can be initiated. The skier/snowboarder who is physically unfit can make gains in all areas from a generalized training program; however, the elite athlete needs more specific training and practice of highly coordinated tasks to notice improvement. It is generally thought that the type of training undertaken directly correlates only with performance of that specifically trained task, with regard to the type and pattern of movement, the velocity of training, and the range of motion and angle at which the exercise is performed. However, recent evidence suggests that eccentric training can increase both concentric and eccentric strength,[65] and can reduce the risk of muscle injury.[66–68]

In skiers and snowboarders, the quadriceps maintains body positioning and sustains constant concentric and eccentric stresses during activities such as carving, skiing moguls, and landing jumps; therefore, strengthening of this muscle group is paramount. In addition, lower extremity strengthening should include the hamstrings and hip groups. It has been postulated that hamstring dominance can stabilize the ACL-deficient knee and may decrease the risk of ACL injury.[69] Closed kinetic chain exercises are often recommended, particularly in the case of rehabilitation after ACL injury or reconstruction, after early research indicated anterior displacement of the tibia with open chain exercises.[70] However, more recent studies indicate that this may not be well founded.[71–73] Lower extremity strengthening exercises can be both ski specific and functional; some examples include squats, lunges, leg press, step-ups, and bicycling with toe clips.

Upper body strengthening is also important, to help with balance, turning and rotational activities, and effective use of the ski pole, for example to push off during a race or when traversing flat areas. Closed kinetic chain exercises target multiple muscle groups simultaneously, and upper body strengthening should include push-ups (triceps), push-ups with a plus (adding protraction of the scapulae at the end of a pushup, strengthening the serratus anterior), pull-downs (latissimus dorsi), pull-backs and reverse flies (rhomboids), and shoulder shrugs (trapezius).

The muscular "core" is considered the foundation of all limb movement, and recent evidence contends that those with poor core stability are more prone to back and lower extremity injury, and that exercise to address such deficiencies may reduce injury.[74–76] Impaired core proprioception has been specifically linked to increased risk of knee injury in females.[77] Therefore, it is important that skiers and snowboarders incorporate a core stabilization program into their training regimen.

Speed and Power

Speed and power are essential in skiing/snowboarding, and must be incorporated into any comprehensive rehabilitation program. Plyometric exercises represent the power component, and should be initiated as the athlete recovers.[78] Plyometric training has been shown to improve vertical jumping,[79] sprinting, running economy, and joint stability, and to reduce the risk of knee injuries.[80] Initially, low-level exercises are safer, with high-level plyometrics prescribed under supervision only as the athlete prepares to return to full activity after injury. Appropriate exercises for skiing/snowboarding include bounding, box jumps (Fig. 16-15), hopping, skipping, and tuck jumps.

Proprioceptive and Sport-Specific Training

Proprioceptive retraining should be an integral component of any rehabilitation program and can often be initiated immediately after injury. Retraining the afferent–efferent neuromuscular control arc during both static and dynamic phases is important in both prevention and rehabilitation of

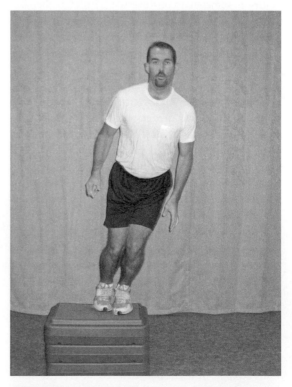

FIGURE 16-15 "Box jumping" plyometric exercise.

injuries,[81,82] particularly those involving the knee or ankle joint. These exercises can be as simple as single-legged stance, with or without the eyes closed, progressing to more challenging activities such as single-legged squats or catching a medicine ball while standing on one leg. Throwing and catching a medicine ball while balancing on a wobble board or semispherical exercise ball (Fig. 16-16), or while bouncing on a mini-trampoline, represent higher-level proprioceptive retraining activities that are relatively easy to implement and can be performed by the athlete independently for the most part.

Sport-specific training is the final but very important step when returning to skiing or snowboarding, as many of the motions involved are quite specific to these sports and, as noted above, exercise gains are specific to the training undertaken. Some examples include running or in-line skating through a slalom course, lateral squats (Fig. 16-17), use of a sliding board for hip adductor and abductor strengthening, balance training, and plyometric exercises to incorporate the explosive nature of many of the movements involved in skiing and snowboarding. Skateboarding and wakeboarding use many of the same muscle groups

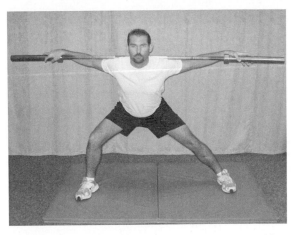

FIGURE 16-17 Ski-specific exercise: lateral squats with a weight bar.

and activation patterns as snowboarding, and can be incorporated, particularly during the off-season. Roller skis are available for ski cross-training during the off-season (Fig. 16-18), either for preseason training or when returning from injury.

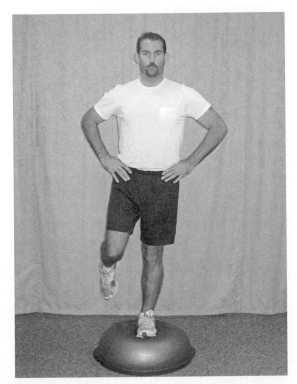

FIGURE 16-16 A semispherical exercise ball can be used for proprioceptive exercise.

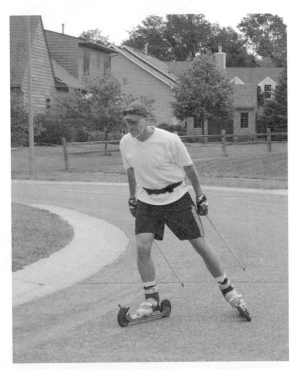

FIGURE 16-18 Ski-specific exercise: roller skiing is an effective simulation exercise that can be undertaken in the off-season or before returning from injury.

SUMMARY

Skiing and snowboarding are two very popular winter sports, with a relatively high risk of injury, and injury patterns unique to each sport. Appropriate conditioning and choice of equipment can have a significant impact on the risk of injury. Rehabilitation programs should emphasize flexibility, sport-specific strengthening, power, agility, proprioception, and cardiovascular fitness, and should be tailored to the individual, to ensure a successful return to the slopes.

REFERENCES

1. Tuggy ML. Telemark skiing injuries. *J Sports Med Phys Fitness.* 1996;36:217–222.
2. Made C, Borg H, Thelander D, et al. Telemark skiing injuries: an 11-year study. *Knee Surg Sports Traumatol Arthrosc.* 2001;9:386–391.
3. Moeller JL, Rifat SF. *Winter Sports Medicine Handbook.* New York: McGraw-Hill; 2004.
4. Langran M, Selvaraj S. Increased injury risk among first-day skiers, snowboarders, and skiboarders. *Am J Sports Med.* 2004;32:96–103.
5. Idzikowski JR, Janes PC, Abbott PJ. Upper extremity snowboarding injuries. Ten-year results from the Colorado snowboard injury survey. *Am J Sports Med.* 2000;28:825–832.
6. Bladin C, McCrory P, Pogorzelski A. Snowboarding injuries: current trends and future directions. *Sports Med.* 2004;34:133–139.
7. Ronning R, Gerner T, Engebretsen L. Risk of injury during alpine and telemark skiing and snowboarding. The equipment-specific distance-correlated injury index. *Am J Sports Med.* 2000;28:506–508.
8. Koehle MS, Lloyd-Smith R, Taunton JE. Alpine ski injuries and their prevention. *Sports Med.* 2002;32:785–793.
9. Pino EC, Colville MR. Snowboard injuries. *Am J Sports Med.* 1989;17:778–781.
10. Chow TK, Corbett SW, Farstad DJ. Spectrum of injuries from snowboarding. *J Trauma.* 1996;41:321–325.
11. Davidson TM, Laliotis AT. Snowboarding injuries, a four-year study with comparison with alpine ski injuries. *West J Med.* 1996;164:231–237.
12. Hackam DJ, Kreller M, Pearl RH. Snow-related recreational injuries in children: assessment of morbidity and management strategies. *J Pediatr Surg.* 1999;34:65–68.
13. O'Neill DF, McGlone MR. Injury risk in first-time snowboarders versus first-time skiers. *Am J Sports Med.* 1999;27:94–97.
14. Sacco DE, Sartorelli DH, Vane DW. Evaluation of alpine skiing and snowboarding injury in a northeastern state. *J Trauma.* 1998;44:654–659.
15. Matsumoto K, Miyamoto K, Sumi H, et al. Upper extremity injuries in snowboarding and skiing: a comparative study. *Clin J Sport Med.* 2002;12:354–359.
16. Prall JA, Winston KR, Brennan R. Severe snowboarding injuries. *Injury.* 1995;26:539–542.
17. Morrow PL, McQuillen EN, Eaton LA Jr, et al. Downhill ski fatalities: the Vermont experience. *J Trauma.* 1988;28:95–100.
18. Xiang H, Stallones L. Deaths associated with snow skiing in Colorado 1980–1981 to 2000–2001 ski seasons. *Injury.* 2003;34:892–896.
19. Xiang H, Stallones L, Smith GA. Downhill skiing injury fatalities among children. *Inj Prev.* 2004;10:99–102.
20. Smith M, Matheson GO, Meeuwisse WH. Injuries in cross-country skiing: a critical appraisal of the literature. *Sports Med.* 1996;21:239–250.
21. Laskowski ER, Murtaugh PA. Snow skiing injuries in physically disabled skiers. *Am J Sports Med.* 1992;20:553–557.
22. Schmid A, Huring H, Huber G, et al. Injury risk of competitive, handicapped cross-country skiers in training and competition. *Sportverletz Sportschaden.* 1998;12:26–30.
23. Torjussen J, Bahr R. Injuries among competitive snowboarders at the national elite level. *Am J Sports Med.* 2005;33:370–377.
24. Sasaki K, Takagi M, Ida H, et al. Severity of upper limb injuries in snowboarding. *Arch Orthop Trauma Surg.* 1999;119:292–295.
25. Takagi M, Sasaki K, Kiyoshige Y, et al. Fracture and dislocation of snowboarder's elbow. *J Trauma.* 1999;47:77–81.
26. Bonvin F, Montet X, Copercini M, et al. Imaging of fractures of the lateral process of the talus, a frequently missed diagnosis. *Eur J Radiol.* 2003;47:64–70.
27. Boon AJ, Smith J, Laskowski ER. Snowboarding injuries—general patterns, with a focus on talus fractures. *Phys Sportsmed.* 1999;27:94–104.
28. Boon AJ, Smith J, Zobitz ME, et al. Snowboarder's talus fracture. Mechanism of injury. *Am J Sports Med.* 2001;29:333–338.
29. Funk JR, Srinivasan SC, Crandall JR. Snowboarder's talus fractures experimentally produced by eversion and dorsiflexion. *Am J Sports Med.* 2003;31:921–928.
30. Valderrabano V, Perren T, Ryf C, et al. Snowboarder's talus fracture: treatment outcome of 20 cases after 3.5 years. *Am J Sports Med.* 2005;33:871–880.
31. Paletta GA, Warren RF. Knee injuries and alpine skiing. Treatment and rehabilitation. *Sports Med.* 1994;17:411–423.
32. Warme WJ, Feagin JA Jr, King P, et al. Ski injury statistics, 1982 to 1993, Jackson Hole Ski Resort. *Am J Sports Med.* 1995;23:597–600.
33. Steadman JR, Scheinberg RR. Skiing injuries. In: Nicholas JA, Hershman EB, eds. *The Lower Extremity and Spine in Sports Medicine.* St. Louis: Mosby; 1995:1376–1380.
34. St-Onge N, Chevalier Y, Hagemeister N, et al. Effect of ski binding parameters on knee biomechanics: a three-dimensional computational study. *Med Sci Sports Exerc.* 2004;36:1218–1225.
35. Johnson RJ, Ettlinger CF, Shealy JE. Skier injury trends. In: Skiing Trauma and Safety: Seventh International Symposium. Philadelphia: American Society for Testing and Materials; 1989:25–31.
36. Yamakawa H, Murase S, Sakai H, et al. Spinal injuries in snowboarders: risk of jumping as an integral part of snowboarding. *J Trauma.* 2001;50:1101–1105.

37. Tarazi F, Dvorak MF, Wing PC. Spinal injuries in skiers and snowboarders. *Am J Sports Med.* 1999;27:177–180.
38. Seino H, Kawaguchi S, Sekine M, et al. Traumatic paraplegia in snowboarders. *Spine.* 2001;26:1294–1297.
39. Wakahara K, Matsumoto K, Sumi H, et al. Traumatic spinal cord injuries from snowboarding. *Am J Sports Med.* 2006;34:1670–1674.
40. Kip P, Hunter RE. Cervical spinal fractures in alpine skiers. *Orthopedics.* 1995;18:737–741.
41. Nakaguchi H, Fujimaki T, Ueki K, et al. Snowboard head injury: prospective study in Chino, Nagano, for two seasons from 1995 to 1997. *J Trauma.* 1999;46:1066–1069.
42. Levy AS, Hawkes AP, Hemminger LM, et al. An analysis of head injuries among skiers and snowboarders. *J Trauma.* 2002;53:695–704.
43. Geddes R, Irish K. Boarder belly: splenic injuries resulting from ski and snowboarding accidents. *Emerg Med Australas.* 2005;17:157–162.
44. Sartorelli KH, Pilcher DB, Rogers FB. Patterns of splenic injuries seen in skiers. *Injury.* 1995;26:43–46.
45. Bouter LM, Knipschild PG, Volovics A. Personal and environmental factors in relation to injury risk in downhill skiing. *Int J Sports Med.* 1989;10:298–301.
46. Jlrgensen U, Fredensborg T, Haraszuk JP, et al. Reduction of injuries in downhill skiing by use of an instructional ski-video: a prospective randomised intervention study. *Knee Surg Sports Traumatol Arthrosc.* 1998;6:194–200.
47. Benoit DL, Lamontagne M, Greaves C, et al. Effect of Alpine ski boot cuff release on knee joint force during the backward fall. *Res Sports Med.* 2005;13:317–330.
48. Finch CF, Kelsall HL. The effectiveness of ski bindings and their professional adjustment for preventing alpine skiing injuries. *Sports Med.* 1998;25:407–416.
49. Giacobetti FB, Sharkey PF, Bos-Giacobetti MA, et al. Biomechanical analysis of the effectiveness of in-line skating wrist guards for preventing wrist fractures. *Am J Sports Med.* 1997;25:223–225.
50. Greenwald RM, Janes PC, Swanson SC, et al. Dynamic impact response of human cadaveric forearms using a wrist brace. *Am J Sports Med.* 1998;26:825–830.
51. Machold W, Kwasny O, Eisenhardt P, et al. Reduction of severe wrist injuries in snowboarding by an optimized wrist protection device: a prospective randomized trial. *J Trauma.* 2002;52:517–520.
52. O'Neill DF. Wrist injuries in guarded versus unguarded first time snowboarders. *Clin Orthop Relat Res.* 2003:91–95.
53. Ronning R, Ronning I, Gerner T, et al. The efficacy of wrist protectors in preventing snowboarding injuries. *Am J Sports Med.* 2001;29:581–585.
54. Chew KTL. Current evidence and clinical applications of therapeutic knee braces. *Am J Phys Med Rehabil.* 2007;86:678–686.
55. Wright RW, Fetzer GB. Bracing after ACL reconstruction: a systematic review. *Clin Orthop Relat Res.* 2007;455:162–168.
56. Macnab AJ, Smith T, Gagnon FA, et al. Effect of helmet wear on the incidence of head/face and cervical spine injuries in young skiers and snowboarders. *Inj Prev.* 2002;8:324–327.
57. Sulheim S, Holme I, Ekeland A, et al. Helmet use and risk of head injuries in alpine skiers and snowboarders. *JAMA.* 2006;295:919–924.
58. Bauman J. Returning to play: the mind does matter. *Clin J Sport Med.* 2005;15:432–435.
59. Smith AM, Scott SG, Wiese DM. The psychological effects of sports injuries. Coping. *Sports Med.* 1990;9:352–369.
60. Hubbard TJ, Denegar CR. Does cryotherapy improve outcomes with soft tissue injury? *J Athl Train.* 2004;39:278–279.
61. Mattiello-Sverzut AC, Carvalho LC, Cornachione A, et al. Morphological effects of electrical stimulation and intermittent muscle stretch after immobilization in soleus muscle. *Histol Histopathol.* 2006;21:957–964.
62. Housh TJ, Housh DJ, Weir JP, et al. Effects of eccentric-only resistance training and detraining. *Int J Sports Med.* 1996;17:145–148.
63. Hartig DE, Henderson JM. Increasing hamstring flexibility decreases lower extremity overuse injuries in military basic trainees. *Am J Sports Med.* 1999;27:173–176.
64. Krivickas LS, Feinberg JH. Lower extremity injuries in college athletes: relation between ligamentous laxity and lower extremity muscle tightness. *Arch Phys Med Rehabil.* 1996;77:1139–1143.
65. Vikne H, Refsnes PE, Ekmark M, et al. Muscular performance after concentric and eccentric exercise in trained men. *Med Sci Sports Exerc.* 2006;38:1770–1781.
66. Askling C, Karlsson J, Thorstensson A. Hamstring injury occurrence in elite soccer players after preseason strength training with eccentric overload. *Scand J Med Sci Sports.* 2003;13:244–250.
67. Brooks JH, Fuller CW, Kemp SP, et al. Incidence, risk, and prevention of hamstring muscle injuries in professional rugby union. *Am J Sports Med.* 2006;34:1297–1306.
68. Gabbe BJ, Branson R, Bennell KL. A pilot randomised controlled trial of eccentric exercise to prevent hamstring injuries in community-level Australian football. *J Sci Med Sport.* 2006;9:103–109.
69. Ahmad CS, Clark AM, Heilmann N, et al. Effect of gender and maturity on quadriceps-to-hamstring strength ratio and anterior cruciate ligament laxity. *Am J Sports Med.* 2006;34:370–374.
70. Yack HJ, Collins CE, Whieldon TJ. Comparison of closed and open kinetic chain exercise in the anterior cruciate ligament-deficient knee. *Am J Sports Med.* 1993;21:49–54.
71. Morrissey MC, Hudson ZL, Drechsler WI, et al. Effects of open versus closed kinetic chain training on knee laxity in the early period after anterior cruciate ligament reconstruction. *Knee Surg Sports Traumatol Arthrosc.* 2000;8:343–348.
72. Perry MC, Morrissey MC, King JB, et al. Effects of closed versus open kinetic chain knee extensor resistance training on knee laxity and leg function in patients during the 8- to 14-week post-operative period after anterior cruciate ligament reconstruction. *Knee Surg Sports Traumatol Arthrosc.* 2005;13:357–369.
73. Perry MC, Morrissey MC, Morrissey D, et al. Knee extensors kinetic chain training in anterior cruciate ligament deficiency. *Knee Surg Sports Traumatol Arthrosc.* 2005;13:638–648.
74. Leetun DT, Ireland ML, Willson JD, et al. Core stability measures as risk factors for lower extremity injury in athletes. *Med Sci Sports Exerc.* 2004;36:926–934.

75. Peate W, Bates G, Lunda K, et al. Core strength: a new model for injury prediction and prevention. *J Occup Med Toxicol.* 2007;2:3.

76. Willson JD, Dougherty CP, Ireland ML, et al. Core stability and its relationship to lower extremity function and injury. *J Am Acad Orthop Surg.* 2005;13:316–325.

77. Zazulak BT, Hewett TE, Reeves NP, et al. The effects of core proprioception on knee injury: a prospective biomechanical–epidemiological study. *Am J Sports Med.* 2007;35:368–373.

78. Chu D. *Jumping into Plyometrics.* Champaign, IL: Leisure Press; 1992.

79. Markovic G. Does plyometric training improve vertical jump height? A meta-analytical review. *Br J Sports Med.* 2007;41:349–355; discussion, 55.

80. Impellizzeri FM, Castagna C, Rampinini E, et al. Effect of plyometric training on sand versus grass on muscle soreness, jumping and sprinting ability in soccer players. *Br J Sports Med.* 2008;42:42–46.

81. Laskowski ER, Newcomer-Aney K, Smith J. Proprioception. *Phys Med Rehabil Clin N Am.* 2000;11:323–340, vi.

82. Lephart SM, Pincivero DM, Giraldo JL, et al. The role of proprioception in the management and rehabilitation of athletic injuries. *Am J Sports Med.* 1997;25:130–137.

Gymnastics Injuries

E valuating and diagnosing injuries that result from the sport of gymnastics can be a very difficult and challenging task. As with other sports, injuries can occur in the upper or lower extremity, can affect the spine, and can either be acute or chronic in nature. However, because the injuries from gymnastics are often "masked" by overuse, it is sometimes difficult to diagnose an underlying problem. For example, shoulder pathology may present as rotator cuff tendonitis or impingement syndrome, but the cause of the pain may ultimately be due to either the labrum or os acromiale.

With the large number of participants that are training at advanced levels at adolescent ages, it is common for injuries to occur.[1] Trends show participants to be ever younger and to have an ever increasing number of training hours. For example, the average junior elite female gymnast (ages 10–14) has been reported to train an average of 5.36 days per week and 5.04 hours per day. As these numbers increase, it can be expected that the number of sport-related injuries will increase.[1]

The three most common injuries in 50 young elite female gymnasts were (i) nonspecific pain, (ii) sprains, and (iii) strains.[1] Examples of nonspecific pain were patello-femoral pain, ankle arthralgia, overuse syndromes, and general pain found in the ankle, wrist, and elbow. Unlike nearly all other youth sports, the most injured body part was the lumbar spine, followed by the knee, ankle, and wrist.

With these unique characteristics of gymnastics injuries in mind, this chapter will describe the techniques of evaluation, whether clinical examination or radiologic imaging should be used, and the most frequently observed injuries. Also included are, where applicable, selected differential diagnoses.

In order to better understand the sport of gymnastics, it is important to have a knowledge of the events and the body parts most affected by those events. In men's gymnastics, there are six events: floor exercise, vault, high bar, pommel horse, parallel bars, and still rings. Women's gymnastic competitors compete and train on four events: floor exercise, vault, uneven bars, and balance beam. Although the events are different, many areas are stressed on more than one event. For example, both the vault and the floor exercise place a high demand on the lower limbs. Landing from various events places the ankle and foot under large amounts of stress. The still rings place a great amount of stress on the shoulder, due to the strength skills that must be performed (Fig. 17-1). The pommel horse places high demands on the forearms and wrists due to the static contractions that are required.

It is important to know the terminology used within the sport, as it will help in obtaining a history and in coming to a diagnosis. A "tumbling pass" is performed on the floor exercise; this is when a participant runs and performs a series of tumbling skills—somersaults, round-offs, handsprings, and other skills. A "dismount" is when the athlete releases from an apparatus and lands on the mat, usually accompanied by a twisting or flipping element.

UPPER LIMB INJURIES

The upper limb is used for weight-bearing in gymnastics. As such, injuries to the shoulder and elbow are very common. A wide range of injuries can occur to these joints, but there are a number that are more frequently seen. In the shoulder, we will focus on tears of the superior labrum, symptomatic os acromiale, and short head biceps tears. For the elbow, we will focus on dislocations, ulnar collateral ligament tears, osteochondritis dissecans lesions of the capitellum, and olecranon stress fractures.

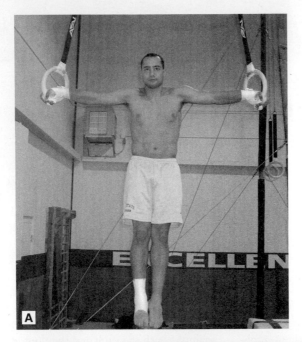

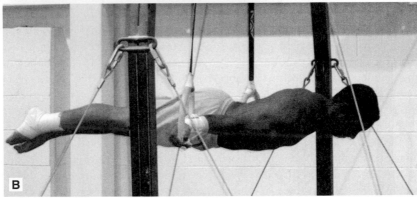

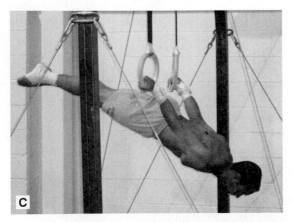

FIGURE 17-1 A. The iron cross. **B.** The Maltese cross. **C.** A reverse lever.

Superior Labral Tears (SLAP Lesions)

SLAP tears may occur during any gymnastic exercise, but the athlete may be particularly vulnerable during ring exercises.[2] In one series of five elite gymnasts with labral pathology, four of the athletes complained of an acute onset of pain during ring exercises in suspension while one suffered a slower onset of pain with parallel bar exercises.[2] In an effort to determine why these injuries occurred, an electromyographic study was performed on three normal gymnasts during exercises on the parallel bars and rings. There was noted to be a "critical phase" during ring exercises in suspension, in which the muscle activity around the shoulder was very low. This low level of muscle activity could potentially lead to greater stress on the articular cartilage and labrum.[2]

Athletes with a SLAP tear most commonly complain of pain, but clicking and/or instability also occur.[3] On physical examination, the patients may have biceps tenderness, positive Hawkins and Neer impingement signs, a positive Speed test, and/or a positive Yergason test.[3] Specialized tests such as the active compression test of O'Brien and the compressive-rotation test may also be positive.[3,4] However, a recent systematic review of the literature demonstrated that specialized tests for labral tears are not very specific or sensitive.[5] Magnetic resonance arthrography (MRA) can be very helpful in establishing the diagnosis, with a 93% sensitivity rate (Fig. 17-2).[3]

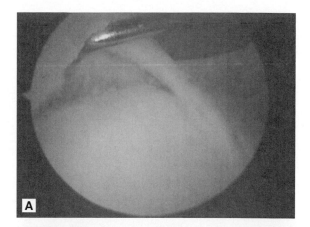

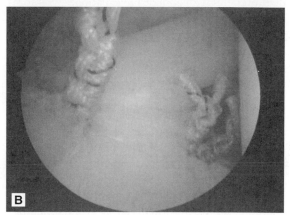

FIGURE 17-3 A. Arthoscopic picture of a displaceable superior labral tear. **B.** Arthroscopic repair of a superior labral tear.

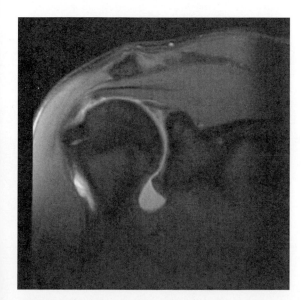

FIGURE 17-2 MR-arthrogram of a collegiate gymnast's shoulder demonstrating a superior labral tear.

The definitive treatment for symptomatic unstable SLAP lesions is arthroscopic labral repair (Fig. 17-3). One study showed that the overall success rate for this procedure for return to sport is 76%, but nonthrowing athletes (11 of 17 of these athletes were gymnasts) do significantly worse than throwing athletes.[3] The authors theorize that gymnastic events, particularly rings and parallel bar exercises, place greater stresses on the labral repair than do other sports, making the repair more vulnerable to reinjury.[2,3]

Symptomatic Os Acromiale

The acromion apophysis develops from four separate ossification centers; the basi-acromion fuses to the spine of the scapula by 12 years of age while the other centers fuse between 15 and 25 years of age.[6-9] Os acromiale occurs when there is a failure of union of these centers, and has an incidence of 1% to 15%.[6-9] The presence of an os acromiale on plain radiographs is usually an incidental finding that is not associated with pain in the shoulder.[9] However, in competitive athletes, such as gymnasts, repetitive use of the upper extremity may result in symptomatic instability of the os acromiale and the development of impingement-type symptoms and/or pain at the site of the nonunion.[6-9]

These athletes usually present with persistent shoulder pain over the deltoid or over the acromion that interferes with athletic participation.[6] Symptoms may also include impingement-type pain with overhead activities, night pain, and inability to sleep on the affected side.[6] Physical examination reveals pain with impingement testing, pain and weakness with resisted abduction of the shoulder, and tenderness over the nonunion site.[6] Plain radiographs, specifically the outlet and axillary views, will show the nonunion site while magnetic resonance imaging (MRI) will reveal the presence of edema at the site of an unstable os acromiale (Fig. 17-4).[6]

Initial treatment consists of activity limitation, a rehabilitation program including rotator cuff and scapular stabilizing exercises, anti-inflammatory medications, and corticosteroid injections.[6-9] Those athletes who do not respond to at least 3 to 6 months of nonsurgical management are considered for surgical intervention.[6-9] Surgical treatment consists of either open reduction and internal fixation of the os acromiale or arthroscopic excision of the unstable anterior portion of the acromion.[6-9] Peckett et al.[9] reported a union rate of 96% and a clinical success rate of 92% with open reduction and internal fixation of the os acromiale. In contrast, Abboud et al.[8] had a clinical success rate of only 37.5% with open reduction and internal fixation despite a successful fusion rate of 100%. Pagnani et al.[6] performed an arthroscopic excision of the unstable fragment in nine competitive athletes who each had persistent shoulder pain that interfered with athletic participation. All of the patients were able to return to full participation by 14 weeks after surgery, and none of the patients had any significant deficits in abduction, internal rotation, or external rotation compared with the opposite side.[6] An unstable os acromiale may be associated with an underlying rotator cuff tear that is repaired at the same time the os acromiale is addressed (Fig. 17-5).[8]

Short Head Biceps Muscle Tear

Another injury that these authors have seen almost exclusively in male gymnasts in the collegiate athletic population is a tear of the muscle belly of the short head of the biceps. Isolated rupture of the short head

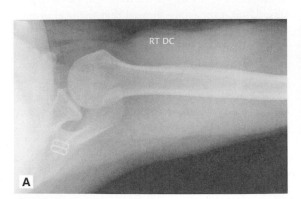
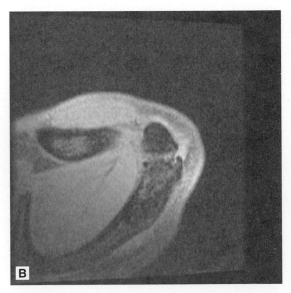

FIGURE 17-4 **A.** Plain radiograph (axillary view) demonstrating an os acromiale in a collegiate gymnast. **B.** MRI (T2—axial image) showing edema at the os acromiale, indicating an unstable os acromiale.

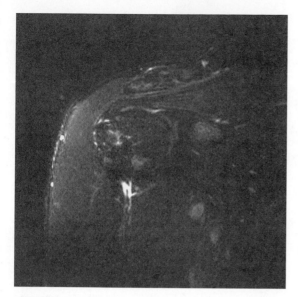

FIGURE 17-5 MRI (T2—coronal image) demonstrating a full-thickness supraspinatus tendon tear in a collegiate gymnast with a concomitant unstable os acromiale.

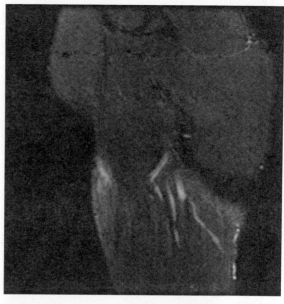

FIGURE 17-6 MRI (T2—sagittal image) of a collegiate gymnast's arm with a superficial tear of the short head biceps muscle belly.

muscle belly is a rare injury with few reported cases in the literature.[10–13] The mechanism is thought to be forced abduction of the arm with an eccentric load on the medial or short head of the biceps.[13] The injured athlete presents with complaints of pain, swelling, bruising, and a defect over the medial aspect of the proximal to middle part of the arm after a traumatic injury.[10] On physical examination, the patient will have a transverse depression of the biceps in this area (which may be masked by a large hematoma) with a sizable bulge proximal and distal to the defect due to proximal and distal retraction of the muscle belly.[10] Active contraction of the muscle will accentuate the defect.[10] MRI will demonstrate the short head muscle belly defect and show that the long head and distal biceps tendons are intact (Fig. 17-6).[10]

Treatment for these tears is controversial. The authors of this chapter treat these injuries in gymnasts nonsurgically with a period of rest in the acute phase (1 to 2 weeks) followed by a gradual return to sport over a 4- to 6-week time period. Except for the persistence of the cosmetic defect in the muscle belly, these gymnasts do well long-term with return to full participation without limitations. Other authors recommend surgical repair of the muscle

tear with protection in a hinged brace for 6 weeks postoperative with gradually increasing extension, followed by a rehabilitation program and return to full activities at 5 to 6 months.[10–13] These patients also fully recover from their treatment with full return to activities.[10–13]

Elbow Dislocation

Elbow dislocations in athletes occur most frequently in wrestling, gymnastics, and fieldball.[14] The pathoanatomy of an elbow dislocation involves a torn joint capsule, a ruptured medial collateral ligament, a tear of the brachialis muscle, and a lateral collateral ligament injury.[14,15] Avulsion fractures of the coronoid process, radial head, and medial epicondyle are also relatively common in elbow dislocations.[14,15]

A gentle closed reduction with traction can be attempted at the athletic event after a careful neurovascular examination. If the elbow does not reduce easily, the arm should be immobilized, and the athlete should be sent to the emergency room by Emergency Medical Services. In the emergency room, plain radiographs should be obtained to

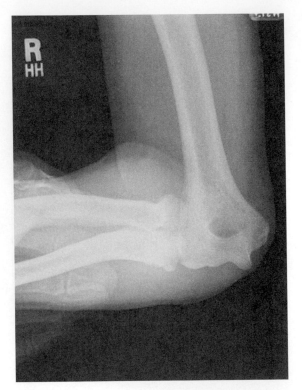

FIGURE 17-7 Plain radiograph of an elbow dislocation in a female collegiate gymnast.

document the dislocation and to evaluate for any associated fractures (Fig. 17-7). A closed reduction is then performed under sedation, and the elbow is immobilized in a splint.

A "simple" dislocation (no large fracture fragments) is generally stable after closed reduction and can be treated with early supervised range of motion.[14] The primary complication after a "simple" dislocation is loss of elbow extension, which can be minimized with early motion.[14,15] The authors of this chapter immobilize the elbow for 5 to 7 days and then initiate a supervised rehabilitation program. Ross et al.[14] advocate immediate motion without any immobilization. In a series of 20 U.S. Naval Academy athletes with elbow dislocations treated with immediate motion, all patients attained final extension within 5 degrees of the contralateral side within an average of 19 days postreduction, and only one patient had a redislocation episode.[14] Sport-specific activities can be initiated when near full range of motion and strength are obtained.

Ulnar Collateral Ligament (UCL) Injury

The primary stabilizer of the elbow to valgus stress is the anterior oblique portion of the UCL, which can be injured either in an acute traumatic event or due to repetitive microtrauma.[16] This injury has been well studied in high-level baseball players,[17] but a recent study has described the presentation and treatment of UCL injuries in 19 female athletes, including 4 gymnasts.[16] All patients presented with pain on the medial aspect of the elbow, and some patients complained of elbow instability. A majority of patients described an acute sudden pain or feeling of a "pop" that started the pain, while a minority of patients described a more insidious onset of symptoms. On physical examination, patients had tenderness medially either at the medial epicondyle or distally over the UCL midsubstance. A valgus stress to the elbow reproduced the patient's pain and, occasionally, resulted in opening of the medial joint line. Anterior–posterior (AP) valgus stress radiographs sometimes demonstrated opening of the medial joint line while an MRI scan often showed a midsubstance tear or avulsion of the UCL.[16]

Nonsurgical management, including elbow and wrist flexor-pronator strengthening, bracing, and anti-inflammatory medications, is the initial treatment of choice. Surgical intervention is indicated in those athletes who have persistent pain or instability limiting their ability to return to their sport after a minimum of 3 months of appropriate nonsurgical management.[16] Surgical management options include either direct repair or reconstruction of the UCL.[6,17] Argo et al.[16] reported successful return to sports in 17 of 18 female athletes at a mean of 2.5 months following UCL repair.

Osteochondritis Dissecans (OCD) of the Radial Capitellum

Osteochondritis dissecans of the capitellum is defined as a separation of the cartilage and subchondral bone from the main portion of the capitellum in patients from early adolescence to the early twenties.[18–20] OCD should be distinguished from Panner disease, which is an osteochondrosis of the capitellum that usually affects the dominant extremity in children younger than 10 years of age and that usually resolves with reduction of stressful activities of the elbow.[21] Patients with OCD of the elbow complain of pain, swelling, and limitation of motion in adolescence

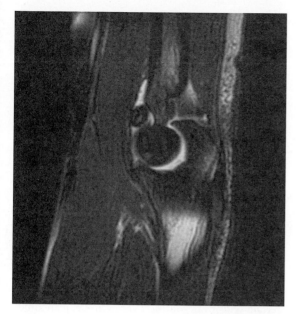

FIGURE 17-8 MRI (T2—sagittal view) of a loose body in an elbow joint.

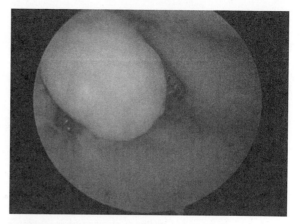

FIGURE 17-9 Arthroscopic removal of a loose body in an elbow joint.

through early adulthood.[18] In more advanced cases, the athletes will complain of catching, clicking, giving away, and crepitation due to irregular radio-capitellar joint surfaces and true locking episodes if loose bodies are present.[18] OCD lesions are usually the result of repetitive microtrauma. The lateral elbow joint (radio-capitellar joint) is subjected to repetitive compressive forces from valgus stresses in throwing and upper extremity weight-bearing athletes.[18]

The diagnosis is established by plain radiographs and MRI, which demonstrate the osteochondral lesion and occasionally loose bodies in the elbow joint (Fig. 17-8). Initial treatment consists of avoidance of the offending exercise, anti-inflammatory medications, and rehabilitation, including range-of-motion and strengthening exercises. For those athletes who do not respond to this treatment or for those who have mechanical symptoms, the treatment is elbow arthroscopy with debridement of the osteochondral lesion, removal of loose bodies, and/or microfracture chondroplasty of the capitellum (Fig. 17-9).[18–20] Krijnen et al.,[18] Baumgarten et al.,[19] and Bojanic et al.[20] all reported on gymnasts who underwent elbow arthroscopy for this disorder and found overall good to excellent results with a high return to sports participation in this population.

Olecranon Stress Injuries

Olecranon epiphyseal stress injuries are relatively common in young gymnasts and comprise a spectrum of disorders ranging from widening and fragmentation of the epiphysis to frank fracture and nonunion of the growth plate.[22–24] The olecranon ossification center fuses with the metaphysis between 15 to 17 years of age.[22] Repetitive strenuous elbow extension activities in adolescence result in a traction injury to the olecranon epiphysis as the forceful contraction of the triceps brachii continually stresses the growth plate.[22] This leads to inflammation, weakening, and widening of the olecranon growth plate and then eventually to fracture and nonunion of the epiphyseal plate.[22] Plain radiographs are obtained to assess for olecranon fragmentation, physeal widening, delayed fusion of the growth plate, and/or displacement of the olecranon epiphysis.

The initial treatment is rest and avoidance of the stressful activity, occasional use of anti-inflammatory medications, and physical therapy. Surgery is indicated in those athletes who have persistent pain with a delayed closure of the growth plate (nonunion) or a displaced olecranon epiphysis.[22–24] Treatment consists of open reduction and internal fixation of the olecranon with the goal of obtaining closure of the growth plate.[22–24]

Wrist Injuries

Due to the number of skills that require repetitive loading and long static contractions of the upper extremity, injuries to the wrist are very common in gymnasts. It is estimated that 46% to 79% of youth age gymnastics participants complain of wrist pain.[25] In addition, more than 50% of young participants who are considered to be beginner or midlevel competitors experience wrist pain. One of the problems with diagnosing wrist pain is that the majority of wrist injuries in gymnastics are chronic in nature. It is also common that it is generally viewed as being "part of the sport," and acute wrist pain is usually not brought to the attention of medical personnel. This delays evaluation and diagnosis and likely contributes to ongoing problems and disability.

Evaluating the injured wrist can be a difficult procedure in any patient due to the complex anatomic structure of the joint. Couple that with the ongoing pain and adaptive changes to gymnasts' wrists and the presentation is often as a chronic overuse injury that makes diagnosis even more challenging. Therefore, an understanding of the sport of gymnastics and of the loads and motions that are placed on the wrist is vitally important. The constant static contraction that occurs during the pommel horse is different than the quick explosive force experienced during the vault or floor exercise. Knowing which event/skill either causes or intensifies the discomfort to the area may be helpful when performing an evaluation and designing a management plan after a diagnosis has been made.

The most common description of chronic wrist pain is dorsal wrist pain while in extension that is provoked by weight-bearing activities.[25] The events that make up gymnastics for both genders (vault, balance beam, floor exercise, rings, pommel horse, etc.) all require significant time with the gymnasts weight-bearing on their hands, therefore making it easy to understand why wrist pain is so prevalent. When performing an evaluation on a skeletally immature gymnast who presents with pain in this area, it is necessary to obtain plain radiographs (AP, lateral) to evaluate the distal radial growth plate and to measure ulnar variance.[25] The distal radial growth plate bears the most of the load applied to the extended wrist and is therefore an at-risk area. MRI can also be used to identify any physeal injury. As mentioned earlier, with the young age at which participants enter the sport of gymnastics, growth plates are sites for potential injury.

When gymnasts present with generalized chronic wrist pain, conservative treatment of the symptoms is the best management. An understanding of the skills in gymnastics makes designing a return to participation plan easier. If possible, removing the participant from painful activities for a period of time allows the inflammation to resolve. Then, focusing on grip, wrist, and forearm strengthening exercises would be advised. Depending on the skill level and time of season for the gymnast, this is not always an option. Therefore, placing the injured wrist in a wrist/forearm immobilizer while not participating in gymnastics can help reduce the stress placed on the joint during activities of daily living. If this type of management plan is followed, it is also recommended that the patient perform range-of-motion and strengthening exercises several of times a day to decrease stiffness and possible atrophy caused by the immobilizer.

As a part of the management plan, it is important to see if there is a biomechanical issue causing the pathology and to try to fix the flaw or remove certain skills from routines. For example, if an athlete complains of distal ulnar wrist pain on the lead hand while performing cartwheel or round-off skills, it may be in the athlete's best interests to either discontinue or modify that skill for a period of time. By changing the forces or loads placed on the wrist one may be able to prevent long-term overuse issues from developing. If pain persists after this conservative plan for a period of time, a referral to an orthopedic or hand and wrist specialist is recommended.

Triangular Fibrocartilage Complex Tears

The differential diagnosis for ulnar-sided wrist pain includes tears affecting the triangular fibrocartilage complex (TFCC); (Fig. 17-10). The patient will complain of ulnar-sided wrist pain that can be accompanied by clicking during pronation/supination movements.[26] Common elements in the patient's history may be (i) fall onto a pronated outstretched extremity, (ii) a rotational injury to the forearm, (iii) an axial load to the wrist, or (iv) a distraction injury to the ulnar aspect of the wrist.[26] All of these forces commonly occur in the sport of gymnastics, therefore putting gymnasts at increased risk for this disorder.

After diagnosing an acute injury to the TFCC, management includes immobilization. The duration of the immobilization depends on the severity of the symptoms and how the injured athlete responds to initial treatment. If immobilization of the affected area does not lead to improvement, referral to an orthopedic or hand and wrist specialist is recommend to decide if arthroscopy is needed.

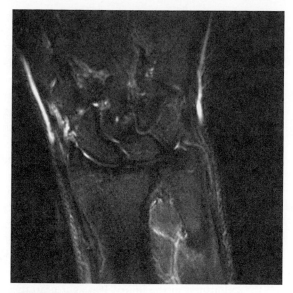

FIGURE 17-10 MRI (coronal image) of a TFCC tear.

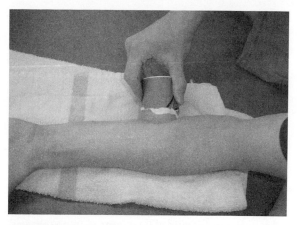

FIGURE 17-11 Ice massage has been found to be an effective means of pain control when treating the symptoms of forearm splints.

Forearm Splints

Forearm splints are a rare injury in the general athletic population but have the greatest prevalence in men's gymnastics, especially in those who specialize in the pommel horse.[27] Forearm splints are caused by a severe static contraction that is sustained and repeated. This injury is very similar to medial tibial stress syndrome (MTSS) in the lower leg, and as is the case with MTSS, is often very difficult to manage. Upon examination, athletes will complain of a dull ache between the extensor muscles on the back of the forearm.[27] This dull pain is caused by an irritation of the interosseus membrane and surrounding soft tissue. Often there is a lack of adequate conditioning, coupled with overuse. Athletes who begin the season without proper preseason conditioning and who start at too high a training level are susceptible for this injury. On the other hand, overuse and fatigue can also lead to this injury becoming a nuisance during the competitive season or at the end of a training period.

Care and treatment of forearm splints is symptomatically based. Massage techniques can also be used, along with ice massage (Fig. 17-11) after a workout to help control pain. As pain decreases it is very important to try to utilize strengthening exercises to rebuild the musculature throughout the forearm.

Practice with Upper Limb Injuries

Because the majority of gymnastics events and skills place stress on the upper limb, it is often difficult to keep the injured athlete involved in practice. For men, this is even more significant, as the majority of men's events place stress upon the shoulder, elbow, and wrist. Women can work on dance elements for the floor exercise and on the balance beam. Apart from gymnastics-specific skills, however, athletes with upper limb injuries can continue to work on core strengthening and cardiovascular training. Once the pain and inflammation of the injury has subsided, the athlete can slowly return to gymnastics activity, starting with basic skills and progressing back into their competitive routines.

LOWER LIMB INJURIES

Whereas previous studies by Kolt and Kirby[28] and Caine et al.[1] suggested that the knee was not a highly injured area in elite young female gymnasts, the Injury Surveillance System (ISS) by the National Collegiate Athletic Association (NCAA) shows the opposite to be true for collegiate gymnasts.[29] For NCAA gymnasts, the knee was the second most commonly injured joint, behind only the ankle for injuries reported from the fall of 1999 to the spring of 2004; the NCAA data also showed that the most common type of knee injury was a sprain.[29] Therefore, the examination of an acute injury needs to include special tests of the soft-tissue structures and their integrity. Overuse injuries to the knee include, but are not limited to, patello-femoral syndrome and iliotibial band friction syndrome. Therefore, a patellar grind test as well as the Renne test and the Noble test will help in the examination of an injury that presents with more of a chronic nature.

Tibial Plateau Fracture

One particular injury to include in the differential diagnosis for an acute knee injury in the gymnast is a tibial plateau fracture. The patient may present with anterior knee pain after performing a dismount that caused a hyperextension moment at the knee. A useful sign for this injury is difficultly in obtaining a clinical examination due to pain over the anterior inferior knee. This is because the hand placement for most special orthopedic tests is on or around the area of the fracture. Firm grasping of the area will cause pain and significant muscle guarding. If this occurs, plain radiographs (AP, lateral) followed by an MRI or other advanced radiographic tests should be obtained, both to rule out fracture and to check the integrity of the ligaments and other soft-tissue structures.

Ankle Sprains

Ankle sprains are the most common injury across all sports, accounting for 10% to 15% of all sports-related injuries.[30] Ankle sprains are the most common injury seen in gymnasts.[1,28] Acute ankle injury in a gymnast is often superimposed on chronic damage. This makes evaluating and diagnosing ankle pain in a competitive gymnast more difficult than might typically be expected. Ankle injuries can occur in gymnastics from a variety of exposures. Whether it is a dismount, a vault landing, or a tumbling pass, these skills must be performed correctly or an injury to the ankle can easily occur. These activities produce forces and movement velocities at the ankle that are very large and difficult to overcome if the gymnast lands with the ankle in an awkward position. The most common mechanism of injury to the ankle is that the athlete reports "rolling" over the outside of the ankle as a result of incorrectly landing a dismount; the participant's weight causes an inversion stress to the joint.[30] While this is a common mechanism in many sports, the added velocity and magnified impact force in gymnastics means that a minor mistake can produce an injury whereas a similar mistake might not produce an injury in another sport.

If a fracture is suspected, plain radiographs must be obtained prior to further evaluation. If a fracture is not suspected and the ankle is able to be examined immediately after injury, special tests for soft-tissue structures can be performed. Interestingly, the clinical evaluation of the ligamentous structures utilizing stability tests are actually best performed between days 4 and 7 postinjury.[30] Waiting for this time period allows the acute pain and swelling to subside, therefore enabling the athlete to relax the lower leg musculature during examination. Two special tests for lateral ankle stability include the anterior drawer test for the anterior talo-fibular ligament and the talar tilt test for the calcaneo-fibular ligament.

The management of an injured ankle depends on the seriousness of the injury. If weight-bearing is difficult, the athlete can be placed on crutches and/or in a walking boot. The authors prefer to not use crutches for a long period of time. Once the athlete can walk with a normal gait, their use is terminated. As pain decreases and range of motion and strengthening improve, the athlete can be placed into a medial/lateral stabilizing ankle brace to allow for greater locomotion. When prescribing a rehabilitation plan, focusing on range-of-motion and strengthening exercises is a necessary foundation. If the patient does not have full range of motion, isometric strengthening exercises can be started and likely will help with pain and "joint stiffness." Due to the importance of balance and proprioception in this sport, exercises of this type are very important components of a return to participation rehabilitation plan for gymnasts. Skills and routines are often based and judged upon the person's ability to show balance; if this is not challenged in rehabilitation exercises, athletes may struggle as they return to competitive activity.

Osteochondral Defects

If after a period of rest and rehabilitation, the patient still complains of pain in the ankle, there may be other injuries that are present. An osteochondral defect (OCD) or chronic ankle instability should be suspected if there is continued chronic pain along with instability episodes. If plain radiographs have already been performed and were negative, more specific imaging may be needed, including a bone scan, computed tomography (CT) scan, or an MRI. However, arthroscopy is the best and most definitive test for not only diagnosis but also treatment of this injury.

An OCD of the talar dome is most commonly caused by "landing short." Landing short is when the athlete does not fully complete the skill he or she is attempting to perform, and lands with the majority of the weight in front. This causes the ankle joint to be forced into extreme dorsiflexion, causing the tibia and talar dome to become compressed, resulting in injury to the talar dome. This injury may be acute, but over a long period of training and many exposures, an OCD can also be a chronic injury.

Ankle Instability

If an athlete has had multiple traumatic events to the lateral ankle and has not taken the necessary time off for rehabilitation and rest, lateral ankle instability may begin to cause difficulty. Athletes with this disorder will often complain of pain, not only while practicing but also during activities of daily living—these activities can be as complicated as playing another sport to as simple as walking around a shopping mall. Recommendations for an athlete with chronic ankle instability would be to rest as much as possible, to wear a medial/lateral ankle brace while not training or competing, and to continue to perform a rehabilitation program that includes both strengthening and balance exercises. If this does not help with the symptoms, surgery may be indicated and therefore a referral to an orthopedic surgeon or foot and ankle specialist would be the next step.

Achilles Tendon Rupture

Due to the nature of the explosive movements common in gymnastics, Achilles tendon ruptures are prevalent. Even though this injury normally occurs in people over the age of 30, gymnasts are at risk due to the stop-and-go action and the plyometric contractions that are required to perform certain skills, especially on the floor exercise.[27] Another factor that can predispose a person to having an Achilles tendon rupture is a history of chronic tendon inflammation. This leads to tendinosis of the soft tissue due to repeated stress placed on the structure.[27] As stated earlier, the young starting age and intensity of gymnastics training places this population at a higher risk than the nonathlete of the same age group.

An Achilles tendon rupture is the result of the pushing-off action of the forefoot with the knee forced

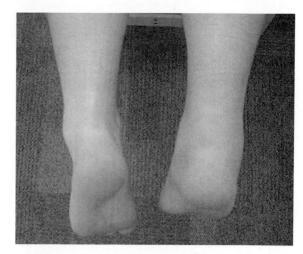

FIGURE 17-12 Right Achilles tendon rupture in a female gymnast. Notice the lack of plantar flexion in the resting position and deformity as compared bilaterally.

into full extension.[27] When this occurs, the three most common complaints the athlete will have are (i) a "pop" in the back of the lower leg described as if someone hit him or her with a baseball bat, (ii) pain and tenderness over the Achilles tendon insertion on the calcaneus, and (iii) lack of plantar flexion or weight-bearing on the affected limb. Diagnosis can be made with a clinical examination after a full history. Typically, a defect is present at the insertion point of the Achilles tendon on the calcaneus. With the patient laying supine on an examination table and the feet off the table, the affected limb will rest in a neutral position, whereas the unaffected side will rest in slight plantar flexion (Fig. 17-12). In addition, Thompson's test will be positive.[31] Management of Achilles tendon ruptures usually requires surgical repair for the general population and almost always requires repair for the competitive athlete. Therefore, immediate referral to an orthopedic surgeon is recommended.

Practice with Lower Limb Injuries

With lower limb injuries, vault, floor exercise, and balance beam practice will be difficult. However, significant portions of the routines from the remaining events can still be practiced. Bar and ring routines should be practiced over a pit of foam cubes. Dismounts are not attempted until the athlete is cleared to do so. Cardiovascular training may be maintained with an upper body ergonometer.

LUMBAR SPINE INJURIES

When dealing with back pain in gymnasts, several key factors need to be taken into account. First, in the general population it is estimated that 20% of people suffer from low back pain at any given time. Second, lifetime incidence of back pain in any individual is estimated to be 60% to 90%.[32] Finally, an individual who has had a previous episode of low back pain has a 50% chance for reoccurrence. With such high incidence and prevalence in the general public, it is reasonable to expect that sports medicine teams will have to deal with low back issues. In individuals who participate in activities or movements that place their backs at greater risk of injury, incidence is increased. Movements that cause jarring or repetitive loading—specifically, hyperextension movements—tend to lead to the greatest number of injuries.

Statistics show that approximately 90% of low back pain is musculoskeletal in nature. It has also been shown that the majority of low back pain resolves within 6 to 12 weeks without any medical intervention.[32] The key is to be able to diagnose the 10% of low back pain patients who will not improve, as well as identify the causes of potentially malevolent back pain.

When dealing with low back pain, the anatomy of the spine should be taken into account. The lumbar spine is broken down into the basic spinal segment, which is made up of two vertebral bodies, one intervertebral disc, and two facet joints. The interface of the vertebra and the facet joints combines to configure the three-joint complex.[32] This complex, along with anterior and posterior muscle groups of the abdominal and lumbar spine, allows specific motions to occur in the low back region. Flexion, extension, left and right side-bending, and rotation make up the cardinal planes of movements in the back. Due to the orientation of the facet articulation in the sagittal plane, flexion and extension are the predominant movement, especially in the lower lumbar segments. Because of this anatomy, it is believed that combined movements, such as extension with rotation, carry the highest potential for injury. Additionally, repetitive movements in this region can lead to fatigue and eventually overwhelm the protective support mechanism of the spinal segment, leading to injury. Finally, it is important to remember that the lumbar spine is the link between the lower limbs and the torso and the upper limbs, allowing the transfer of power through the body via the kinetic chain. Any weakness in the extremities may put undue stress across the low back, increasing the chance for injury.

The exact cause of most low back pain is usually not found; in only about 15% of cases is a firm diagnosis given. The differential diagnosis of low back pain is extensive (Table 17-1). Fewer then 2% of patients have disc herniation. To make a proper diagnosis, a thorough history must be obtained. The health care team must remember to look for red flag symptoms during the diagnosis of low back pain that will require immediate management (Table 17-2). The

TABLE 17-1	Extended Differential Diagnosis in Low Back Pain

Mechanical

Lumbar strain/sprain
Spondylolysis
Spondylolisthesis
Herniated disc
Spinal stenosis
Osteoporosis
Compression fracture
Congenital disease
Paget disease

Nonmechanical

Neoplasm
Infection
Inflammatory arthritis

Visceral Disease

Pelvic
Renal
Vascular
Gastrointestinal

TABLE 17-2	Red Flag Symptoms Associated with Low Back Pain That Indicate Further Immediate Evaluation and Management

- Fever
- Malaise
- Inability to establish a position of comfort
- Bowel or bladder issues
- Saddle anesthesia
- Progressive neurologic deficits

TABLE 17-3	Special Tests for Low Back Pain

- Stork (single-legged hyperextension) test
- Straight leg raise test
- Modified straight leg raise test
- Patrick or FABER (Flexion-ABduction-External Rotation) testing

history, along with a detailed physical examination—including attention to movement, strength, palpation of the anatomic region, and special tests (Table 17-3)—will help identify a more specific diagnosis in low back pain.[32,33] Radiographic tests and/or electrodiagnostic studies may also be of benefit.

Spondylolysis and Spondylolisthesis

In gymnastics, the most common cause of low back pain is overuse or stress-related. This type of injury manifests itself as spondylolysis (acute) or spondylolisthesis (chronic) injury. Spondylolysis is a defect in the pars interarticularis of the lumbar vertebral body. This injury is usually seen in younger patients and is related to stress from repetitive hyperextension movements.

Spondylolysis is associated with pain that progressively worsens with activity (specifically extension) and typically shows improvement with rest. This injury is most commonly found in the L5 level of the lumbar spine.[34] To make the diagnosis of spondylolysis, the history and examination reveal important clues. Positive findings such as pain with one-legged hyperextension (Stork testing) raise suspicion of spondylolysis. The diagnosis is confirmed by positive radiographic imaging including five-view radiographic films of the lumbar spine and single photon emission computed tomography (SPECT) bone-scan; the radiographic images should include oblique views to identify any fracture at the pars interarticularis.[34]

Spondylolisthesis is defined as bilateral spondylolysis with progressing forward displacement of the superior vertebral body on the inferior vertebral body. Spondylolisthesis is graded into four stages; increasing in severity. Grades 1 and 2 are treated with conservative measures including traditional rehabilitation centered on core strengthening. Grades 3 and 4 are referred for surgical evaluation and possible posteriolateral fusion.

OTHER INJURIES

This chapter has discussed the most common injuries that can occur in the sport of gymnastics. However, many other injuries can occur. Due to the nature of the sport, if a grip breaks or the competitor slips off the apparatus and falls landing on the head or neck, serious injury to these areas is possible; thankfully, these injuries are rare. On the other hand, injuries to the skin are quite common from hitting an apparatus or as a result of wear and tear on the palms of the hands. Further discussion of these injuries is beyond the scope of this chapter.

CONCLUSION

The evaluation process of gymnastics injuries can be a very difficult and frustrating task for both the athlete and the health care provider. The most important step to take is to determine if there is an underlying anatomic problem that is causing the pain. You can treat an athlete for rotator cuff tendonitis, but if the true problem is an anatomic os acromiale, the treatment plan will likely not work in the long-term. Because many gymnastics injuries present in the same fashion, one must recognize when the initial treatment plan has failed, and then consider what other factors might be playing a role in the athlete's ongoing symptoms.

REFERENCES

1. Caine D, Cochrane B, Caine C. An epidemiologic investigation of injuries affecting young competitive female gymnasts. *Am J Sports Med.* 1989;17:811–820.
2. Caraffa A, Cerulli G, Buompadre V, et al. An arthroscopic and electromyographic study of painful shoulders in elite gymnasts. *Knee Surg Sports Traumatol Arthrosc.* 1996;4: 39–42.
3. Yong GR, Lee DH, Chan TL. Unstable isolated SLAP lesion: clinical presentation and outcome of arthroscopic fixation. *Arthroscopy.* 2005;21:1099.e1–1099.e7.
4. O'Brien SJ, Pagnani MJ, Fealy S, et al. The active compression test (a new and effective test for diagnosing labral tears and acromioclavicular joint abnormality). *Am J Sports Med.* 1998;26:610–613.
5. Jones GL, Galluch DB. Clinical assessment of superior glenoid labral lesions: a systematic review. *Clin Orthop Rel Res.* 2007;455:45–51.
6. Pagnani MJ, Mathis CE, Solman G. Painful os acromiale (or unfused acromial apophysis) in athletes. *J Shoulder Elbow Surg.* 2006;15:432–435.

7. Mudge MK, Wood VE, Frykman GK. Rotator cuff tears associated with os acromiale. *J Bone Joint Surg.* 1984;66: 427–429.

8. Abboud JA, Silverberg D, Pepe M, et al. Surgical treatment of os acromiale with and without associated rotator cuff tears. *J Shoulder Elbow Surg.* 2006;15:265–270.

9. Peckett WRC, Gunther SB, Harper GD, et al. Internal fixation of symptomatic os acromiale: a series of 26 cases. *J Shoulder Elbow Surg.* 2004;13:381–385.

10. Shah AK, Pruzansky ME. Ruptured biceps brachii short head muscle belly: a case report. *J Shoulder Elbow Surg.* 2004;13:562–565.

11. DiChristina DG, Lustig KA. Rupture through the short head of the biceps muscle belly. A case report. *Clin Orthop Relat Res.* 1992;277:139–141.

12. Postacchini F, Ricciardi-Pollini PT. Rupture of the short head tendon of the biceps brachii. *Clin Orthop Relat Res.* 1977;124:229–232.

13. Heckman JD, Levine MI. Traumatic closed transaction of the biceps brachii in military parachutists. *J Bone Joint Surg Am.* 1978;60:369–372.

14. Ross G, McDevitt ER, Chronister R, et al. Treatment of simple elbow dislocations using an immediate motion protocol. *Am J Sports Med.* 1999;27:308–311.

15. Mehlhoff TL, Noble PC, Bennett JB, et al. Simple dislocation of the elbow in the adult. Results after closed treatment. *J Bone Joint Surg Am.* 1988;70:244–249.

16. Argo D, Trenhaile SW, Savoie FH, et al. Operative treatment of ulnar collateral ligament insufficiency of the elbow in female athletes. *Am J Sports Med.* 2005;34:431–437.

17. Azar FM, Andrews JR, Wilk KE, et al. Operative treatment of ulnar collateral ligament injuries of the elbow in athletes. *Am J Sports Med.* 2000;28:16–23.

18. Krijnen MR, Lim L, Willems WJ. Arthroscopic treatment of osteochondritis dissecans of the capitellum: report of 5 female athletes. *Arthroscopy.* 2003;19:210–214.

19. Baumgarten TE, Andrews JR, Satterwhite YE. The arthroscopic classification and treatment of osteochondritis dissecans of the capitellum. *Am J Sports Med.* 1998;26:520–523.

20. Bojanic I, Ivkovic A, Boric I. Arthroscopy and microfracture technique in the treatment of osteochondritis dissecans of the humeral capitellum: report of three adolescent gymnasts. *Knee Surg Sports Traumatol Arthrosc.* 2005;14: 491–496.

21. Kobayashi K, Burton KJ, Rodner C, et al. Lateral compression injuries in the pediatric elbow: Panner's disease and osteochondritis dissecans of the capitellum. *J Am Acad Orthop Surg.* 2004;12:246–254.

22. Tavares JO. Nonunion of the olecranon epiphysis treated with sliding bone graft and tension band wire. *Am J Sports Med.* 1998;26:725–728.

23. Maffulli N, Chan D, Aldridge MJ. Overuse injuries of the olecranon in young gymnasts. *J Bone Joint Surg Br.* 1992;74: 305–308.

24. Wilkerson RD, Johns JC. Nonunion of an olecranon stress fracture in an adolescent gymnast: a case report. *Am J Sports Med.* 1990;18:432–434.

25. DiFiori JP, Caine DJ, Malina RM. Wrist pain, distal radial physeal injury, and ulnar variance in the young gymnast. *Am J Sports Med.* 2006;34:840–849.

26. Ahn AK, Chang MD, Plate A. Triangular fibrocartilage complex tears, a review. *Bull NYU Hosp Joint Dis.* 2006;64: 114–118.

27. Arnheim DD, Prentice WE. *Principles of Athletic Training.* Burr Ridge, IL: McGraw Hill; 2000.

28. Kolt GS, Kirby RJ. Epidemiology of injury in elite and subelite female gymnasts: a comparison of retrospective and prospective findings. *Br J Sports Med.* 1999;33:312–318.

29. NCAA research. Injury surveillance system, gymnastics 2003-04. Available at: http://www1.ncaa.org/membership/ ed_outreach/health-safety/iss/Injury_Reports_2004/ Gymnastics_Summary_2004.pdf. Accessed April 11, 2007.

30. Lynch SA. Assessment of the injured ankle in the athlete. *J Athletic Training.* 2002;37:406–412.

31. Konin JG, Wiksten DL, Isear JA, et al. *Special Tests for Orthopedic Examination.* Thorofare, NJ: Slack; 2006.

32. Drezner JA, Herring SA. Managing low-back pain. Steps to optimize function and hasten return to activity. *Physician Sportsmed.* 2001;29:37–43.

33. Patel AT, Ogle AA. Diagnosis and management of acute low back pain. *Am Fam Phys.* 2000;61:1779–1786, 1789–1790.

34. Moeller JL, Rifat SF. Spondylolysis in active adolescents: expediting return to play. *Physician Sportsmed.* 2001;29: 27–32.

Basketball Injuries

This chapter will highlight the evaluation and management of musculoskeletal injuries common to basketball players. Lower limb injuries will be emphasized, as injury trends at all levels reveal that the majority of injuries sustained in basketball involve the lower limb, with ankle ligament sprains being the most common.[1,2] Injuries to the upper limb most commonly involve the hand and wrist, followed by the shoulder.

EPIDEMIOLOGY

Since its creation in the late 1800s, basketball has largely been considered a noncontact sport; however, it is also one of the leading causes of sports-related injuries in the United States.[3] This may be due in part to the number of high school, collegiate, and professional basketball players, as well as to the popularity of the sport recreationally. Basketball remains the most popular sport at the high school level, with over 35,000 boys and girls basketball programs in U.S. high schools.[4]

Epidemiologic studies suggest varying rates of injury among basketball players at different levels of competition. A recent large-scale review of high school basketball injuries suggests injury rates near 30% in both males and females; however, other reviews report injury rates from 15% to 56%.[5]

At the collegiate level, much of the data on injuries is available through the National Collegiate Athletic Association (NCAA) Injury Surveillance System. Recent reviews of basketball injury rates in men and women participating in collegiate basketball encompass data available from the 1988 to 1989 season through the 2003 to 2004 season.[6,7] Injury rates were expressed as incidence per 1,000 athlete-exposures, with each athlete-exposure representing a practice or game in which an athlete participated and had a risk of athletic injury. These injury rates were further classified according to season (preseason, in season, or postseason), activity (game or practice), and NCAA division. Across all divisions and all seasons, female basketball players demonstrated practice incidence rates of 3.99 and game injury incidence rates of 7.68. A similar analysis for male basketball players revealed a practice injury rate of 4.3 and game injury rate of 9.9.

Professional basketball players have higher rates of injury among Women's National Basketball Association (WNBA) players relative to male players in the National Basketball Association (NBA).[8] The WNBA game-related incidence was 24.9 and the NBA game-related injury incidence rate was 19.3. Distribution of injury types was similar between both leagues, with lateral ankle sprains being the most common diagnosis.

FOOT/ANKLE

An analysis by McKay et al. suggests that ankle injuries are sustained during landing, cutting, and twisting maneuvers.[9] Risk factors identified for ankle injury include a history of prior ankle injury, use of shoes with air cells in the heels, and lack of stretching during warm-up. Basketball players with a prior history of ankle injury were nearly five times more likely to sustain a repeat injury. Athletic taping of the ankle has been shown to decrease the risk of repeat injury in those basketball players with prior ankle injury.

LisFranc Sprains

With their repetitive landing movements, basketball players are susceptible to midfoot injuries such as LisFranc sprains. LisFranc injuries are a result of

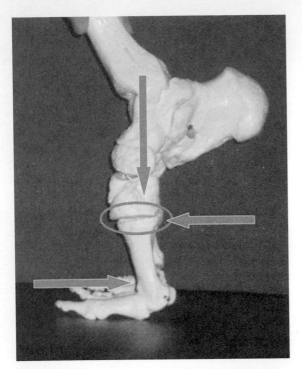

FIGURE 18-1 Mechanical forces leading to LisFranc injury. Jumping repetitively stresses the marked areas, leading to ligamentous strain and possible joint dislocation.

mechanical forces (Fig. 18-1) that stress the first and second tarsometatarsal joints, which leads to ligamentous sprain and possible joint dislocation. These frequently missed or misdiagnosed midfoot injuries typically present with regional pain and swelling, as well as with difficulty bearing weight. Pain may be elicited on exam by placing an abduction stress on the forefoot. Malalignment demonstrated by bilateral weight-bearing foot radiographs often necessitates surgical correction.[10] Either a trial of nonweight-bearing immobilization with casting or the use of a walking boot for 3 to 6 weeks may be considered for the acute, aligned LisFranc injury.[11] However, the physician should keep in mind that outcomes are best when the injury is addressed within 4 weeks of the injury, and may be poor if surgery is delayed beyond 8 weeks postinjury.

Jones Fractures

Jones fractures (acute fractures at the base of the fifth metatarsal) are of particular concern as they occur near the metaphyseal–diaphyseal junction. When treated nonoperatively, these fractures are associated with a high rate of malunion/nonunion or recurrent fracture. However, when a trial of nonoperative immobilization is attempted, outcome may be optimized with nonweight-bearing for 6 to 8 weeks, followed by use of a walking boot once union has been demonstrated radiographically.[12] Operative treatment may shorten return-to-play time and improve outcome.[13]

Navicular Stress Fractures

Navicular stress fractures present with persistent midfoot pain, often exacerbated by push-off or landing activities. Patients may demonstrate classic tenderness in the "N" spot on exam, or have pain reproduced with single-leg toe hop on the affected foot.[14] Initial weight-bearing foot radiographs may be negative; however, a positive bone scan may detect the presence of fracture, followed by computed tomography (CT) scan to help classify the extent of injury. Many clinicians recommend nonweight-bearing immobilization for management of these injuries. Open reduction with internal fixation has been utilized for those patients with fractures extending through the plantar cortex or in those with poor outcomes following conservative management.[12]

Ankle Sprains

Ankle sprains comprise the majority of acute injuries encountered in basketball. The mechanism of injury and examination help distinguish the ligaments involved; radiographs may help exclude fracture if the suspicion exists. Ligaments providing support for the lateral ankle (Fig. 18-2) may be injured through an inversion injury. Clinical examination tests such as

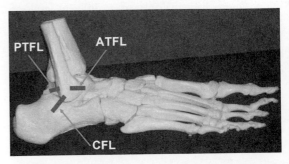

FIGURE 18-2 The ligaments of the lateral ankle: anterior talofibular ligament (ATFL), posterior talofibular ligament (PTFL), and calcaneofibular ligament (CFL).

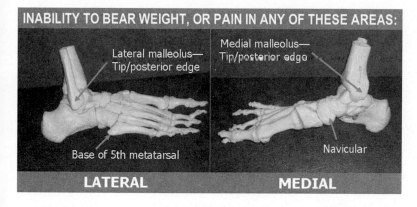

INABILITY TO BEAR WEIGHT, OR PAIN IN ANY OF THESE AREAS:

Lateral malleolus—
Tip/posterior edge

Medial malleolus—
Tip/posterior edge

Base of 5th metatarsal

Navicular

LATERAL   **MEDIAL**

FIGURE 18-3 The Ottawa Ankle Rules. Plain radiographs are indicated when the athlete is unable to bear weight or has bony tenderness at any of the points indicated.

the anterior drawer test and talar tilt test help determine which ligamentous structures may be injured. The Ottawa Ankle Rules (Fig. 18-3) have been advocated as a tool to help the clinician determine the need for radiographs.

Grading lateral ankle sprains (Table 18-1) by clinical exam may help determine the treatment strategy. Initial treatment of all sprains includes the immediate use of ice, nonsteroidal anti-inflammatory drugs (NSAIDs) if tolerated, compression, and elevation. An early rehabilitative program is started within the first 48 to 72 hours after injury, gradually progressing the athlete from early range of motion (ROM), strengthening, and biking to sport-specific activities.[15] While the immediate care and early functional rehabilitation of all lateral ankle sprains may be similar, recommendations for bracing and immobilization differ.[11] Grade I lateral ankle sprains, presenting with mild symptoms and stretching of the anterior talofibular ligament without tearing, may be rehabilitated with use of a lace-up or stirrup brace to assist with ligamentous healing and to prevent further disability. Grade II and III lateral ankle sprains may be treated with a walking boot for the first 1 to 3 weeks both day and night, with subsequent transition to daytime bracing and nighttime boot wear during weeks 4 and 5. Beynnon et al., in a randomized controlled clinical trial, determined

that when compared to either element alone, the combination of an Air-Stirrup brace and elastic wrap optimizes return to preinjury function for first-time, mild to moderate lateral ankle sprains.[16]

Syndesmotic Sprains

A thorough examination of an ankle injury includes efforts to detect the presence of a tibial-fibular syndesmotic injury ("high ankle" sprain). The mechanism of injury typically involves forced external rotation of the foot with or without dorsiflexion. Structures affected may include the tibial-fibular syndesmosis, anterior tibio-fibular ligament, and the posterior tibio-fibular ligament. Athletes typically complain of pain extending up the anterolateral leg, and they usually have difficulty bearing weight. In addition to checking for tenderness to palpation over the involved structures, physical exam could include the calf squeeze test and the external rotation stress test (Fig. 18-4) to see if pain in the involved area is elicited.[17] The proximal fibula should be evaluated for tenderness, which could indicate an underlying Maissoneuve fracture. Radiographs are indicated when syndesmotic injury is suspected. Weight-bearing and bilateral ankle radiographs with AP and mortise views should evaluate the tibial-fibular and medial clear spaces for any abnormal widening (Fig. 18-5).[10]

TABLE 18-1	**Clinical Grading of Lateral Ankle Sprains**		
	Grade I	**Grade II**	**Grade III**
Ligament injury	No ligament tear	Partial ligament tear	Complete ligament tear
Pain/swelling	Mild	Moderate	Severe
Special tests	− Anterior drawer	+ Anterior drawer	+ Anterior drawer
			+ Talar tilt

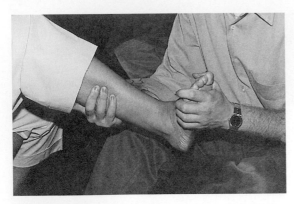

FIGURE 18-4 External rotation stress test. (From Cohen AR, Metzl JD. Sports-specific concerns in the young athlete: basketball. *Pediatr Emerg Care.* 2000;16:462–468.)

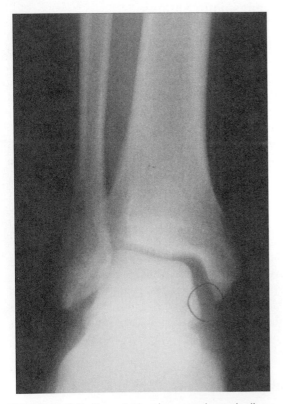

FIGURE 18-5 Radiograph showing a syndesmotic disruption, with increased medial clear space and decreased overlap of the tibia and fibula. (From Amendola A, Williams G, Foster D. Evidence-based approach to treatment of acute traumatic syndesmosis [high ankle] sprains. *Sports Med Arthrosc Rev.* 2006;14:232–236.)

Stability of the sprain needs to be determined. Unstable sprains include any grade II or III sprain or those associated with fracture, widening of the mortise, or persistent pain and/or instability. These unstable high-ankle sprains should undergo evaluation promptly for surgical intervention.

While much debate exists on an appropriate treatment protocol for stable high-ankle sprains, rehabilitation is generally understood to be more extensive than that for lateral ankle sprains. Treatment includes immobilization in a high-top walking boot (to stabilize both the proximal and distal lower leg) used both during the day and at night for 2 to 12 weeks. An initial period of nonweight-bearing and frequent follow-up allows individualization of the treatment course for the athlete. Rehabilitation exercises progress from ROM exercises to general strengthening exercises with emphasis on the posterior tibial tendon. Use of a short-articulating ankle–foot orthosis such as a stirrup brace provides additional stability when the athlete is returned to sport.

Chronic Ankle Injuries

Chronic ankle injuries may result from serious underlying pathology. Differentiating between chronic pain and persistent instability aids in the treatment of the injury. Chronic ankle instability can be accompanied by a history of frequent ankle sprains or poor rehabilitation efforts after acute injuries. Chronic ankle instability can be classified as functional or mechanical. Functional instability may indicate underlying neurologic disease, weakness, or inflexibility. Physical therapy (PT) may improve functional instability by addressing peroneal muscle strengthening, Achilles stretching, and proprioceptive training. Mechanical instability involves persistent ligament laxity and may improve with a similar rehabilitative program over a period of a few months. Athletes who fail conservative treatment may benefit from surgical intervention.

Osteochondral lesions may be present in patients with chronic ankle pain or instability. Persistent pain or instability in athletes during rehabilitation of an acute ankle sprain may warrant evaluation for osteochondral lesions of the talus or tibia. Many patients with these lesions have had a history of an ankle injury. The lesion may be seen radiographically, but may require CT imaging to delineate the extent of the injury. If radiographs do not demonstrate any suspicious lesion yet clinical suspicion remains, further assessment with MRI may be warranted.[10] Treatment

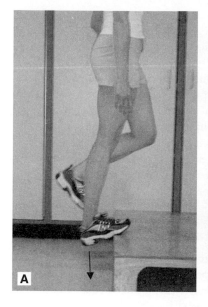
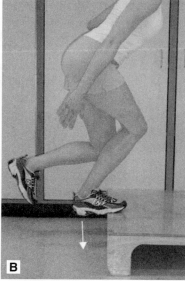

FIGURE 18-6 Eccentric calf strengthening, focusing on the gastrocnemius **(A)** with the leg straight, and the soleus **(B)** with the knee bent. (From Sorosky B, Press J, Plastaras C, et al. The practical management of Achilles tendinopathy. *Clin J Sports Med.* 2004;14:40–44.)

options vary based on clinical symptoms and the extent of the lesion. Conservative management consists of immobilization followed by PT. If conservative treatment fails, or if there is significant effusion, catching, locking, or painful instability, the athlete may need to be referred for operative treatment.

Achilles Tendinopathy

Tendonous pain in the Achilles is often described as having an insidious onset. It may diminish during activity but recur following activity. Localized tenderness on exam supports the diagnosis. Activity modification, ice therapy, and temporary bilateral heel lifts with a thickness of 0.5 to 1.0 cm may assist with pain control in a midportion Achilles tendinopathy. Chronic tendinopathy is not considered to be an inflammatory problem and the role of nonsteroidal anti-inflammatory drugs in its treatment is debatable.[18,19] Some advocate use of therapeutic ultrasound for increasing tensile strength and the promotion of collagen synthesis within the tendon.[20,21] Corticosteroid injections may or may not be helpful in treatment of Achilles tendinopathy. Tendon rupture has been a reported serious complication of intratendinous injection.[22]

Addressing any underlying biomechanical issues is an important aspect of conservative treatment for Achilles tendinopathy.[18] Footwear should be evaluated to ensure adequate support for foot type. Additionally, patients should begin a calf/Achilles stretching program to improve flexibility. Eccentric calf strengthening

(Fig. 18-6) can be attained through a heel drop rehabilitation program.[23,24] Some studies support use of topical glyceryl nitrate and sclerosing injections in treatment of Achilles tendinopathy.[25] Patients should improve with conservative treatment; persistence of pain despite 3 to 6 months of activity modification and rehabilitation should prompt further workup or surgical referral.

Achilles Rupture

Athletes who have ruptured the Achilles tendon may describe sudden pain accompanied by a "pop," or they may describe feeling as if they have been kicked. Physical examination can reveal a void in the area or deformity within the tendon. If the Achilles is ruptured, there will be no plantar flexion when the gastrocsoleus muscle is squeezed during the Thompson test. Partial rupture may be suspected if there is minimal movement during testing.[26]

Haglund Deformity

In addition to insertional Achilles tendinosis, patients may have a prominent posterior calcaneal process (bone spur) known as a Haglund deformity, which may irritate the distal Achilles tendon. The pain or tenderness is localized near the insertion of the Achilles on the calcaneus. A Haglund deformity may be most apparent on lateral radiographs of the ankle (Fig. 18-7). The deformity may also lead to chronic impingement of the retrocalcaneal bursa, which is located between the Haglund deformity and the distal Achilles tendon.

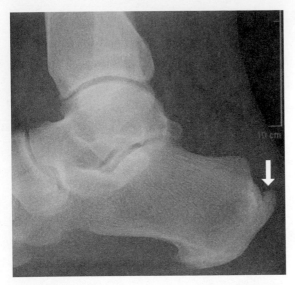

FIGURE 18-7 Haglund deformity, indicated by the *arrow* on this lateral radiograph.

Retrocalcaneal Bursitis

Retrocalcaneal bursitis may also develop from repetitive trauma or overuse. Its location just deep to the distal Achilles tendon helps to distinguish it on exam from the subcutaneous Achilles bursa, which lies superficial to the tendon. Achilles bursitis may also present as insertional Achilles pain that develops from the external friction of tight, large, or stiff shoes. Swelling and erythema in the region may be present on exam.

Treatment of Achilles Pain

Initial management of insertional Achilles pain—whether due to underlying distal Achilles tendinopathy with or without Haglund deformity, retrocalcaneal bursitis, or Achilles bursitis—is similar to conservative management of midportion Achilles pain. Patients may utilize ice therapy, progressive Achilles stretching, heel cups, and open-backed shoes. Insertional Achilles pain without known precipitating factors (Haglund deformity, overuse activities, poorly fitted footwear, or sudden change in shoe heel height) should prompt investigation of rheumatic disease such as gout, seronegative spondylarthropathies, and rheumatoid arthritis.[27] Recalcitrant pain in the calcaneus may indicate underlying calcaneal stress fracture. Persistent pain despite conservative treatment may require resection of Haglund deformity or debridement of bursitis.

KNEE

Knee injuries encountered in basketball include contusions, muscle-tendon strains and tendinopathies involving the muscles about the knee, and internal derangements of the knee. In the collegiate basketball reviews, internal derangement of the knee was the most frequent injury that led to a loss of more than 10 days of participation.[6,7] Of these, anterior cruciate ligament injuries are most concerning, given the related loss of participation and the likely need for surgical intervention.

Patellofemoral Pain

Chronic anterior knee pain may be due to a patellofemoral pain syndrome (PFPS). Pain and/or stiffness can be exacerbated by repeated knee flexion or periods of prolonged knee flexion. Pain tends to be worse while climbing stairs and performing squatting activities. Physical exam may reveal crepitus in the patellofemoral compartment, positive compression sign (retropatellar pain with compression of the patella against the femoral groove while the athlete actively contracts the quadriceps), and abnormal patellar tracking (such as that found in a J-sign where the patella moves laterally at terminal extension of the knee).[30,31] Persistent effusion or mechanical symptoms such as locking or catching may be indicative of other etiology such as osteochondral lesion, meniscal tear, or loose body and warrants evaluation with imaging and occasionally arthroscopy. Exclusionary diagnoses include quadriceps tendinopathy, iliotibial band syndrome, patellar tendinopathy, and infrapatellar fat pad syndrome.[32] Radiographs should be ordered in younger patients with chronic symptoms, those with a history of prior knee surgery, or patients with pain recalcitrant to an initial trial of conservative management. Views obtained should include weight-bearing posterior–anterior, Merchant/Sunrise, lateral, and possibly tunnel views. These may be normal in early disease, but in more advanced cases may demonstrate changes of lateral patellar subluxation or narrowing/sclerosis in the lateral patellar compartment.[33]

Treatment of PFPS is conservative, particularly in the competitive athlete. Ice, NSAIDs, and activity modification may help manage acute flares of pain. Physical therapy focuses on treatment and prevention, with exercises for core strengthening (hip flexors and internal/external rotators, transversus abdominus, gluteals), quadriceps strengthening (emphasizing vastus medialis oblique development), and lower limb flexibility.[34] Bracing, McConnell taping of the patella, and foot orthoses may also be considered when indicated, although evidence for these interventions are limited; these interventions do not substitute for an appropriate rehabilitative program.[35–37] Intractable pain in the minority of patients not responding to conservative treatment may be an indication to consider various surgical options.[38]

Patellar Tendinopathy

Another common cause of anterior knee pain in basketball players is patellar tendinopathy. Athletes usually relate a history of symptoms that increase with jumping and squatting activities. Basketball players may be particularly at risk for this condition if they have poor quadriceps or hamstring flexibility, or if they train on certain court surfaces.[39,40] Examination usually reveals tenderness (with or without associated swelling or erythema) along the patellar tendon, particularly at the inferior patellar pole. Resisted knee extension or a single-legged decline squat test (Fig. 18-8) may elicit pain. Imaging is usually unnecessary unless significant tendon tears or ruptures are suspected; if imaging is desired, options include gray-scale ultrasound, Doppler ultrasound, and magnetic resonance imaging (MRI). Warden et al. demonstrated similar specificities of these modalities, although ultrasound was found to be significantly more sensitive than MRI; the best imaging option may be a combination of gray-scale and Doppler ultrasound.[41]

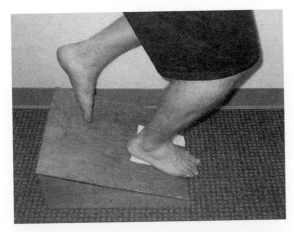

FIGURE 18-8 The single-legged decline squat test may cause pain in cases of patellar tendinopathy.

A 3- to 6-month trial of conservative treatment may involve a variety of options. Significant tendinopathy, or that which impacts quality of athletic performance, may benefit from a 3-to 6-week period of relative rest from activity. A cho-pat strap, ice therapy, iontophoresis, lower limb stretching exercises, and eccentric strength training may be useful in the treatment of patellar tendinopathy, although there is little agreement as to the effectiveness of these strategies.[42–44] Some recent studies indicate therapeutic roles for extracorporeal shock wave therapy, ultrasound-guided dry needling with autologous blood injection, and ultrasound-guided polidocanol sclerosing treatment.[45–47]

Pain recalcitrant to an adequate trial of conservative treatment may indicate the need for further workup for underlying lesions with imaging and/or possible surgical intervention. Surgical options include debridement, tenotomy, or resection of the inferior pole with reattachment of the patellar tendon.

Medial Collateral Ligament Sprain

The most common ligament sprains of the knee are of the medial collateral ligament (MCL) and of the anterior cruciate ligament (ACL). Injury to the MCL usually occurs after a collision or forceful misstep that places a significant valgus stress on the knee.[48] Athletes usually experience immediate pain over the medial aspect of the knee, and may have a sense of instability or buckling upon attempted walking or pivoting. Examination typically reveals tenderness along the course of the MCL, swelling, and pain (with or without laxity) during valgus stress testing of the knee.[49] If there is a concern for fracture, a suspicion for ACL or meniscal injury, an inability to bear weight, a joint effusion, limitation of knee flexion, or if a complete MCL tear is suspected, an MRI evaluation is recommended. Treatment for isolated MCL injury is conservative and consists of ice therapy, NSAIDs for pain, short-term use of crutches to assist with weight-bearing, and activity restriction.[50] Athletes can be placed in a hinged knee brace and started on a progressive rehabilitation program that focuses on normalizing range of motion (ROM) and strengthening the knee joint stabilizers.[51,52] Return to sport typically takes 1 to 5 weeks depending upon the degree of injury.

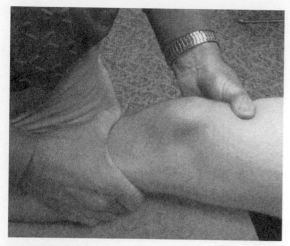

FIGURE 18-9 Lachman test for anterior cruciate ligament injury. (From McKeag DB, Mueller JL, eds. *ACSM's Primary Care Sports Medicine.* 2nd ed. Philadelphia: Lippincott Williams & Wilkins; 2007.)

Anterior Cruciate Ligament Sprain

Injury to the ACL typically occurs with noncontact deceleration forces, hyperextension, or pivoting/cutting movements. Athletes report immediate pain, often rapidly develop an effusion, and are unable to continue sport participation. They may report having heard a "pop" during the injury, a sense of instability, or giving-away/buckling episodes.[53] Physical examination reveals effusion and laxity with the Lachman maneuver (an anteriorly directed force on the tibia relative to a stabilized femur while the knee is slightly flexed) compared to the uninjured knee (Fig. 18-9).[54] The sense of instability may be reproduced by the pivot shift test, in which the examiner applies a valgus force to the knee and subtly internally rotates the tibia as the flexed knee is passively extended.[54] Treatment for the competitive basketball player typically involves surgical reconstruction, with preoperative therapy utilized to maximize active knee extension prior to surgery.[49] Postoperative rehabilitation may extend for a full year, with cautious return to play as early as 3 months after surgery. Recently, the role of balance and neuromuscular training programs has been investigated in prevention of ankle sprains and ACL injuries.[28,29]

Meniscus Injuries

Meniscal injury in basketball most commonly involves the medial meniscus after a sudden twisting motion upon a planted foot. Athletes may experience sudden pain, although this is variable and may not restrict continued play. Pain, swelling, and stiffness may gradually develop over the next 24 hours.[53] There may or may not be mechanical symptoms such as locking or catching. Pain is usually reproduced by weight-bearing, squatting, or twisting motions. Examination reveals joint line tenderness and a palpable joint line popping may be noted in early to mid extension during the McMurray test.[54] MRI is generally indicated when suspicion for concomitant ligamentous injury is present, in the presence of significant mechanical symptoms or effusion, or when there is locking of the knee that prevents terminal extension. Conservative therapy may be attempted initially to see if symptoms resolve. Persistent symptoms, often associated with large or complex tears, usually warrant referral for surgical treatment.[55] Postoperative rehabilitation and return to play typically depends on the type of meniscal injury and surgical intervention. Generally, a progressive return to basketball may be allowed when there is full range of motion (as compared bilaterally), no effusion, and near-normal strength.[49]

HAND

The most common upper limb injuries in basketball players involve the hand. Common basketball injuries involve the proximal interphalangeal (PIP) joint, the collateral ligaments of the thumb metacarpophalangeal (MCP) joint, and the extensor mechanism of the fingers. Injuries to the digits present with pain, stiffness, and swelling. Examination should confirm intact neurovascular status, and assess for deformity, bony tenderness, joint instability, and tendon rupture. Radiographs are recommended in most acute injuries to assess for fractures.

PIP Injuries

Proximal interphalangeal joint stability is created by the volar plate and collateral ligaments. Injuries involving the PIP joint typically involve hyperextension and axial loading forces, and may injure the volar plate. Volar plate injuries commonly include plate avulsions from the middle phalanx, either proximally or distally. Left untreated, distal plate avulsions may lead to swan neck deformities that are characterized by hyperextension at the PIP joint and

Pseudoboutonniere deformity

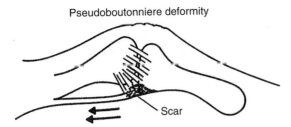

Scar

FIGURE 18-10 Pseudoboutonniere deformity. (From McKeag DB, Mueller JL, eds. *ACSM's Primary Care Sports Medicine.* 2nd ed. Philadelphia: Lippincott Williams & Wilkins; 2007.)

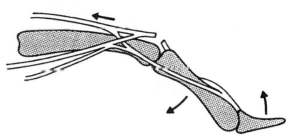

FIGURE 18-11 Boutonniere deformity. (From McKeag DB, Mueller JL, eds. *ACSM's Primary Care Sports Medicine.* 2nd ed. Philadelphia: Lippincott Williams & Wilkins; 2007.)

usually require surgical repair.[56] Proximal volar plate avulsions may result in flexion contracture of the PIP from scar tissue with associated mild hyperextension of the distal interphalangeal (DIP) joint, these are known as pseudoboutonniere deformities (Fig. 18-10). Mild flexion contractures may benefit from splinting, while more significant contractures will likely require surgical release.[57]

Proximal interphalangeal joint dislocations most commonly occur dorsally; they are usually stable. These injuries may be associated with avulsion fractures of the middle phalanx where the volar plate attaches. Such fracture/dislocation injuries should be carefully evaluated for stability through clinical exam and imaging. Conservative treatment suffices for stable injuries, with repeat radiographs obtained 1 week postinjury to monitor stability.[56] They may be buddy taped or splinted after closed reduction. Early ROM is emphasized to attain rapid return to play. Surgical repair may be needed for irreducible dislocations, for unstable injuries involving a deformity of greater than 20 degrees, or for a fracture of greater than one-third of the articular surface.[58] Return to play in these situations may take as long as 8 weeks.

Partial rupture of the PIP collateral ligaments usually involves the radial collateral ligament and may be associated with minor instability; complete tears occur infrequently. Treatment generally involves buddy taping, splinting, and ROM exercises. Once the athlete has regained full ROM, return to play typically occurs within 1 to 3 weeks for mild injuries or 4 to 6 weeks for injuries with greater ligamentous laxity.

Boutonniere Deformity

Injuries to the extensor mechanism of the fingers may occur at the distal or middle phalanx. PIP joint

dislocation or forced DIP flexion can result in rupture of the central slip at its middle phalanx insertion. A true boutonniere deformity involving PIP joint flexion and hyperextension at the DIP may result (Fig. 18-11). Exam reveals loss of active PIP extension or extension lag (the loss of active extension range of motion, in the face of normal passive extension). Most injuries resolve well with extension splinting of the PIP while allowing the DIP to remain in flexion. Basketball players can be taped with the PIP in extension, reserving the splint for nonplay time. Surgical repair is considered when large avulsion fractures are found.

Mallet Finger

Flexion force to the DIP joint, such as when an athlete's fingertip directly impacts a basketball, may injure the terminal extensor tendon at its distal phalanx insertion. Examination may reveal a mallet finger, which is characterized by at least 40 degrees of flexion of the DIP joint at rest (Fig. 18-12). These injuries are usually treated with continuous extension splinting of the DIP joint with a Mallet finger

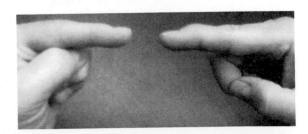

FIGURE 18-12 A chronic Mallet finger deformity on the right.

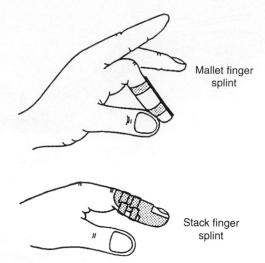

FIGURE 18-13 Splinting for mallet finger. (From McKeag DB, Mueller JL, eds. *ACSM's Primary Care Sports Medicine*. 2nd ed. Philadelphia: Lippincott Williams & Wilkins; 2007.)

splint or Stack splint (Fig. 18-13).[61] If associated fractures are present, surgical repair may be considered.

Metacarpophalangeal Injuries

Metacarpophalangeal injuries of the thumb seen in basketball include dislocations and ulnar collateral ligament sprains. MCP dislocations from a hyperextension force should be splinted for up to 4 weeks following a closed reduction. Unstable or nonreducible dislocations may require surgical intervention.

Acute tears of the MCP joint's ulnar collateral ligament, or "skier's thumb," may result from a radial force on an abducted thumb. Most injuries involve partial tears that may respond to immobilization of the MCP joint with thumb spica splinting.[59] Physical examination should attempt to identify complete tears with Stenar lesions (adductor aponeurosis interposition between the distally avulsed UCL and its phalangeal insertion), as these injuries may necessitate surgical intervention.[56] When a complete tear is suspected, stress testing of the UCL (Fig. 18-14) in full extension and in 30 degrees of flexion can help to determine ligamentous instability. There may also be a mass over the ulnar aspect of the MP joint.[60] Stress radiographs may be needed to help diagnose unstable injuries.

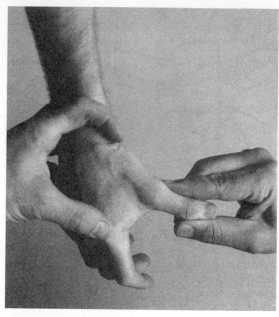

FIGURE 18-14 Ulnar collateral ligament stress test. (From McKeag DB, Mueller JL, eds. *ACSM's Primary Care Sports Medicine*. 2nd ed. Philadelphia: Lippincott Williams & Wilkins; 2007.)

WRIST

Injuries to the wrist are less common in basketball players than are injuries to the hand. However, because of the position of the hands when shooting, these injuries can significantly impact an athlete's ability to play. After an injury to the wrist, an athlete must regain 120 degrees of flexion/extension in the shooting wrist and 32 degrees of flexion/extension in the nonshooting wrist.

Scaphoid Fractures

The mechanism of injury for a scaphoid fracture results from a loaded extension force at the wrist with radial deviation, such as that resulting from a fall on an outstretched hand. Athletes may present with radial-sided wrist pain that is exacerbated by wrist extension, as well as point tenderness in the anatomic snuffbox or at the scaphoid tubercle.[62] Initial radiographs with AP, lateral, oblique, and scaphoid views of the wrist may be negative, despite the presence of a fracture. If clinical suspicion of a fracture persists, repeat plain films may be obtained; however, bone

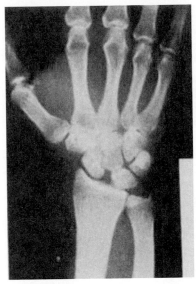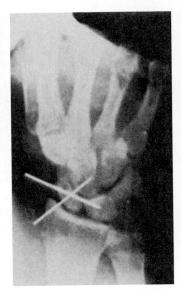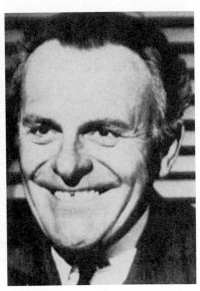

FIGURE 18-15 The Terry-Thomas sign: widening of the joint space between the scaphoid and lunate. (From Frankel VH. The Terry-Thomas sign. *Clin Orthop.* 1977;129:321–322.)

scan or MRI may be the better follow-up diagnostic imaging modalities.[63,64] The main objective of treatment is to obtain healthy union, and treatment options vary depending on the location and stability of the fracture. Most commonly, fractures occur in the mid-third of the scaphoid and are nondisplaced. These tend to obtain union either with casting or with internal surgical fixation. While both treatment options tend to obtain adequate union, surgical fixation may be associated with a more rapid return to play or work.[65] If casting is chosen, the average healing time is 8 to 10 weeks if the fracture is stabilized within the first few weeks after injury.[66] Initially, the athlete is placed in a long arm thumb spica cast for 4 weeks, followed by a short arm thumb spica cast. Fractures at the proximal pole or that are displaced or unstable have a poor prognosis for union with conservative management, and thus are usually addressed surgically.[67]

Scapholunate Ligament Injury

Scapholunate ligament injury may result from a fall onto a pronated hand. Acutely, the athlete may present with decreased ROM, tenderness, and swelling on the dorsal aspect of the wrist. Chronic cases may demonstrate a positive scaphoid shift test (or Watson test) that

is characterized by pain or a "pop" that occurs as pressure is applied to the dorsal distal pole of the scaphoid while moving the wrist from ulnar to radial deviation. Radiographs should include bilateral posterior-to-anterior (PA), lateral, and clenched fist views.[65–67] Widening of the scapholunate junction on plain films is called the Terry-Thomas sign and supports the diagnosis of scapholunate dissociation (Fig. 18-15). MR-arthrogram may be helpful if needed, though may be falsely negative in cases of incomplete ligament tears. Wrist arthroscopy confirms the diagnosis and allows for surgical repair.

SHOULDER

Glenohumeral instability is a term that describes a variety of pathologies, including atraumatic multidirectional instability and traumatic unidirectional instability. Underlying tears of the anterior glenoid labrum associated with detachment of the inferior glenohumeral ligament are known as Bankart lesions.[69] These are shoulder injuries that may be seen in basketball as a result of a fall, from a collision, or (in the case of multidirectional instability) with an insidious onset.

Traumatic unidirectional instability typically occurs in an anterior direction after a force is applied to an upper limb held in abduction and external rotation. The injury may spontaneously reduce or require manual reduction. In contrast, multidirectional instability usually presents without history of trauma; congenital laxity may be present throughout most joints, or shoulder capsular laxity may be present specifically in the overhead athlete with a history of repetitive motion.[68] These athletes may complain of "looseness" or vague pain in their shoulder with extremes of motion. They may also relate a history of minor subluxation episodes.

Examination includes neurovascular status, strength, range of motion, direction of glenohumeral laxity, and presence of any generalized joint laxity. Special examination tests such as the load-and-shift test, anterior apprehension test, relocation test, and sulcus test may be used. Athletes who have experienced a traumatic dislocation often describe a "pop"; displacement may be elicited during the anterior apprehension test.

Recommended radiographic imaging includes AP views with the humerus in slight external rotation and internal rotation, an axillary view, and a Stryker notch view.[70,71] Radiographs obtained after an initial episode of instability can help visualize the anterior glenoid rim and posterolateral surface of the humeral head. These structures can abut during traumatic anterior instability, leading to a bony Bankart lesion (fracture of the anterior glenoid rim); (Fig. 18-16) or Hill-Sachs defect (osteochondral lesion on the humeral head). Both of these lesions may be associated with recurrent instability due to decreased bony

support for the glenohumeral articulation, and typically necessitate surgical repair. MRI, especially MR-arthrogram, may be helpful if needed to help diagnose labral pathology.

Treatment of glenohumeral instability largely depends on the patient's age and athletic involvement. Treatment is geared toward preventing the recurrence of instability. For the patient with a history of atraumatic instability, a rehabilitation program emphasizing rotator cuff strengthening may be the mainstay of treatment for several months prior to considering surgical intervention.[68,69,72] For acute anterior instability, conservative treatment involves rehabilitation to regain motion and strengthening of the rotator cuff musculature. Some recommend a 2- to 6-week period of rest prior to beginning a course of rehabilitation.[69] Athletes may return to contact sport once range of motion and strength allow performance of athletic tasks without significant risk of recurrent instability. Supportive braces, such as the Sulley brace or glenohumeral taping, may be utilized to provide additional support. Conservative therapy in the younger active patient has been linked to higher rates of recurrent instability when compared to open primary repair of first-time traumatic anterior dislocations.[73] Both arthroscopic and open repair procedures have been utilized for recurrent anterior shoulder instability; however, a recent review of the literature suggests that arthroscopic approaches are not as effective as open repair.[74] Additionally, the presence of bony lesions usually prompts primary surgical intervention.

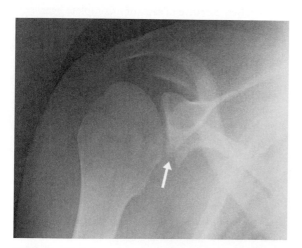

FIGURE 18-16 Bony Bankart lesion on radiograph. The anterior glenoid labrum is torn, with associated detachment of the inferior glenohumeral ligament.

CONCLUSION

Basketball is a popular sport, played by thousands at all skill levels. It is a fast-moving game, involving running, jumping, and cutting. It is a game of skill, with dribbling, passing, and shooting as key skills. It is a noncontact sport that has a great deal of incidental (or not-so-incidental) contact.

With all of these facets of the game, basketball is a sport in which we can encounter a wide variety of injuries. Excellent physical examination skills for the entire musculoskeletal system are important to possess, in order to obtain the correct diagnosis for an injury. Certain conditions do require surgical management; however, many of the injuries will benefit from a careful, conservative approach to rehabilitation.

REFERENCES

1. Hoffman JR. Epidemiology of basketball injuries. In: McKeag DB, ed. *Basketball.* Malden, MA: Blackwell Science; 2003:1–10.
2. Meeuwisse, WH, Sellmer R, Hagel BE. Rates and risks of injury during intercollegiate basketball. *Am J Sports Med.* 2003;31:379–385.
3. Cohen AR, Metzl J. Sports-specific concerns in the young athlete: basketball. *Pediatr Emerg Care.* 2000;16:462–468.
4. 2006-07 High School Athletics Participation Survey. Available at: http://www.nfhs.org/core/contentmanager/uploads/2006-07_Participation_Survey.pdf. Accessed December 2, 2007.
5. Powell JW, Barber-Foss KD. Sex-related injury patterns among selected high school sports. *Am J Sports Med.* 2000;28:385–391.
6. Agel J, Olson DE, Dick R. Descriptive epidemiology of collegiate women's basketball injuries: National Collegiate Athletic Association injury surveillance system 1988–1989 through 2003–2004. *J Athlet Train.* 2007;42:202–210.
7. Dick R, Hertel J, Agel J. Descriptive epidemiology of collegiate men's basketball injuries: National Collegiate Athletic Association injury surveillance system 1988–1989 through 2003–2004. *J Athlet Train.* 2007;42:194–201.
8. Deitch JR, Starkey C, Walters S, et al. Injury risk in professional basketball players: a comparison of Women's National Basketball Association and National Basketball Association athletes. *Am J Sports Med.* 2006;34:1077–1083.
9. McKay GD, Goldie PA, Payne WR, et al. Ankle injuries in basketball: injury rate and risk factors. *Br J Sports Med.* 2001;35:103–108.
10. Clanton TO, Porter DA. Primary care of the foot and ankle. *Clin Sports Med.* 1997;16:435–466.
11. Porter DA. Ligament injuries of the foot and ankle. In: Fitzgerald RH, Kaufer H, Malkani AL, eds. *Orthopaedics.* St. Louis: Mosby; 2002:1607–1621.
12. Chen RC, Shia DS, Kamath GV, et al. Troublesome stress fractures of the foot and ankle. *Sports Med Arthrosc Rev.* 2006;14:246–251.
13. Reese K, Litsky A, Kaeding C, et al. Cannulated screw fixation of Jones fractures: a clinical and biomechanical study. *Am J Sports Med.* 2004;32:1736–1742.
14. Fitch K, Blackwwell J, Gilmour W. Operation for non-union of stress fracture of the tarsal navicular. *J Bone Joint Surg.* 1989;71:105–110.
15. Ivins D. Acute ankle sprain: an update. *Am Fam Physician.* 2006;74:1714–1720, 1723–1726.
16. Beynnon BD, Renstrom PA, Haugh L, et al. A prospective, randomized clinical investigation of the treatment of first-time ankle sprains. *Sports Med.* 2006;34:1401–1412.
17. Amendola A, Williams G, Foster D. Evidence-based approach to treatment of acute traumatic syndesmosis (high ankle) sprains. *Sports Med Arthrosc Rev.* 2006;14:232–236.
18. Alfredson H, Cook J. A treatment algorithm for managing Achilles tendinopathy: new treatment options. *Br J Sports Med.* 2007;41:211–216.
19. Almekinders L, Temple J. Etiology, diagnosis, and treatment of tendinitis: an analysis of the literature. *Med Sci Sports Exer.* 1998;30:1183–1190.
20. Enwemeka CS. The effects of therapeutic ultrasound on tendon healing: a biomechanical study. *Am J Phys Med Rehabil.* 1989;68:283–287.
21. Jackson B, Schwane J, Starcher B. Effect of ultrasound therapy on the repair of Achilles tendon injuries in rats. *Med Sci Sports Exerc.* 1991;23:171–176.
22. Shrier I, Matheson G, Kohl H. Achilles tendonitis: are corticosteroid injections useful or harmful? *Clin J Sports Med.* 1996;6:245–250.
23. Alfredson H, Pietiln T, Jonsson P. Heavy-load eccentric calf muscle training for the treatment of chronic Achilles tendinosis. *Am J Sports Med.* 1998;26:360–366.
24. Fahlstrom M, Jonsson P, Lorentzon R. Chronic Achilles tendon pain treated with eccentric calf muscle training. *Knee Surg Sports Traumatol Arthrosc.* 2003;11:327–333.
25. Paoloni J, Appleyard R, Nelson J, et al. Topical glyceryl trinitrate treatment of chronic noninsertional Achilles tendinopathy. *J Bone Joint Surg Am.* 2004;86A:916–922.
26. Mazzone MF, McCue T. Common conditions of the Achilles tendon. *Am Fam Physician.* 2002;65:1805–1810.
27. Aldridge T. Diagnosing heel pain in adults. *Am Fam Physician.* 2004;70:332–338.
28. Emery CA, Rose MS, McAllister JR, et al. A prevention strategy to reduce the incidence of injury in high school basketball: a cluster randomized controlled trial. *Clin J Sports Med.* 2007;17:17–24.
29. Hewett TE, Ford KR, Myer GD. Anterior cruciate ligament injuries in female athletes. Part 2. A meta-analysis of neuromuscular interventions aimed at injury prevention. *Am J Sports Med.* 2006;34:490–498.
30. Dixit S, DiFiori J, Burton M, Mines B. Management of patellofemoral pain syndrome. *Am Fam Physician.* 2007;75:194–202.
31. Fredericson M, Yoon K. Physical examination and patellofemoral pain syndrome. *Am J Phys Med Rehabil.* 2006;85:234–243.
32. Gerbino P, Griffin E, Hemecourt P, et al. Patellofemoral pain syndrome: evaluation and location and intensity of pain. *Clin J Pain.* 2006;22:154–159.
33. Haim A, Yaniv M, Dekel S, et al. Patellofemoral pain syndrome. *Clin Orthop.* 2006;451:223–228.
34. Crossley K, Bennell K, Green S, et al. A systematic review of physical interventions for patellofemoral pain syndrome. *Clin J Sports Med.* 2001;11:103–110.
35. Lun V, Wiley P, Meeuwisse W, et al. Effectiveness of patellar bracing for treatment of patellofemoral pain syndrome. *Clin J Sports Med.* 2005;15:235–240.
36. McConnell J. The management of chrondomalacia patella: a long-term solution. *Aust J Physiother.* 1986;32:215–223.
37. Crossley K, Bennell K, Green S, et al. Physical therapy for patellofemoral pain. *Am J Sports Med.* 2002;30:857–865.
38. Fulkerson JP. Diagnosis and treatment of patients with patellofemoral pain. *Am J Sports Med.* 2002;30:447–456.
39. Witvrouw E, Bellemans J, Lysens R. Intrinsic risk factors for the development of patellar tendinitis in an athletic population: a two-year prospective study. *Am J Sports Med.* 2001;29:190–195.
40. Ferretti A. Epidemiology of jumper's knee. *Sports Med.* 1986;3:289–295.
41. Warden SJ, Kiss ZS, Malara FA, et al. Comparitive accuracy of magnetic resonance imaging and ultrasonography

in confirming clinically diagnosed patellar tendinopathy. *Am J Sports Med*. 2007;35:427–436.

42. Bahr R, Fossan B, Loken S, et al. Surgical treatment compared with eccentric training for patellar tendinopathy (jumper's knee). *J Bone Joint Surg Am*. 2006;88A:1689–1698.

43. Visnes H, Bahr R. The evolution of eccentric training as treatment for patellar tendinopathy (jumper's knee): a critical review of exercise programmes. *Br J Sports Med*. 2007;41:217–223.

44. Peers KH, Lysens RJ. Patellar tendinopathy in athletes. *Sports Med*. 2006;35:71–87.

45. Wang CJ, Ko JY, Chan YS, et al. Extracorporeal shock wave for chronic patellar tendinopathy. *Am J Sports Med*. 2007;35:972–978.

46. James S, Ali K, Robertson C, et al. Ultrasound guided dry needling and autologous blood injection for patellar tendinosis. *Br J Sports Med*. 2007;41:518–521.

47. Hoksrud A, Ohberg L, Alfredson H, et al. Ultrasound-guided sclerosis of neovessels in painful chronic patellar tendinopathy. *Am J Sports Med*. 2006;34:1738–1746.

48. Calmbach WL, Hutchens M. Evaluation of patients presenting with knee pain: part II. Differential diagnosis. *Am Fam Physician*. 2003;68:917–922.

49. Swenson EJ. Knee injuries. In: McKeag DB, Moeller JL, eds. *ACSM's Primary Care Sports Medicine*. Philadelphia: Lippincott; 2007:461–490.

50. Reider B, Sathy MR, Talkington K, et al. Treatment of isolated medial collateral ligament injuries in athletes with early functional rehabilitation. A five-year follow-up study. *Am J Sports Med*. 1994;22:470–477.

51. Albright JP, Powell JW, Smith W, et al. Medial collateral ligament knee sprains in college football. Effectiveness of preventive braces. *Am J Sports Med*. 1994;22:12–18.

52. Jackson MD. Rehabilitation. In: McKeag DB, Moeller JL, eds. *ACSM's Primary Care Sports Medicine*. Philadelphia: Lippincott; 2007:563–593.

53. Calmbach WL, Hutchens M. Evaluation of patients presenting with knee pain: part I. History, physical examination, radiographs, and laboratory tests. *Am Fam Physician*. 2003;68:917–922.

54. Malanga GA, Andrus S, Nadler S, et al. Physical examination of the knee: a review of the original test descriptions and scientific validity of common orthopedic tests. *Arch Phys Med Rehabil*. 2003;84:592–603.

55. Walsh WM, Vanicek JJ. Knee injuries. In: Mellion MB, Walsh WM, Madden C, et al., eds. *Team Physian's Handbook*. 3rd ed. Philadelphia: Hanley & Belfus; 2002: 490–509.

56. Rettig AC. Athletic injuries of the wrist and hand. Part II: overuse injuries of the wrist and traumatic injuries to the hand. *Am J Sports Med*. 2004;32:262–273.

57. McCue FC, Honner R, Gieck JH, et al. A pseudo-boutonniere deformity. *Hand*. 1975;7:166–170.

58. Lang J, Counselman F. Common orthopedic hand and wrist injuries. *Emerg Med*. 2003;35:20–38.

59. Lillegard W. Wrist, hand, and finger injuries. In: McKeag DB, Moeller JL, eds. *ACSM's Primary Care Sports Medicine*. Philadelphia: Lippincott; 2007:563–593.

60. Abrahamsson SO, Sollerman C, Lunborg G, et al. Diagnosis of displaced ulnar collateral ligament of the metacarpophalangeal joint of the thumb. *J Hand Surg (Am)*. 1990;15:457–460.

61. Wang Q, Johnson B. Fingertip injuries. *Am Fam Physician*. 2001;63:1961–1966.

62. Phillips TG, Reibach AM, Slomiany WP. Diagnosis and management of scaphoid fractures. *Am Fam Physician*. 2004;70:879–884.

63. Brydie A, Raby N. Early MRI in the management of clincial scaphoid fracture. *Br J Radiol*. 2003;76:296–300.

64. Thorpe A, Murray A, Smith F, et al. Clincially suspected scaphoid fracture: a comparison of magnetic resonance imaging and bone scintigraphy. *Br J Radiol*. 1996;69:109–113.

65. Bond C, Shin A, McBride M, et al. Percutaneous screw fixation or cast immobilization for nondisplaced scaphoid fractures. *J Bone Joint Surg Am*. 2001;83A:483–488.

66. Cooney W, Dobyns J, Linscheid R. Nonunion of the scaphoid: analysis of the results from bone grafting. *J Hand Surg Am*. 1980;5:343–354.

67. Rettig AC. Athletic injuries of the wrist and hand. Part I: traumatic injuries of the wrist. *Am J Sports Med*. 2003;31:1038–1048.

68. Nelson B, Arciero R. Arthroscopic management of glenohumeral instability. *Am J Sports Med*. 2000;28:602–614.

69. Mahaffey B, Smith P. Shoulder instability in young athletes. *Am Fam Physician*. 1999;59:2773–2782, 2787.

70. Friedman R, Blocker E, Morrow D. Glenohumeral instability. *J South Orthop Assoc*. 1995;4:182–199.

71. Gusmer PB, Potter HG. Imaging of shoulder instability. *Clin Sports Med*. 1995;14:777–795.

72. Castagna A, Nordenson U, Garofalo R, et al. Minor shoulder instability. *Arthroscopy*. 2007;23:211–215.

73. Jakobsen B, Johannsen H, Suder P, et al. Primary repair versus conservative treatment of first-time traumatic anterior dislocation of the shoulder: a randomized study with 10-year follow-up. *Arthroscopy*. 2007;23:118–123.

74. Lenters TR, Franta AR, Wolf FM, et al. Arthroscopic compared with open repairs for recurrent anterior shoulder instability: a systematic review and meta-analysis of the literature. *J Bone Joint Surg Am*. 2007;89A:244–254.

Volleyball Injuries

Volleyball is an immensely popular sport. Part of its popularity stems from its high appeal as a casual sport for both men and women. Beyond the casual player, it is estimated that some 800 million people participate in volleyball at a recreational level on a regular basis worldwide.[1] In addition to these recreational participants, volleyball has a large professional contingent. The Fédération Internationale de Volleyball (FIVB) is the international governing body representing 500 million elite and professional players, with 218 affiliated national federations.[2] In 1964, volleyball became an Olympic sport; in 1996, beach volleyball was added as an event.[1,2]

In the course of a match, a player may jump 150 times.[3] A professional player may practice and play for such an extensive amount of time that he or she performs 40,000 spikes per year.[4] A number of injuries in volleyball result from the repetitive stresses this sport places upon the athlete. Volleyball is considered a noncontact sport because the two teams are separated by a net; however, in reality, contact does occur beneath the net and plays a role in the nature of the injuries encountered. The ankle, knee, and hand are among the most commonly injured areas.

SPORT SKILLS

Volleyball is played on a court measuring 18 meters long by 9 meters wide. A center line and net divide the court into two equal square areas. Three meters from the net on either side of the court, the attack line demarcates the front (or attack) zone and the service zone. The net height for men is 2.43 meters (7' 11 5/8"); for women it is 2.24 meters (7' 4 1/8").[3,5] At social levels, a variety of rules may apply, with any number players being on a side. Recreational leagues tend to formalize the number of players allowed on the court and follow the official rules more closely. Professional games played on hard courts use six-player teams that rotate through all positions on the court; substitutions may occur.[1]

The basic premise of the game is to win a rally by having the ball drop to the ground on the opponent's side of the net. A team can touch the ball only three times on its side of the net before it must be hit over. Volleyball is a rebound sport—the ball may not be held. The ball is rallied back and forth over the net until the ball hits the ground, a team hits it too many times on its side of the net, or some other fault is made (hitting the net during a play on the ball, one player hitting the ball twice in succession, catching the ball, etc.).[5]

Game play starts with one team serving the ball to the other team. The player serving the ball generally tosses the ball up into the air and strikes it with the dominant hand while it is overhead; this may be done while standing or while jumping. The opposing team then receives the serve, usually as a *bump*, played off of both forearms simultaneously. The ball is then *set*—hit with both hands held overhead—to direct it forward to the net in preparation for a *spike*. In a spike (also called an attack or smash), the player jumps into the air, ideally contacting the ball overhead while at the highest point of the jump. The hand or fist is used to strike the ball down onto the court on the other side of the net. At professional levels, a spike may travel at speeds of 90 miles per hour.[1] During a spike, the other team attempts to defend against the spike by jumping with outstretched arms and hands to *block* the spike (a block does not count as one of the team's three hits, and the player who contacts the ball during the block may hit the ball consecutively as the team's first hit). Should the block fail, other team members attempt to *dig* (bump the ball into the air just before it hits the ground) the spiked ball up into play so that their team may rally it back over the net. This pattern of bump–set–spike is repeated until a rally ends and a point is won.

Recent rule changes have been made to make the game more exciting, with faster-paced scoring and longer rallies. For the Sydney Olympic Games in 2000, the scoring system was changed to "rally scoring." Instead of a team scoring a point only when they served and won a rally, a point is now scored by whichever team wins a rally, even if they did not serve. Also in 2000, the "libero" position was added; this defensive specialist is allowed to substitute into the back row, but may not serve or spike the ball. The libero position allows shorter athletes to play a vital role for their teams.[6]

Injury rates are the highest with blocking. These injuries are often finger or hand injuries from contact with the ball, or ankle injuries from landing on another player's foot.[1,7] The act of spiking is also associated with a large number of injuries, primarily to the knee and ankle. Serving, bumping, and setting have relatively lower rates of injury.[1] Digging is not associated with a high level of risk among high-level players, except for when they are first learning to dive. Then, there is an increased risk of chin laceration or contusion.[3] Injury rates are also related to position on the court. Those playing close to the net have a threefold greater risk of injury than those playing away from the net (Fig. 19-1).[3]

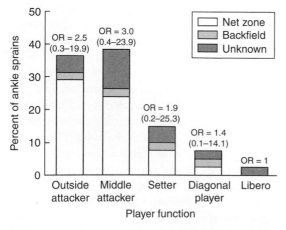

FIGURE 19-1 Example of injuries—in this case, ankle sprains—by position on the court. (From Verhagen EAL, Van der Beek A, Bouter L. A one season prospective cohort study of volleyball injuries. *Br J Sports Med.* 2004;38:477–481.)

ANKLE INJURIES

The most common acute volleyball injury is the ankle sprain. In some series, it accounts for up to 55% of all injuries.[8] Ankle injuries are usually of the plantar-flexion inversion type and involve the lateral ligaments.[3] They can occur in any situation in this fast-moving game, but most often are a result of a blocker landing on the foot of an attacker from the opposite team under the net.[1]

Treatment of the acutely injured ankle depends upon the severity and the setting. If a fracture is suspected, if there is excessive swelling, or if the athlete is incapable of bearing weight, the player is held from further play/practice and radiographs are obtained. In the midst of a tournament, the ankle sprain may be treated with ice water immersion between matches and electrical stimulation twice daily. Play may continue using an ankle air stirrup brace over a tubular compression dressing; slow, gradual warm-up prior to play is recommended.[7] Relative rest, ice, compression, and elevation may be utilized if the injury occurs during practice.

In the longer term, ankle taping, high-top shoes, or semirigid ankle supports may be of benefit, as is proprioceptive and coordination training. Attention should be paid to proper jump technique to emphasize vertical rather than horizontal travel.[1]

KNEE INJURIES

The most commonly seen knee injury in volleyball is patellar tendinitis, or jumper's knee. It is a condition that typically has an insidious onset; the condition is often persistent. In most cases, it does not cause a significant loss of time from play. Jumper's knee has been shown to have a 45% prevalence among professional male players; those with greater leg strength and jumping ability are at greater risk to develop this condition.[9,10]

The symptoms of patellar tendonitis include pain at the inferior pole of the patella; less frequently, pain is at the superior pole or at the tibial tuberosity (Fig. 19-2).[1] Treatment includes ice and compression with a neoprene sleeve; nonsteroidal anti-inflammatory medications may be of benefit. Strengthening the vastus medialis muscle should be a part of the long-term treatment, and shoe orthotics may need to be considered.[7] Surgery is reserved for recalcitrant cases.

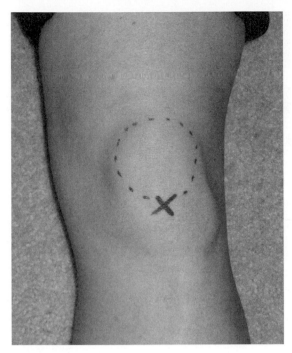

FIGURE 19-2 The most common site of pain with patellar tendonitis is the inferior patellar pole (*marked*). Less common sites include the superior patellar pole and the tibial tuberosity.

Injury to the ligaments of the knee occurs less frequently than patellar tendonitis, but obviously has more serious consequences. They generally occur near the net in the attack zone, usually during some phase of a jump.[1] These injuries occur more frequently in females than males (for unclear reasons), and during spikes more than blocks.[11] Immediate treatment includes ice and removal from play; further management of these injuries is beyond the scope of this text.

In adolescent volleyball players, one may encounter pain, swelling, and tenderness over the tibial tubercle. This condition, commonly referred to as Osgood-Schlatter syndrome, is a traction apophysitis at the tibial tubercle and may be seen in sports where jumping is common. Radiographs may confirm the diagnosis. Most cases respond to relative rest, ice, activity modification, and low-intensity quadriceps strengthening exercises; surgery may be necessary in refractory cases once skeletal maturity is attained.[12]

FINGER, HAND, AND WRIST INJURIES

Injuries to the finger, hands, and wrists are fairly common in volleyball, with most occurring as a result of contact with the ball during play near the net.[13] Sprains and strains are most frequently seen, followed by fracture, contusion, and dislocation.[1] Although these are common injuries, they are often perceived as being minor, and the athlete may continue to play without seeking treatment. Immediate treatment of a finger injury includes a thorough evaluation; radiographs should be obtained when indicated. Play can usually resume with splinting and/or buddy taping of the affected digits.[1] Despite their seemingly minor nature, these injuries should not simply be ignored. In one series, more than one in four volleyball players with prior finger injuries complained of ongoing problems, including pain, stiffness, deformity, movement limitations, and discomfort with the use of the hand.[13]

De Quervain stenosing tenosynovitis may be encountered in volleyball players. This is an inflammatory synovitis in the tendon sheaths of the extensor pollicis brevis and abductor pollicis longus muscles within the first dorsal compartment of the wrist. It is due, in part, to the frequent forceful contact of the ball on the radial forearms in the process of bumping. Symptoms of pain and tenderness may be noted along these tendons as they run along the radial aspect of the wrist; a positive Finkelstein maneuver may be elicited (Fig. 19-3). This condition may be more severe in professional players as a result of the increased training time required of elite athletes.[14]

Less frequently seen injuries to this area include pisiform fracture and blunt-force injuries to the radial and ulnar arteries.[1] Players should not be allowed to wear rings or other jewelry due to the potential for avulsion injury should the items become caught in the net.[13]

SHOULDER INJURIES

The majority of shoulder injuries in volleyball are related to chronic overuse, especially of the rotator cuff and long-head biceps tendons. Many of the skills necessary for volleyball play involve the forceful use of the arms in an overhead position. In particular, they are often rapidly and forcefully moved from a position of abduction and external rotation

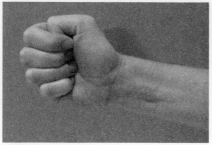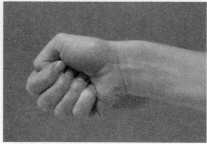

FIGURE 19-3 Finkelstein maneuver. A fist is made with the thumb inside the fingers. The hand is then deviated in an ulnar direction, either actively (as shown) or passively. Pain along the radial aspect of the wrist is a positive finding.

into a position of extension and internal rotation.[1] Because these injuries are often chronic, they usually do not cause an athlete to lose playing time. In a game setting, provided the athlete can abduct the arm, play may continue with ice application between the matches and twice daily electrical stimulation; if the athlete has significant pain or is unable to abduct the arm, play should not be allowed.[7] A formal shoulder rehabilitation program should begin in either case.

Studies have attempted to identify the features most closely associated with shoulder injury in volleyball players. Muscle weakness, impaired shoulder mobility, and scapular asymmetry play some role, but muscle strength imbalance between the muscles of internal rotation and the muscles external rotation appears to be the most strongly associated factor. The act of spiking the ball requires a dynamic balance between these muscle groups to allow for a strong, fast, powerful movement of the limb, followed immediately by a controlled deceleration.[15] Strengthening of the muscles of external rotation to balance the typically better-developed muscles of internal rotation may help lessen symptoms, or may help prevent players from developing problems later in their careers.[4]

In elite volleyball players, isolated atrophy of the infraspinatus muscle is encountered on a surprisingly frequent basis. Between 13% and 32% of elite players may be found to have atrophy in the infraspinatus muscle, but the majority are asymptomatic.[1] This condition is thought to be due to an entrapment and compression of the suprascapular nerve at the spinoglenoid notch, resulting in the partial paralysis of the terminal motor branch of the nerve (Fig. 19-4).[16]

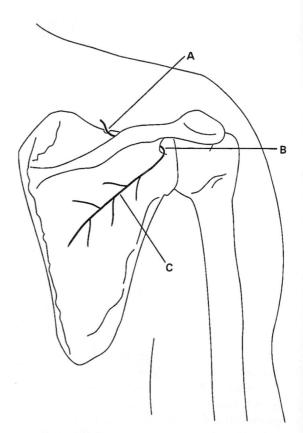

FIGURE 19-4 The suprascapular nerve as it travels along the scapula. **A.** Suprascapular notch. **B.** Spinoglenoid notch. **C.** Suprascapular nerve (in infraspinatus muscle). (From Wang DH, Koehler SM. Isolated infraspinatus atrophy in a collegiate volleyball player. *Clin J Sports Med.* 1996;6:255–258.)

LOW BACK INJURIES

Low back injuries occur with reasonable frequency in volleyball players. The most commonly reported diagnosis is mechanical low back pain with onset while landing from a jump.[1] Although these injuries may be seen regularly, they are usually not severe. In one series, none of those players with low back injuries missed more than one day of play.[3] Ice, electrical stimulation, massage, and stretching are utilized for treatment. In cases of low back pain with radiating leg symptoms, the athlete should be held from play and undergo appropriate further evaluation and management.[7]

OTHER INJURIES

Traumatic brain injury is reported only infrequently in volleyball players. In one series, an injury rate of 0.14 per 100 player-seasons was reported.[18] Neck injuries are also quite rare in this sport, with the majority being muscular in nature.[1] Isolated case reports exist of a traumatic myocardial infarction after being struck in the chest by a spiked ball and of a spontaneous pneumomediastinum occurring during volleyball practice.[19,20]

BEACH VOLLEYBALL

There are a number of differences between indoor and beach volleyball. Most obvious is that the latter game is played on a sand court rather than a hard surface. The court size is slightly smaller for beach volleyball—16 meters by 8 meters. Athletes play barefoot in beach volleyball, unless permitted to wear shoes by the official for an appropriate reason. Instead of six-on-six competition, beach volleyball is played as a two versus two game. Substitution is not allowed in beach volleyball. In beach volleyball, a blocking attempt is counted as one of the team's three hits. Finally, the air pressure in the beach volleyball is reduced roughly by half.[5,21]

Despite the differences in play, injury types and causes are similar between beach and indoor volleyball. Of the injuries reported in beach volleyball, overuse injuries of the knee, shoulder, and low back are the most commonly seen.[22] For acute injuries, field defense and spiking are considered the most

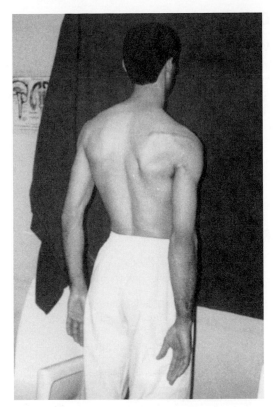

FIGURE 19-5 Wasting of the right infraspinatus muscle. (From Ravindran M. Two cases of suprascapular neuropathy in a family. *Br J Sports Med.* 2003;37:539–541.)

Examination findings may include atrophy of the infraspinatus muscle and loss of external rotation strength (Fig. 19-5). Needle electromyography may be helpful in documenting denervation in the infraspinatus. For most, rehabilitative exercises aimed at strengthening the muscles of external rotation are sufficient treatment; for those with persistent pain, surgery may be considered, as ganglion cysts may be present at the spinoglenoid notch.[16]

One final shoulder-region problem that may be seen more frequently in volleyball players is the development of a posterior circumflex humeral artery aneurysm. This rare condition is characterized by ischemia-related symptoms, such as forearm pain and tightness, hand cramping, pallor, and paresthesias. Evidence of distal emboli may be found. Arterial evaluation is required, and surgical repair may be necessary.[17]

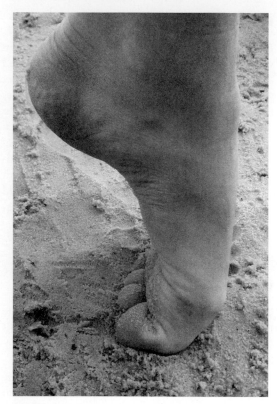

FIGURE 19-6 "Sand toe." A hyperplantar-flexion injury of the metatarsophalangeal joint, caused when the body's weight lands on plantar-flexed toes.

common causes.[23] Although data vary, there appear to be slightly fewer time-loss injuries in beach volleyball, possibly as a result of the softer playing surface.[1,22]

One injury unique to beach volleyball is the condition known as "sand toe"—a hyperplantar-flexion injury to the metatarsophalangeal joint (Fig. 19-6). This differs from "turf toe"—a hyperdorsiflexion injury to the metatarsophalangeal joint. In sand toe, pain is the main symptom, with difficulty reported in activities such as pushing off, running, and jumping. Treatment is conservative, with relative rest, ice, and anti-inflammatory medications. The affected joint may be taped, and shoe wear may need modification. In the longer term, a "toe-strengthening" program may be of benefit, including toe squeezes, toe pulls (against rubber bands), golf ball rolls, marble pick-ups, and towel curls. In one series, sand toe injuries averaged 6 months to recover.[24]

CONCLUSION

Volleyball is a popular sport, both socially and recreationally due to its widespread availability and appeal, and professionally due to its fast-paced action. Although it is a noncontact sport, some of the most significant injuries occur as a result of contact with other players. Overuse injuries are also common. Close attention paid to technique, and efforts to follow a balanced training regimen, have potential to reduce the number of injuries encountered.

REFERENCES

1. Briner WW Jr., Kacmar L. Common injuries in volleyball: mechanisms of injury, prevention and rehabilitation. *Sports Med*. 1997;24:65–71.
2. FIVB today. Available at: http://www.fivb.org/EN/FIVB/Cp_fivbToday.htm. Accessed November 10, 2007.
3. Schafle MD, Requa RK, Patton WL, et al. Injuries in the 1987 national amateur volleyball tournament. *Am J Sports Med*. 1990;18:624–631.
4. Kugler A, Krüger-Franke M, Reininger S, et al. Muscular imbalance and shoulder pain in volleyball attackers. *Br J Sports Med*. 1996;30:256–259.
5. 2005 Official Volleyball Rules. Available at: http://www.fivb.org/en/volleyball/Rules/FIVB.2005.VB.RulesOfThe Game.Eng-Fre.pdf. Accessed November 10, 2007.
6. The Game. Available at: http://www.fivb.org/TheGame/TheGame_Volleyballl.htm. Accessed November 10, 2007.
7. Schafle MD. Common injuries in volleyball: treatment, prevention and rehabilitation. *Sports Med*. 1993;16:126–129.
8. Watkins J, Green BN. Volleyball injuries: a survey of injuries of Scottish National League male players. *Br J Sports Med*. 1992;26:135–137.
9. Lian ØB, Engebretsen L, Bahr R. Prevalence of jumper's knee among elite athletes from different sports: a cross-sectional study. *Am J Sports Med*. 2005;33:561–567.
10. Lian Ø, Refsnes PE, Engebretsen L, et al. Performance characteristics of volleyball players with patellar tendinopathy. *Am J Sports Med*. 2003;31:408–413.
11. Ferretti A, Papandrea P, Conteduca F, et al. Knee ligament injuries in volleyball players. *Am J Sports Med*. 1992;20:203–207.
12. Gholve PA, Scher DM, Khakharia S, et al. Osgood-Schlatter syndrome. *Curr Opin Pediatr*. 2007;19:44–50.
13. Bhairo NH, Nijsten MWN, von Dalen KC, et al. Hand injuries in volleyball. *Int J Sports Med*. 1992;13:351–354.
14. Rossi C, Cellocco P, Margaritondo E, et al. De Quervain disease in volleyball players. *Am J Sports Med*. 2005;33:424–427.
15. Wang HK, Cochrane T. Mobility impairment, muscle balance, muscle weakness, scapular asymmetry, and shoulder injury in elite volleyball athletes. *J Sports Med Phys Fitness*. 2001;41:403–410.

16. Ferretti A, De Carli A, Fontana M. Injury of the supras-capular nerve at the spinoglenoid notch: the natural history of infraspinatus atrophy in volleyball players. *Am J Sports Med.* 1998;26:759–763.

17. McIntosh A, Hassan I, Cherry K, et al. Posterior circumflex humeral artery aneurysm in 2 professional volleyball players. *Am J Orthop.* 2006;35:33–36.

18. Powell JW, Barber-Foss KD. Traumatic brain injury in high school athletes. *JAMA.* 1999;282:958–963.

19. Grossfeld PD, Friedman DB, Levine BD. Traumatic myocardial infarction during competitive volleyball: a case report. *Med Sci Sports Exerc.* 1993;25:901–903.

20. Nichols AW. Spontaneous pneumomediastinum in a collegiate volleyball player. *Clin J Sport Med.* 1999;9:97–99.

21. Official Beach Volleyball Rules 2007–2008. Available at: http://www.fivb.org/EN/BeachVolleyball/Rules/RulesOf theGames2007_2008_EN.pdf. Accessed November 10, 2007.

22. Bahr R, Reeser JC. Injuries among world-class professional beach volleyball players: the Fédération Internationale de Volleyball beach volleyball injury study. *Am J Sports Med.* 2003;31:119–125.

23. Aagaard H, Scavenius M, Jørgensen U. An epidemiological analysis of the injury pattern in indoor and in beach volleyball. *Int J Sports Med.* 1997;18:217–221.

24. Frey C, Andersen GD, Feder KS. Plantarflexion injury to the metatarsophalangeal joint ("sand toe"). *Foot Ankle Int.* 1996;17:576–581.

Weight-Training Injuries

H istorically, soldiers in ancient Rome lifted heavy stones to prepare for battle and performed feats of strength for sport. Since the 1950s, weight lifting has been popularized by body-building professionals such as Steve Reeves, Reg Park, Arnold Schwarzenegger, and Dorian Yates. Today, weight training has become a very important part of a comprehensive fitness program in the quest for optimal health for all ages. Weight training is also an essential component of cross-training, which has become an integral part in preparing for and improving performance in most sports.[1]

In general, weight training is repetitive in nature, and most injuries that are seen are chronic.[2] Improper training techniques and overtraining are associated with the development of these injuries. This chapter will focus on proper weight-lifting techniques, common injuries in weight lifters, and the management of those injuries.

COMMON WEIGHT LIFTING TECHNIQUES

Squat

In the squat, the bar should rest on the trapezius muscles with the head straight forward and facing slightly upward (Fig. 20-1). The feet should be positioned approximately shoulder width apart to increase the base of support. The hips and knees should be slightly flexed and the spine should be in neutral. Then with a fluid, controlled movement, the hips and knees are flexed until the knees come to a 90-degree angle to the floor. The body weight should fall onto the gluteals, hamstrings, and quadriceps. The hips and knees are then extended, back to the

initial position and the exercise is repeated. The core stabilizer muscles should be activated isometrically throughout the exercise. These muscles include the abdominal muscles (transversus abdominus, internal and external obliques, rectus abdominus), quadratus lumborum, pelvic floor muscles, and hip and pelvic muscles (glutei); as well as a tightening of the thoracolumbar fascia (connecting lower extremity to upper extremity) and the diaphragm; working in multiple planes to provide a "rigid cylinder for trunk support."[3,4] Many exercises, including the squat, call for the spine to be in an anatomically neutral position. Excessive extension of the spine can produce excessive shearing forces and strain on the erector musculature and on posterior spinal elements.

Bench Press

The bench press is one of the most widely used weight-training exercises. The bench press is done primarily to strengthen the pectorals with secondary deltoid and triceps involvement. The exercise is done correctly with the athlete in a supine position with the spine in neutral and feet planted on the floor with the knees at approximately 90 degrees (Fig. 20-2). The bar should be held approximately two finger-breadths wider than shoulder width. The scapulae should be retracted slightly. The weight should be lowered until the elbows come to a 90-degree angle. The weight is then lifted to the starting position using a controlled, fluid movement. The core stabilizer muscles should be activated throughout the movement. Unfortunately, some athletes use excessive weight and compensate by arching the back to produce more leverage to lift the weight, which produces stress on the posterior elements of the spine and can lead to injury.

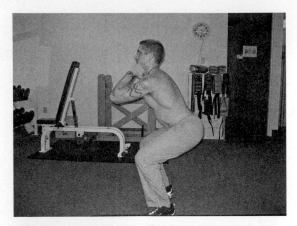

FIGURE 20-1 Squat. Note position of head, back in neutral position, hips, and knees.

Shoulder Press

The primary target area of the military or overhead shoulder press is the deltoids, with secondary emphasis on the trapezius muscles, upper pectorals, and triceps. The exercise can be done in the seated or standing position. In the seated position (Fig. 20-3), the athlete sits with the hips and knees at 90 degrees and the spine in neutral. The shoulders should be abducted at a 90-degree angle, and the elbows flexed also to a 90-degree angle. The weight is then lifted above the head until directly over the shoulders. The weight is then

lowered slowly back to the starting position. The core stabilizer muscles should be activated throughout the exercise. Excessive extension of the spine in this exercise (Fig. 20-3) can lead to back pain and injury.

Latissimus ("Lat") Pull-Down

The lat pull-down, as suggested by the name, primarily trains the lastissimus dorsi muscles. The athlete sits with feet flat on the floor and the bar is held above the head, with a grip slightly wider than shoulder width (Fig. 20-4). The spine should be in neutral. The bar is then pulled down until it is in front of the chin, then raised back to its original position. Pulling the bar behind the neck can cause injury to the shoulder and should be avoided.

Chest Fly

Chest fly begins in a supine position, with the dumbbells above the chest and with the elbows slightly flexed (Fig. 20-5). Then in a slow arcing motion, the weights are lowered until the arms are parallel to the floor and the hands are just above ear level. Another version of chest fly using a machine is called the pectoralis ("pec") deck, which is done sitting (Fig. 20-5). A common mistake in pec deck is extending the arms past the plane of the body, which places the pectoralis muscles at an excessive stretch, and which can lead to glenohumeral instability.[5,6]

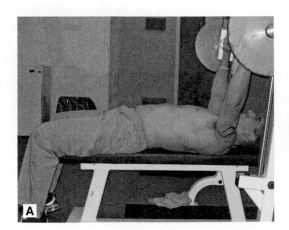
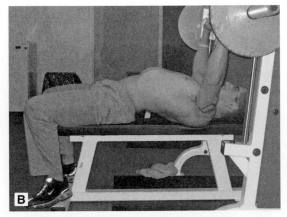

FIGURE 20-2 A. Bench press (correct method). Weight lifter supine with spine in neutral, feet flat on ground with knees bent approximately 90 degrees. **B.** Bench press (incorrect method). Note hyperextension of back with attempt to generate more leverage to lift a heavier weight than what is advisable.

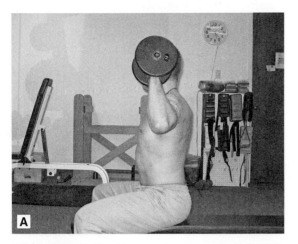

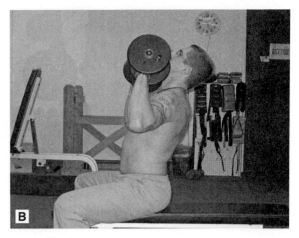

FIGURE 20-3 A. Shoulder press (correct method). Seated position with arms abducted 90 degrees and with elbows flexed 90 degrees. **B.** Shoulder press (incorrect method). Note hyperextension of back with attempt to produce more leverage to lift more weight than what is advisable.

Knee Extension

If knee extension is performed on a machine, the knee joint forms a 90-degree angle with the seat in starting position. The spine should be in neutral and supported by the seat. The leg pads should be located directly above the ankle on the shin. With a controlled motion, the knees are extended to approximately negative 30 degrees (Fig. 20-6). The weight is then lowered in a slow, controlled manner. The knees should not be flexed greater than 90 degrees. Additionally, the knees should never be extended fully to 0 degrees since this may lead to hyperextension of the knees.

Lunge

The starting position for the lunge is with the feet about shoulder width apart and hands (with or without weights) at the sides. The spine should be kept in neutral position. One forward step is taken approximately 2 to 3 feet in front of the body, with the hips and knees flexed until the thigh is almost parallel to the ground (Fig. 20-7). The front knee should be directly over the toes and should not advance past this position. Excessive advancement of the knee (Fig. 20-7B) may lead to increased tibiofemoral and patellofemoral shear forces (see below).

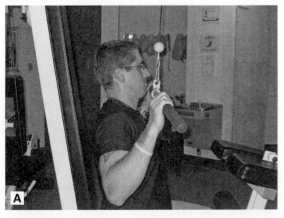

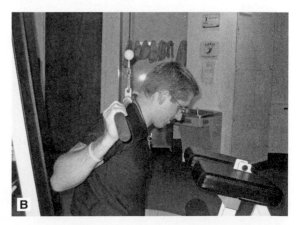

FIGURE 20-4 A. Latissimus pull-down (correct method). Note bar in front of chin. **B.** Latissumus pulldown (incorrect method). Note bar in back of neck with resultant stress on the shoulders.

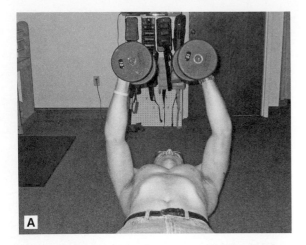

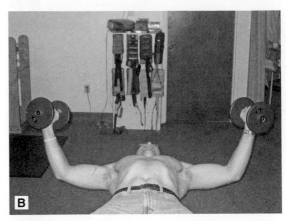

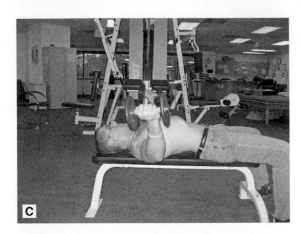

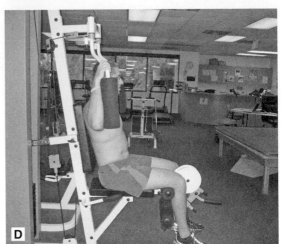

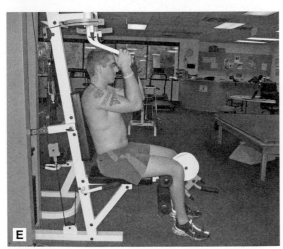

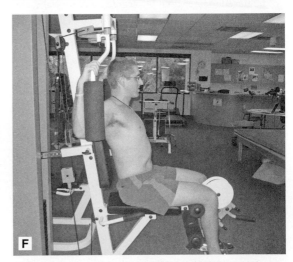

FIGURE 20-5 A. Chest fly, starting position. Note position of dumbbells directly above the chest. **B.** Chest fly, ending position. Arms are almost parallel to ground. **C.** Chest fly, ending position, lateral view. Dumbbells are just above ear level. **D.** Pectoralis deck, starting position (correct method). **E.** Pectoralis deck, ending position (correct method). **F.** Pectoralis deck, starting position (incorrect method). Note hyperextension of the shoulders, placing the pectorals at a stretch.

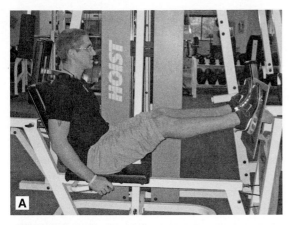 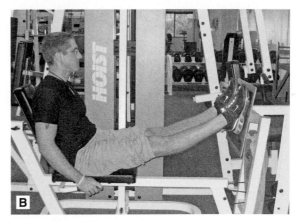

FIGURE 20-6 A. Knee press, ending position (correct method). Knees are extended to negative 30 degrees. **B.** Knee press, ending position (incorrect method). Knees are extended to zero degrees, which over time can lead to hyperextension of the knees.

BODY PARTS INJURED

Low Back Pain

Discogenic Back Pain

It is estimated that the incidence of low back pain is as high as 40% in weight lifters.[7] Lifting weights overhead, such as in the shoulder press, generates large axial compressive forces in the lumbar spine.[7] Axial loading with inadvertent rotation of the lumbar spine may lead to injury to the lumbar intervertebral discs. An example would be doing squats with inadvertant twisting of the lumbar spine instead of maintaining a neutral position, described above. Watkins demonstrated that annular tears can be produced with as little as 3 degrees of high-torque rotation.[7] Currently, there is little literature on disc injury directly attributed to weight training.[8]

The athlete with disc-related injury will typically give a history of pain that is worsened with flexion-based activities of the spine. There may be radiation of symptoms down a leg with flexion movements if there is neural irritation. On examination, muscle

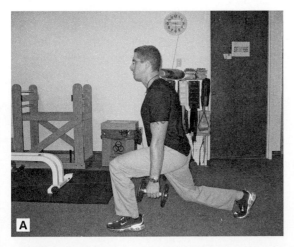 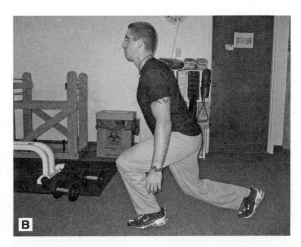

FIGURE 20-7 A. Lunge (correct method). Note position of the thigh almost parallel to ground with the knee directly over the toes. **B.** Lunge (incorrect method). Note position of the knee anterior to the toes.

spasms of the spinal erectors may be noted, resulting in limitations of lumbar spine flexion, rotation, and lateral bending to the affected side. The straight leg raise may be positive if there is neural irritation. Electrodiagnostics (EDX) is the best test to determine nerve and muscle function in radiculopathy, whereas magnetic resonance imaging (MRI) would be the modality of choice in visualizing the intervertebral discs and possible neural encroachment. If EDX or MRI findings are consistent with disc herniation/radiculopathy, treatment will depend on the severity of symptoms and neurologic findings; conservative treatment typically consists of anti-inflammatory medications and starting a therapy program that concentrates on progressive stretching of the hip flexors and hamstrings followed by strengthening of the core muscles, including the gluteals. If symptoms are severe, epidural steroid injections may be necessary to decrease symptoms so that therapy can be implemented. If conservative treatment fails and neurologic symptoms worsen, surgical consultation may be considered.

However, if the workup reveals only annular disc tears without herniation, further testing with discography may be required to confirm pathology. Conservative treatment for annular tears is similar to the treatment program for disc herniations as noted above. If conservative measures fail, intradiscal electrothermal therapy (IDET) may be done to treat the symptomatic disc(s).[9] IDET consists of introducing a flexible catheter into the symptomatic intervertebral disc with fluoroscopic guidance. After successful placement, the disc (annulus) is then heated, thereby destroying nociceptors.[9] Surgical consultation is indicated with intractable pain, muscle weakness, loss of sensation, or bowel and bladder incontinence.

Spondylolysis/Spondylolisthesis

The forces involved in the extension of the spine during weight lifting increase the risk of developing spondylolysis and spondylolisthesis. Isthmic spondylolysis is a fatigue fracture of the neural arch at the pars interarticularis, which can eventually lead to a spondylolisthesis or slipping of one vertebra over another.[10] Namey and Carek showed that 36% of competitive weight lifters have a spondylolytic defect on imaging studies, as compared to 5% of the general population.[11] Improper technique involving hyperextension of the spine is most commonly seen in the bench press (Fig. 20-2B), shoulder press (Fig. 20-3B), and squat.

The weight trainer with suspected spondylolysis usually presents with chronic low-grade back pain with predominantly unilateral pain on extension-based activities. There may be referred pain to the buttock and upper thigh region, but typically not below the knee. Physical examination may reveal a slightly forward-flexed posture and compensatory hamstring and gastrocnemius muscle tightness. Muscle spasms and tenderness in the erector muscles may be seen at the associated level. There may also be limitations in extension-based maneuvers accompanied by reproduction of pain. The stork test is an extension-based maneuver where the athlete stands on the leg on the same side as the back pain and then rotates the extended trunk to the affected side. Reproduction of pain is a positive test; however, other extension-based pathology, such as facet arthropathy, must be excluded.[11,12]

Initial diagnostic imaging for spondylolysis consists of an oblique lumbar plain film where a defect of the pars interarticularis (break in the neck of the "Scottie dog") may be seen. If radiographs do not show any obvious defects, then a bone scan or single-photon emission computed tomography (SPECT) scan may detect the spondylolysis, as well as an MRI. Treatment of spondylolysis varies depending on the acuity of the symptoms. If the symptoms are mild to moderate, relative rest is indicated, with progressive integration of stretching and strengthening of the hamstrings and gluteals, and with core stabilization and relative avoidance of extension-based exercises. If the symptoms are severe, a rigid thoracolumbar brace is recommended until the lesion heals.[13]

In spondylolisthesis, there is a bilateral defect in the pars interarticularis with resultant forward displacement of the affected vertebra relative to the one below it; 90% occur at the L5-S1 level.[13,14] Slippage of L4 on L5 is more common in degenerative spondylolisthesis.[13] Spondylolisthesis is classified using a system developed by Meyerding[15] and is outlined in Table 20-1. Most spondylolistheses are asymptomatic; those that do cause symptoms will typically cause generalized low back pain, especially with transitional flexion/extension movements of the spine. The athlete will most often have tight hamstrings and muscle spasms in the erector spinae muscles. There may be tenderness in the lower lumbar paraspinals, with a step-off on palpation at the level of the defect. There are also commonly range-of-motion limitations with both flexion and extension of the spine, with pain noted mainly in extension.

TABLE 20-1	Meyerding Classification

The most commonly used grading system for spondylolisthesis is the one proposed by Meyerding.[15] The degree of slippage is measured as the percentage of distance the anteriorly translated vertebral body has moved forward relative to the superior end-plate of the vertebra below. Classifications use the following grading system:

- Grade 1: 1–25% slippage
- Grade 2: 26–50% slippage
- Grade 3: 51–75% slippage
- Grade 4: 76–100% slippage
- Grade 5: Greater than 100% slippage

Flexion/extension, oblique and lateral radiographs may show the defects in the pars interarticularis and the coinciding slippage. Treatment of spondylolisthesis varies by the amount of slippage. If the slippage is grade I or II, conservative measures are started and include lumbar bracing, progressive stretching and strengthening of the hip musculature, and core stabilization.[16,17] Medications such as anti-inflammatories and muscle relaxants may also be given acutely. Grades III or IV may need surgical consultation, especially if there is neurologic compromise.

Knee Pain

Patellofemoral Pain Syndrome

Exercises such as the squat, lunges, and knee extensions are essential to overall lower extremity strengthening and are considered routine exercises performed in weight training. The knee is located between two long levers, the femur and the tibia. The development of torque and compressive forces on the knee at the tibiofemoral and patellofemoral joints is large with weight bearing and even higher when weight lifting.[18] Shear forces at the tibiofemoral joint are defined as the anterior displacement of the femur on the tibia during knee flexion. This force must be resisted by the supporting ligaments, tendons, menisci, and other support structures; these forces increase as the angle approaches 90 degrees.[19] Likewise, during knee extension, shear forces at the tibiofemoral joint are greatest during the last 5 to 10 degrees.[20] Hence in exercises such as the squat or seated leg press, it is important not to go past 90 degrees during the eccentric phase and not to lock or hyperextend the knee during the concentric phase (Fig. 20-6B).

There are also compression forces involved at the junction between the patella and the femoral sulcus. The patella acts as a fulcrum point for knee extension. During the squat, the quadriceps contract eccentrically (Fig. 20-1) as the knee flexes, increasing the compressive load on the patellofemoral joint up to seven times body weight.[19] Friction produced from patellar gliding and the compressive force of the patella on the femoral sulcus may produce chondromalacia patella or softening of the retropatellar cartilage. In chondromalacia patella, the weight trainer typically presents with the gradual onset of anterior and/or medial knee pain, especially after doing a lower extremity workout session. The athlete may also complain of anterior knee pain that occurs during prolonged sitting ("theater sign"). The athlete may also complain of clicking of the knee with or without pain during flexion and extension. On physical examination it is important to note the alignment of the knee, as lateral patellar tracking is a common finding in patellofemoral pain. Additionally, excessive external tibial rotation and internal femoral rotation, as well as valgus malalignment, may be seen. The hamstrings and the quadriceps may be tight. The patellofemoral grind test and Clarke sign may be positive (Fig. 20-8). Radiographs may show malalignment of the patella and decreased space between the patella and femur. MRI may reveal thinning of the retropatellar cartilage.

Treatment of patellofemoral pain syndrome in the weight lifter typically begins with the use of anti-inflammatory medications and a therapy program consisting of progressive stretching of the hamstrings and hip flexors. Closed kinetic chain (distal limb is fixed) exercises that incorporate integration of hip muscles down to the ankle/foot are then implemented.

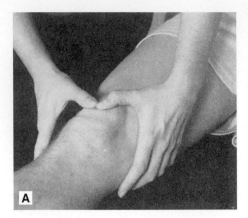 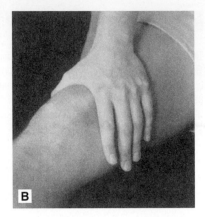

FIGURE 20-8 A. Patellofemoral grind test. Pain on compression of the patella into the groove indicates pathology of the patellar articular cartilage. **B.** Clarke sign. Slight compression is applied proximal to the superior pole of the patella, and the patient is asked to contract the quadriceps. The test is positive if the patient has pain or cannot hold the contraction. False-positive tests are common. (From Anderson MK, Hall SJ, Martin M. *Sports Injury Management*. 2nd ed. Philadelphia: Lippincott Williams & Wilkins; 2000.)

Low-impact aerobic exercises such as elliptical trainers and ski machines should be emphasized, and activities such as running, jumping, or stair climbing should be curtailed. Intra-articular corticosteroid injections may aid in reducing inflammation associated with patellofemoral pain syndrome. Surgery is reserved for refractory cases.

Shoulder Pain

Upper body weight training involves the use of multiple joints in which the shoulder becomes a primary weight-bearing joint.[21] Improper techniques and overtraining can lead to shoulder injuries, such as rotator cuff injury, acromioclavicular (AC) joint pain, and shoulder subluxation.[21] Some of the more common exercises that can lead to shoulder pain include the bench press, shoulder press, lat pull-down, and pec deck.

Rotator Cuff Injury

Rotator cuff injury typically stems from using too much weight and poor technique. Weight trainers tend to overdevelop the pectorals and anterior shoulder musculature and underdevelop the scapular stabilizers, which include the serratus anterior and posterior, trapezius, levator scapulae, rhomboids, and teres major.[22] This creates an inefficient transfer of the forces in the shoulder leading to overloading

of the rotator cuff. The supraspinatus is the most commonly injured of the rotator cuff muscles due to its location closest to the acromion.[23]

The athlete with rotator cuff injury typically presents with pain on lifting the arms above the shoulders, especially in shoulder abduction.[24] On examination, the athlete may have mild atrophy of the rotator cuff musculature on the affected side. There may be guarding of the affected arm, holding it in close approximation to the body as well as tenderness at the insertion of the supraspinatus tendon on the humerus.[25] There may be functional shoulder winging or dyskinesis of the scapula.[22] Limitations in active range of motion in abduction and forward flexion of the shoulder may be found. Shoulder impingement tests, such as the Neer and Hawkins tests, may be positive (Fig. 20-9). The neurologic exam is usually normal and is useful in ruling out other causes of shoulder muscle weakness such as cervical radiculopathy or brachial plexopathy.

Conservative management of rotator cuff injury should include starting anti-inflammatory medication, relative rest, and implementing a therapy program consisting of progressive stretching, range-of-motion, and strengthening exercises with emphasis on the scapular stabilizers.[26] Judicious use of steroid injections can be used to decrease pain so that therapy can be implemented.[27] If conservative treatment fails, then surgical intervention may be required.

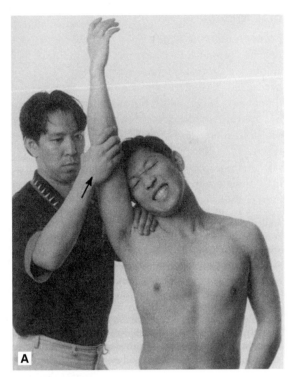
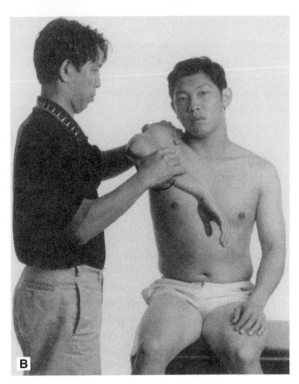

FIGURE 20-9 A. Neer impingement test. The arm is internally rotated and passively flexed forward to impinge the supraspinatus tendon between the greater tuberosity and the coracoacromial arch. **B.** Hawkins impingement test. The shoulder is internally rotated while flexed forward 90 degrees, causing the supraspinatus tendon to impinge between the greater tuberosity and the coracoacromial arch. (From Anderson MK, Hall SJ, Martin M. *Sports Injury Management*. 2nd ed. Philadelphia: Lippincott Williams & Wilkins; 2000.)

Acromioclavicular Joint Pain

Acromioclavicular (AC) joint pain is a common symptom in weight trainers and hence is also known as "weight lifter's shoulder." It is typically seen in athletes who use excessively heavy weights and who also use a wider grip on the bench press.[6] Fees et al.[28] demonstrated that using a narrow grip (approximately 1.5 times the biacromial width) with controlled movement on the descent phase of the shoulder press to approximately 4 to 6 cm above the anterior chest minimized the development of AC pain. Cahill also showed that dropping the elbows below the body line in the descent phase of the bench press excessively stresses the AC joint.[29]

The athlete typically presents with pain in the AC joint area, especially after doing the bench press as well as at night. On examination there may be some swelling of the affected area and tenderness specifically at the AC joint. The cross-body adduction test is positive. This test is done by passively adducting the affected shoulder across the body, with reproduction of pain at the AC joint.

Radiographs of the AC joint may show osteolysis of the distal clavicle, which is a stress fracture of the subchondral bone of the distal clavicle as a consequence of chronic stress from exercises including the bench press and parallel bar dips.[29] Bone scans may show increased uptake in the AC joint; MRI may reveal marrow edema in the AC joint area.[30]

Management of "weight lifter's shoulder" consists of actively modifying the exercise program. Flat barbell bench press and parallel bar dips should be avoided initially. Using dumbbells instead of barbells may reduce stress across the AC joint. Nonsteroidal anti-inflammatory medications and a therapy program including the use of modalities such as ice can be helpful. AC joint injections may be appropriate if conservative measures fail. Surgical intervention with distal clavicular excision may be required in refractory cases.[31]

Shoulder Subluxation

Shoulder instability may be seen with chronic weight training. Anterior instability is the most common type noted in the literature.[21] It has been postulated that performing the shoulder press behind the neck, the lat pull-down behind the neck, and performing the chest fly or bench press incorrectly can all lead to instability.[6,20] Gross et al. showed that the shoulder press behind the neck produces undue stress to the rotator cuff and the inferior glenohumeral ligament, which may exacerbate anterior instability.[5] Additionally, the lat pull-down performed behind the neck produces too much external rotation, stressing the shoulder capsule anteriorly.

The athlete with shoulder instability will typically present with shoulder pain and shoulder laxity. There may be history of clicking in the shoulder. The apprehension and relocation tests may be positive (Fig. 20-10). Management includes physical therapy to strengthen the scapular stabilizers, specifically the posterior deltoids, rhomboids, teres minor, and infraspinatus. Surgical consultation may be needed if pain or instability persists.

Elbow/Forearm

Lateral Epicondylitis

Lateral epicondylitis is a common condition seen among weight trainers, since a stable, powerful grip is needed to repetitively lift and move barbells and dumbbells. This condition is caused biomechanically by overloading the wrist extensor muscles during eccentric contraction.[32] Most weight-lifting activities require resisted wrist extension, which increases the risk of developing lateral epicondylitis. The athlete may present with pain at the lateral epicondyle that may radiate down the dorsal aspect of the forearm. The athlete may also have pain with lifting even light objects, such as a milk jug or bottled water. On examination, there will tenderness at the origin of the extensor musculature at the elbow (lateral epicondyle). Resisted wrist extension and middle-finger extension will stress the extensor carpi radialis brevis, in turn causing pain at the lateral epicondyle. Treatment consists of relative rest, anti-inflammatory medications, ice, counterforce bracing, and therapy. Judicious use of corticosteroid injections would be appropriate if other conservative treatment fails.

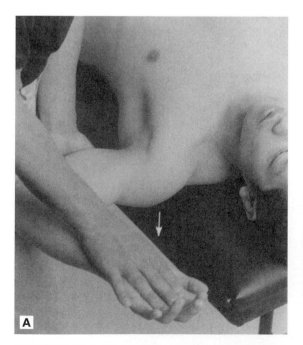
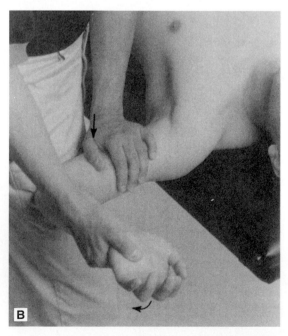

FIGURE 20-10 A. Apprehension test. The athlete lies supine, slowly externally rotating and abducting the arm. The athlete may feel like the "shoulder is going to dislocate"—thus, apprehension. **B.** Relocation test. Posteriorly directed pressure is applied to the athlete's shoulder which gives relief of the athlete's apprehension. (From Anderson MK, Hall SJ, Martin M. *Sports Injury Management.* 2nd ed. Philadelphia: Lippincott Williams & Wilkins; 2000.)

Wrist

Ulnar Neuropathy

In pressing movements such as the bench press and the overhead press, the weight trainer may develop wrist pain by using a "false grip," which is done by placing the thumb under the bar (Fig. 20-11). This places the weight directly over the medial aspect of the wrist at the Guyon canal. Over time, this can lead to ulnar neuropathy, with numbness and tingling in the ulnar nerve distribution.[6] Diagnosis of this condition can be documented by electromyography and nerve conduction studies. Treatment initially consists of anti-inflammatory medication, relative rest, and activity modification. The correct grip would be to have the thumb wrapped in front of the bar and the wrist in neutral position, which minimizes compression of the Guyon canal.[33]

Median Neuropathy

Carpal tunnel syndrome (CTS) is commonly seen in weight-training sports.[34] Improper grip, as well as repeated flexion and extension at the wrists, are postulated to contribute to CTS.[35] The athlete may present with wrist pain and numbness and tingling in the first 3½ digits. A positive "flick sign" is when the athlete awakens at night with the above symptoms and must shake the hands vigorously to alleviate symptoms. On exam, the Phalen test and Tinel sign at the wrist over the median nerve may be positive. There may be a decrease in light touch and pinprick in the median nerve distribution and possibly weakness of thumb abduction. Electrodiagnosis is the diagnostic modality of choice in CTS; its sensitivity approaches 85%, and specificity is greater than 95%.[36] Treatment typically includes wearing wrist splints at night, physical therapy, modification of activity, and judicious use of corticosteroid injections.[37] Overall, 80% of people with carpal tunnel syndrome initially respond to conservative treatment.[34] Gerritsen et al. showed that of patients with CTS who responded to wrist night splints at 6 weeks, 31% also had symptom relief at 12 months.[38] Surgery is indicated if there is significant pain, thenar atrophy, sensory loss, and/or motor weakness.

Wrist Ligamentous Injury

Wrist ligament sprains typically cause swelling, tenderness, and pain. The grading of sprains[39] is based on the degree of laxity to the joint on examination. Grade 1 sprain is relatively painful without joint laxity. Grade 2 involves pain with some laxity compared to the contralateral ligament. Grade 3 lesions typically reveal gross instability. Treatment for grades 1 and 2 begins conservatively with relative rest, ice, nonsteroidal anti-inflammatory drugs (NSAIDs), and splints, whereas grade 3 injuries may require the attention of a hand surgeon.[40] Activity modification such as simply changing equipment or technique may help relieve symptoms. An example is the barbell bicep curl, which can produce high torque on the wrist ligaments if using a straight barbell (Fig. 20-12). Using an angled or cambered bar tends to decrease the stress on these ligaments.

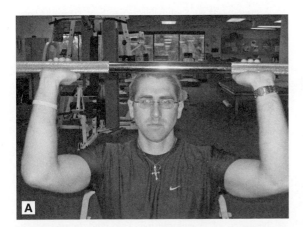
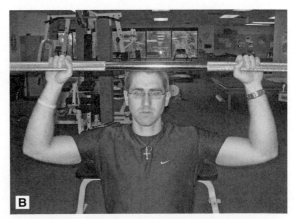

FIGURE 20-11 A. False grip. Note thumb on undersurface of the bar, placing undue force on Guyon canal. **B.** Correct grip. Note thumb completely wrapping around the bar, completing a full grip, lessening pressure on Guyon canal.

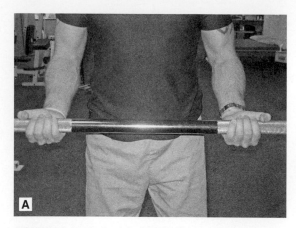 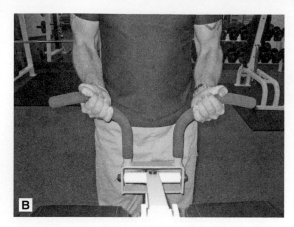

FIGURE 20-12 A. Straight barbell. This can produce high torque on wrist ligaments during bicep curls. **B.** Cambered barbell. This can reduce high torque on wrist ligaments during bicep curls.

SUMMARY

Weight training has become an integral part of healthy lifestyles and fitness programs throughout the world. The importance of proper form and technique, constantly changing the exercises performed for each body part, and getting the appropriate rest for each body part help to decrease the development of ligament and tendon sprains and strains and chronic joint pain symptoms. This helps ensure a lifetime of enjoyment and full health benefits of this sport.

REFERENCES

1. Mazur LJ, Yetman RJ, Risser WL. Weight-training injuries: common injuries and preventative methods. *Sports Med.* 1993;16: 57–63.
2. Hamill BP. Relative safety of weight lifting and weight training. *J Strength Condition.* 1994;8:53–57.
3. Kibler WB, Press J, Sciascia A. The role of core stability in athletic function. *Sports Med.* 2006;36:189–198.
4. Cholewicki J, Panjabi MM, Khachatryan A. Stabilizing function of trunk flexor-extensor muscles around a neutral spine posture. *Spine.* 1997;22:2207–2212.
5. Gross ML, Brenner SL, Esformes I, et al. Anterior shoulder instability in weight lifters. *Am J Sports Med.* 1993;21:599–603.
6. Haupt HA. Upper extremity injuries associated with strength training. *Clin Sports Med.* 2001;20:234–246.
7. Watkins R. Lumbar disc injury in the athlete. *Clin Sports Med.* 2002;21:560–572.
8. Mundt DJ, Kelsey JL, Golden AL, et al. An epidemiologic study of sports and weight lifting as possible risk factors for herniated lumbar and cervical discs: the Northeast Collaborative Group on Low Back Pain. *Am J Sports Med.* 1993;21:854–860.
9. Saal JA, Saal JS. Intradiscal electrothermal treatment for chronic discogenic low back pain: prospective outcome study with a minimum 2-year follow-up. *Spine.* 2002;27:966–973.
10. Farfan JF, Osteria V, Lamy C. The mechanical etiology of spondylolysis and spondylolisthesis. *Clin Orthop.* 1976;117:40–55.
11. Namey TC, Carek JC. Power lifting, weight lifting and bodybuilding. In: Fu FH, Stone DA, eds. *Sports Injuries: Mechanics, Prevention, Treatment.* Baltimore: Williams & Wilkins; 1994:515–529.
12. Reeves RK, Laskowski ER, Smith J. Weight training injuries. Part 2: diagnosing and managing chronic conditions. *Phys Sports Med.* 1998;26:54–70.
13. Cogeni J, McCulloch J, Swanson K. Lumbar spondylolysis: a study of natural progression in athletes. *Am J Sports Med.* 1997;25:567–579.
14. Anderson MJ. Biomechanical aspects of lumbar spine injuries in athletes: a review. *Can J Appl Sport Sci.* 1985;10:1–20.
15. Meyerding HW. Spondylolisthesis. *Surg Gynecol Obstet.* 1932;54:371.
16. Fredrickson BE, Baker D, McHolick WJ, et al. The natural history of spondylolysis and spondylolisthesis. *J Bone Joint Surg.* 1984;66:699–707.
17. Hefti F, Brunazzi M, Morscher E. Natural course in spondylolysis and spondylolisthesis. *Orthopade.* 1994;23:220–227.
18. Lee TQ, Morris G, Csintalan RP. The influence of tibial and femoral rotation on patellofemoral contact area and pressure. *J Orthop Sports Phys Ther.* 2003;33:677–685.
19. Anderson MK, Hall SJ, Martin M. *Sports Injury Management.* 2nd ed. Baltimore: Lippincott Williams & Wilkins; 2000:282–355.
20. Reeves RK, Laskowski ER, Smith J. Weight training injuries. Part 1: diagnosing and managing acute conditions. *Phys Sports Med.* 1998;26:67–96.
21. Neviasser TJ. Weight lifting: risks and injuries to the shoulder. *Clin Sports Med.* 1991;10:615–621.
22. Kibler WB. Role of the scapula in the overhead throwing motion. *Contemp Orthop.* 1991;22:525–532.

23. Janda DH, Loubert P. Basic science and clinical application in the athlete's shoulder. A preventative program focusing on the glenohumeral joint. *Clin Sports Med.* 1991;10:955–971.

24. Neer CS, Welsh RP. The shoulder in sports. *Orthop Clin North Am.* 1977;8:583–591.

25. Jobe FW, Bradley JP. The diagnosis and nonoperative treatment of shoulder injuries in athletes. *Clin Sports Med.* 1989;8:419–438.

26. Malanga GA, Bowen JE, Nadler SF, et al. Non-operative management of shoulder injuries. *J Back Musculoskeletal Med.* 1999;12:179–189.

27. Dixit R. Nonoperative management of shoulder injuries in sports. *Phys Med Rehab Clin N Am.* 1994;5:69–80.

28. Fees M, Decker T, Synder-Mackler L, et al. Upper extremity weight-training modifications for the injured athlete: a clinical perspective. *Am J Sports Med.* 1998;26:732–742.

29. Cahill BR. Osteolysis of the distal part of the clavicle in male athletes. *J Bone Joint Surg Am.* 1982;64:1053.

30. De la Puente R, Boutin RD, Theodorou DJ, et al. Post-traumatic and stress-induced osteolysis of the distal clavicle: MR imaging findings in 17 patients. *Skeletal Radiol.* 1999;28:202–208.

31. Auge WK II, Fischer RA. Arthroscopic distal clavicle resection for isolated atraumatic osteolysis in weight lifters. *Am J Sports Med.* 1987;15:285–289.

32. Kiefhaber TR, Stern PJ. Upper extremity tendonitis and overuse syndromes in athletes. *Clin Sports Med.* 1992;11:39–55.

33. Buterbaugh GA, Brown TR, Horn PC. Ulnar-sided wrist pain in athletes *Clin Sports Med.* 1998;17:567–583.

34. Parmalee-Peters K, Eathorne SW. The wrist: common injuries and management. *Prim Care Clin Office Pract.* 2005;32:114–144.

35. Rettig AC. Wrist and hand overuse syndromes. *Clin Sports Med.* 2001;20:591–611.

36. Norvell JG, Steele M, Carpal tunnel syndrome. *Emedicine* 2006. Available at: http://www.emedicine.com/emerg/topic83.htm. Accessed November 2, 2007.

37. DeStefano F, Nordstrom DL, Vierkant RA. Long-term symptom outcomes of carpal tunnel syndrome and its treatment. *J Hand Surg Am.* 1997;22:200–210.

38. Gerritsen AA, de Vet HC, Scholten RJ. Splinting vs. surgery in the treatment of carpal tunnel syndrome: a randomized controlled trial. *JAMA.* 2002;288:1245–1251.

39. Cohen MS. Ligamentous injuries of the wrist in the athlete. *Clin Sports Med.* 1998;17:533–552.

40. Morgan WJ, Slowman LS. Acute hand and wrist injuries in athletes: evaluation and management. *J Am Acad Orthop Surg.* 2001;9:389–400.

SECTION III

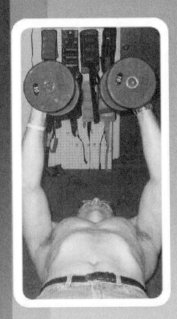

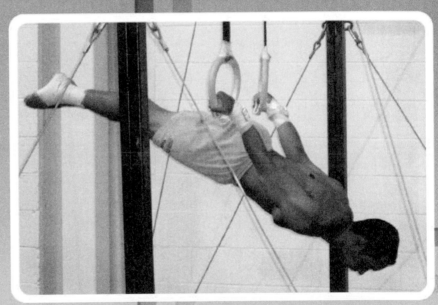

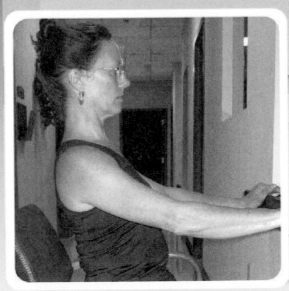

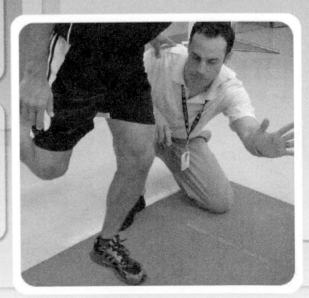

Women's Musculoskeletal Issues

omen have become increasingly more active over the past 35 years. One of the most important landmarks for the increased interest in women's sports was the advent of Title IX legislation in 1972,[1] which was designed to limit sex-based discrimination at federally funded institutions.[2] While this legislation applies to both female and male athletes, and is not limited to athletic programs, likely the most profound effect of this has been the impact on the rates of athletic participation since its enactment.

Since the enactment of Title IX, the rate of female sports participation has increased markedly, with an increase in varsity participation by girls in high school from 1 in 27 to 1 in 3 in 1998.[1] Comparing 1972 to 1996, the percentage of athletes who are female has increased at the high school (from 17.8% to 40.0%), college (16.0% to 39.1%), and Olympic (14.8% to 34.2%) levels. This increase in percentage is almost entirely a function of increasing the level of female participation, as only at the high school level has the absolute number of male athletes competing declined. In achieving the goal of increasing the athletic participation of female athletes, Title IX has clearly been successful. As an obvious consequence of this increase in female sports participation, female athletes have had a concomitant increase in their injury rate.[3] Therefore, clinicians should be aware of those concerns specific to female athletes.

Female athletes have a number of issues specific to them. The first group of these is unique to female anatomy, and includes pregnancy and the peripartum period. The second group of issues concerns those conditions influenced by female hormones and physiology, including the female athlete triad and its components (bone metabolism, menstrual cycle dysregulation, and disordered eating), negative energy balance, ligamentous laxity, spatiomotor processing, and perception of pain. The final class of issues affecting the female athlete relates to gender-specific biomechanics, which can either increase the frequency of a musculoskeletal complaint, as in sacroiliac arthropathy, or predispose women disproportionately to a class of injuries, such as anterior cruciate ligament (ACL) injuries or patellofemoral syndrome.

DIFFERENCES BETWEEN MALE AND FEMALE ATHLETES

Male and female athletes differ in multiple characteristics, including body shape, hormonal profile, and biomechanics. Not all of these are clinically significant, however, and indeed often times the discussion of gender differences obfuscates the quality clinical management of the specific medical needs of female athletes. Therefore, the focus of this discussion on differences between female and male athletes will emphasize those that have clinical correlates that could affect the diagnosis and management of the particular clinical presentations of female athletes.

Anatomy

Female skeletal anatomy differs from that of men in several ways. The most obvious is body size, with the American woman on average weighing 93% of the weight of her male counterpart, and with a height 85% that of his.[4] In addition, women differ from men in body proportions, with proportionately shorter trunks, narrower shoulders, wider hips, and a lower center of gravity.[5-11] Given that women have proportionately wide hips relative to their femur length, the angle of pull of the quadriceps muscle (the Q-angle); (Fig. 21-1) is more oblique in the female than in the male athlete, which has been implicated as a causative factor for a number of knee injuries.

The significance of these differences in body shape is twofold. First, the skeletal anatomy can alter the biomechanics of sports performance. This relationship between body shape and athletic performance is termed kinanthropometry. Second, because of the differences in skeletal anatomy, female athletes are susceptible to injuries in different proportions than men.

Endocrine Differences

The female menstrual cycle is characterized by fluctuating levels of various hormones (Fig. 21-2), whether they be centrally released hormones such as luteinizing hormone (LH) and follicle-stimulating hormone (FSH), female sex hormones (estrogen and its derivatives, progesterone, relaxin), or androgens (testosterone and its derivatives). These hormones are known to have multiple impacts on the female athlete, including ligamentous laxity, but also more subtle findings like spatial cognition, muscular strength, and dynamic neuromuscular control. Therefore, it is an area of great interest to determine the impact of endocrine fluctuations (whether as part of the monthly cycle, the process of pregnancy, or a woman's life cycle) on various aspects of sport, whether it be performance or injury risk.

One area where hormone fluctuation may impact the female athlete is ligamentous laxity. There is an adaptive benefit with ligaments becoming more lax in the presence of female hormones, as this allows the pelvis to widen during birth. This process, however, can become maladaptive in the context of sports performance, where increased ligamentous laxity can make a joint unstable. This has been proposed a potential contributor to injuries like anterior cruciate ligament (ACL) injuries and ankle sprains in female athletes, and indeed there is some literature to suggest that ligamentous laxity and perhaps the incidence of these injuries may be affected by hormone levels.[12–19]

The relationship between hormonal levels and ligamentous laxity are relevant even in the absence of frank ligamentous failure. The primary role of the ligaments is to maintain the stability and to aid in the appropriate articulation of a joint, and ligamentous failure only represents the end-point of inappropriate joint motion. Thus, even if increased laxity is not associated with frank ligamentous failure, it may lead to suboptimal biomechanics, and perhaps force increased loadings onto other structures, including the surrounding bone, cartilage, and muscular tissue.

Female hormones, in addition to their peripheral affects on ligamentous function, may also function centrally on spatial processing. For example, sex hormones are known to have pronounced affects on spatial ability[20] and other aspects of cognition.[21–23]

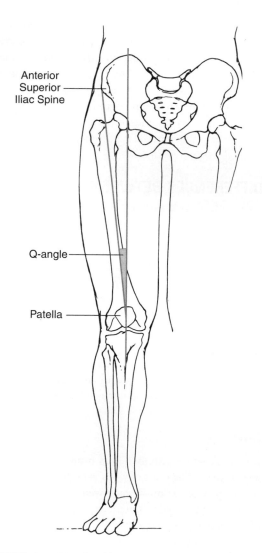

FIGURE 21-1 The Q-angle approximates the pull of the quadriceps muscle. (From Oatis CA. *Kinesiology: The Mechanics and Pathomechanics of Human Movement.* Baltimore: Lippincott Williams & Wilkins; 2004.)

Anterior Superior Iliac Spine

Q-angle

Patella

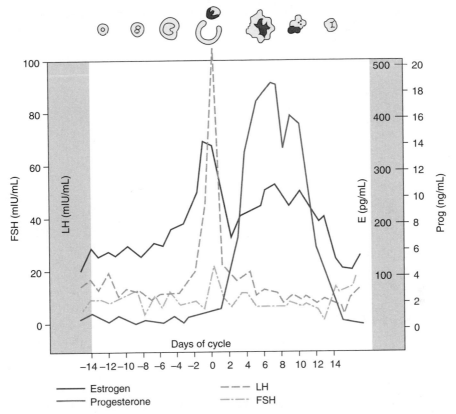

FIGURE 21-2 The menstrual cycle. (From LifeART image. Copyright © [2008] Lippincott Williams & Wilkins. All rights reserved.)

Therefore, it is likely that an individual's hormonal profile will have some affect on her athletic performance, by influencing the spatial substrates used in sport. Sex hormones can affect cognition either by affecting brain organization early in development or by altering performance as a function of the menstrual cycle.[21,24] Finally, another important role of hormones in the presentation of athletic injuries is the direct impact of hormone levels on pain modulation. Estrogens have been demonstrated as pain potentiators, while androgens have been identified as pain suppressors.[25–27]

Therefore, the role of estrogens and female-specific hormones on athletic injuries is likely multimodal. First, hormones may increase ligamentous laxity, potentially creating joint instability and suboptimal biomechanics. Second, circulating hormones may impact spatial perception and perhaps even proprioceptive feedback, which may further alter an athlete's

biomechanics. Finally, estrogens can potentiate pain processes, thus contributing to clinically significant pain presentations in what otherwise might have been incidental nociceptive feedback.

FEMALE ATHLETE TRIAD

The female athlete triad has historically been defined as a syndrome consisting of disordered eating, amenorrhea, and osteoporosis. The existence of the female athlete triad, however, has been a point of significant contention in the recent literature.[28,29] While each component of the triad is a significant health risk for the female athlete, it is debated whether the three truly constitute a syndrome, occurring at a higher incidence collectively than would be anticipated based on each of their frequencies in the general population.[28]

Part of the ambiguity in the existence of the female athlete triad is that each of the three components falls along a spectrum. For example, eating difficulties can range from irregular eating patterns at the mild end of the spectrum, as opposed to DSM-IV classified eating disorders at the most severe end of the spectrum. Similarly, menstrual dysregulation can range from menstrual irregularities to true amenorrhea, and bone density can range from osteopenia to osteoporosis. By definition, the true female athlete triad involves the more severe ends of these spectra, but it is certainly plausible that a female athlete can have less severe manifestations of any or all of these conditions.[29]

One common underlying mechanism that may affect all three components of eating patterns, menstrual regulation, and bone density is energy balance. Because of the increased levels of activity in female athletes, female athletes are potentially at risk for negative energy balance.[29] This is particularly true in sports, where a lean body shape or lower body weight may confer a competitive advantage, since the female athlete may deliberately constrict her caloric intake for a perceived performance advantage. It is these athletes that are most likely to have negative energy balance, and have subsequent risk for each of the components of the female athlete triad, whether separately or collectively as part of a syndrome. It is not entirely clear why negative energy balance is associated with each component of the female athlete triad. Disruption of the hypothalamic–pituitary–adrenal axis is one proposed mechanism, although further research is needed to clarify this relationship.

More importantly, it is unclear how the existence of the female athlete triad should affect exercise recommendations for women in general. One could certainly make the case that for the female population as a whole, lack of exercise is a significantly greater public health problem than overexercising.[28] With that in mind, then, the role of the clinician should primarily be that of health advocate. However, in the active female athlete, it is important to be cognizant of the potential for negative calorie and nutrient balance, and that these may be early signs of disordered eating, osteopenia, or menstrual cycle disregulation.

In addition, whenever a clinician sees a patient with one component of the triad, he or she should be mindful of other aspects of the triad.[30] For example, when examining a young female runner with a stress fracture, the clinician should consider that low bone density may have contributed to the stress fracture, and then further probe for the other aspects of the triad (e.g., disordered eating or menstrual dysregulation).

PREGNANCY

One of the most important questions concerning any female athlete contemplating pregnancy is whether she can exercise safely. To this end, different exercise recommendations have been made by various organizations,[31–35] and one synopsis of these recommendations is presented in Table 21-1. The basis for these guidelines is to maximize and maintain fitness for the mother, while at the same time ensuring a healthy delivery of the fetus.

Given the potentially grave consequences of harm to the fetus, many of the original exercise recommendations have erred toward limiting the mother's exercise regimen. However, it has now been demonstrated that the pregnant mother can actively exercise without compromising the safety of the fetus, and indeed, a regular exercise program may improve the health of the fetus.[30] By following some of the recommendations listed in Table 21-1 and maintaining regular visits with her obstetrician, the female athlete should be able to optimize the health of both herself and her future child.

SPECIFIC MUSCULOSKELETAL COMPLAINTS

In addition to the musculoskeletal conditions experienced by all athletes, there are a number of musculoskeletal conditions that are more commonly experienced by female athletes. Of particular interest with these entities are adjustments that can be made to an athlete's biomechanics to prevent either an initial injury or a reoccurrence.

Anterior Cruciate Ligament Injuries

One of the most common, and devastating, injuries to the female athlete is disruption of the anterior cruciate ligament (ACL). The cruciate ligaments are paired ligaments crossing within the knee joint. The smaller of the two, the ACL, helps track knee joint motion by limiting hyperextension and limiting anterior translation or internal rotation of the tibia.

TABLE 21-1 Exercise Recommendations in Pregnancy

- **Type of exercise**_____
  - Continue preferred mode of prepregnancy exercise
  - Swimming and cycling may be better tolerated
  - Avoid supine exercise (lying on back) for more than a few minutes
  - Standing exercise may be challenging in late pregnancy because of ligamentous laxity from hormones
- **Frequency of exercise**_____
  - American College of Obstetricians Gynecologists recommends daily exercise
  - Other research by Canadian researchers suggests that 3 or 4 days weekly may have the least negative impact on birth weight
- **Duration**_____
  - 30 minutes or more for aerobic benefit
  - Stop when fatigued—do not exercise to exhaustion
  - May exercise to prepregnancy duration if active prior to pregnancy
- **Intensity**
  - Goal: 60–80% of maximum heart rate (HR)

Note: Use of age based formula (220—age) for max HR tends to underestimate fit females and overestimate unfit females.

Prior Fitness Level	Fit HR	Active HR	Unfit HR
Peak HR age 20–29	176.3	171.9	159.7
Target HR (60–80%)	106–142 bpm	103–138 bpm	96–128 bpm
Peak HR age 30–39	175.1	167.7	160.3
Target HR (60–80%)	106–140 bpm	101–134 bpm	96–128 bpm

  - Can use **Borg Scale** or **Talk test** to guide intensity levels
    - **Borg Scale:** should be 12–14 for pregnancy
      - 7 = No exertion at all
      - 8 = Extremely light (7.5)
      - 9 = Very light
      - 10 = Light (40–50% of HR max)
      - 12 = Somewhat hard (50–65% of HR max)
      - 14 = Hard (heavy) (65–80% of HR max)
      - 16 = Very hard
      - 18 = Extremely hard, maximal exertion
    - **Talk test** (should be *moderate* which corresponds to Borg of 13)
      - *Light* **intensity level:** should be able to sing while doing the activity
      - *Moderate* **intensity level:** should be able to carry on a conversation comfortably while engaging in the activity
      - *Vigorous* **intensity level:** person becomes winded or too out of breath to carry on a conversation (AVOID IN PREGNANCY)
- **Exercise precautions**_____
  - Beware of decreased balance in mid to late pregnancy
  - Caution for overheating during exercise, wear light clothing
  - Make sure you have adequate fluid intake

Female athletes injure their ACL 2 to 8 times as frequently as do male athletes,[36–40] and the increased incidence is even higher for noncontact ACL injuries.[37] For example, the National Collegiate Athletic Association (NCAA) surveyed collegiate athletes, and found that the incidence of ACL injuries was 27 per 100,000 female and 8 per 100,000 male athletes. Of these injuries, 85.3% to 87.5% of ACL injuries are noncontact injuries,[37] typically the result of improper landing or other such positioning activities.

There has been considerable effort to understand why female athletes are particularly susceptible to ACL injuries, whether that mechanism is anatomic, hormonal, or biomechanical. The previous sections have discussed how anatomic factors (e.g., the Q-angle), or hormonal patterns may affect ACL injuries. However, this is more descriptive than prescriptive, as the clinician is limited in his or her capacity to alter an athlete's anatomy or hormone profile, and doing so through interventions such as surgery or hormone supplementation is not particularly desirable for most athletes. Fortunately, a growing body of literature demonstrates the dramatic impact biomechanics has on the ACL injury rate, and therefore optimizing biomechanics is an obvious means to making a positive intervention.

As noted earlier, most ACL injuries are noncontact injuries associated with landing and cutting maneuvers, and there are multiple biomechanical factors that may be related to female athletes' increased rates of ACL injury when performing these maneuvers. For example, women tend to overactivate the quadriceps relative to the hamstrings when landing.[36] The quadriceps anteriorly displace the tibia by means of their attachment to the tibial tuberosity, whereas the medial hamstrings displace the tibia posteriorly.

Landing posture may also influence the ACL injury rate in female athletes.[41] Female athletes, as a group, tend to land with a more upright posture, with greater hip extension, adduction, and internal rotation; more forward momentum; and with increased valgus at the knee. Since the foot is fixed during landing, any motion at the hip will be matched by an opposite motion at the knee. Therefore, landing with hip

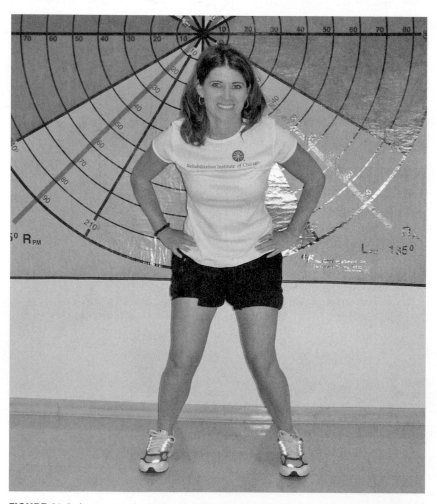

FIGURE 21-3 A squat performed with suboptimal biomechanics, with excessive internal rotation and adduction of the femur.

extension, adduction, and internal rotation will cause knee extension and especially valgus. Eventually, the knee will reach what Mary Lloyd Ireland termed the "point of no return," after which the ACL will tear.

Other studies have confirmed that female athletes, as a group, tend to underutilize their hip and core musculature, and therefore require the knee musculature to bear the bulk of forces during cutting and landing.[41–48] In this scenario, if the knee musculature is unable to withstand the forces required, the ligaments will have to, and this pathway can lead to ligament failure.[49] One approach to prevent ACL failure would be to strengthen the knee musculature (and, indeed, this is beneficial). A more important step is to train the athlete biomechanically so that the knee musculature and ligaments are not asked to bear forces that are better suited for the more powerful hip musculature.

One useful strategy, then, for minimizing the risk of ACL injuries is a prehabilitation program with a focus on optimizing hip biomechanics during squatting, plyometrics, and agility training.[41,46,47,50] In particular, training should focus on maintaining a flexed, externally rotated, and abducted hip throughout the range of motion, which will help prevent an excessive valgus moment from being transmitted to the knee. Examples of these squatting movements are shown in Figures 21-3 (with improper adduction and internal rotation of the femur) and 21-4 (with more proper abduction and external rotation of the femur).

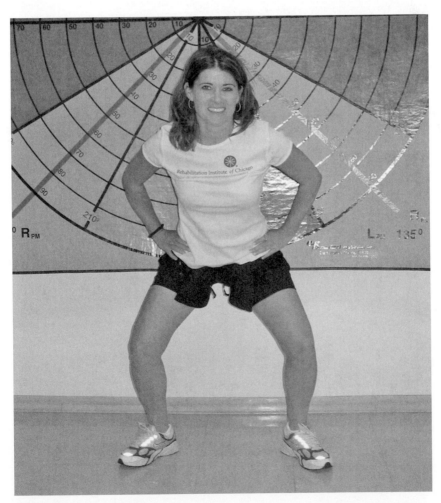

FIGURE 21-4 A more optimal squat, with external rotation and abduction of the femur to better activate the gluteus maximus.

Patellofemoral Pain

Like ACL injuries, patellofemoral pain syndrome (PFPS) is more common in female athletes than in male athletes.[51,52] The main pathokinematics in PFPS is a malalignment between the patella and the femur. Clinicians have historically considered the primary problem with patellofemoral pain syndrome to be related to the patella tracking laterally relative to the femur. However, recent evidence suggests that the main pathology may actually be related to the femur tracking medially relative to the patella.[53]

The significance of these biomechanics is in how to best rehabilitate PFPS. Traditionally, the core part of PFPS rehabilitation has focused on strengthening of the quadriceps. Efforts have been made to strengthen the vastus medialis obliquvs (VMO) in isolation of the other quadriceps muscles, although the ability to isolate VMO has been questioned.[54]

However, because of the importance of correcting excessive internal rotation and adduction of the hip during closed kinetic chain motions, efforts need to be made to correct the femur positioning during these activities. Examples of such exercises include

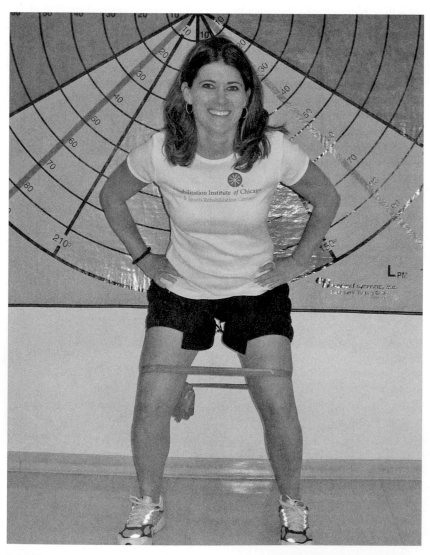

FIGURE 21-5 Squatting with resistance around the knees to encourage greater activation of the hip abductors and external rotators throughout the range of motion.

squatting with a belt around the knees, which forces the hips to be externally rotated during motion throughout the range of motion (Fig. 21-5) and therefore encourages activation of gluteus maximus.

Sacroiliac Joint Pain

One of the most important areas where the differential of a musculoskeletal pain syndrome differs in the genders is in the presentation of sacroiliac (SI) joint pain. The SI joint is thought to be responsible for approximately 15% of low back pain in the general population,[55] but this may be more common in the female athlete population.[52,56]

Diagnosis of the SI joint as a pain generator can be challenging. For example, a study using a double anesthesia block design found that most physical examination maneuvers had limited sensitivity and specificity for diagnosing the SI joint as a source of low back pain.[57] However, using multiple physical examination maneuvers in combination may increase the likelihood of correctly diagnosing SI joint-mediated pain.[58–61]

Management of SI joint-mediated pain should focus on correcting any imbalances about the SI joint, whether they are related to flexibility or strength. Strengthening of core muscles that act across or near the SI joint can often be helpful in SI joint pain. The pelvic floor muscles are often neglected, but since they make up the floor of the core, pelvic floor strengthening exercises should be considered as part of the rehabilitation program.[62] Other measures, such as belts acting across the SI joint to better control joint motion, can be beneficial, and the judicious use of intrarticular injections may be beneficial in cases refractory to conservative management.[63]

Stress Fractures

One consequence of increased activity is the potential to disrupt the equilibrium between bone building and bone remodeling. During normal exercise and activity, the initial response is bone breakdown, and during rest, bone rebuilds in response to loading forces. When this equilibrium is disrupted in periods of increased exercise and/or decreased rest, the net effect is bone breakdown. The clinical end-point of this dysregulation can be osteopenia, osteoporosis, or a stress fracture.

Female athletes are particularly prone to stress fractures. Runners in particular are susceptible to stress fractures, as the pounding of the road may often overload the ability of the musculature to withstand the ground reaction forces, and thus the forces are instead absorbed by the bone. Stress fractures can occur in multiple different locations, including the sacrum and pelvis, the femur, the tibia, and the metatarsals. Most of these stress fractures can be managed with relative rest and alternative exercises (such as water exercise), and possible referral to an endocrinologist or dietician to assess any predisposing factors. An important exception is stress fractures along the superolateral portion of the femur; because of the increased tensile load across the stress fracture, these injuries require surgical referral to limit progression of the fracture.

SUMMARY

As women become increasingly involved in athletic activities, sports medicine clinicians must continue to broaden their knowledge base to account for those domains that specifically pertain to the female athlete. In doing so, clinicians can help all of their patients maintain the healthy and active lifestyle they enjoy.

REFERENCES

1. Lopiano DA. Modern history of women in sports. Twenty-five years of Title IX. *Clin Sports Med.* 2000;19:163–173, vii.
2. Title IX of the education amendments of 1972. www.dol.6ov/oasam/re65/statutes/title ix.htm
3. Sports-related injuries among high school athletes—United States, 2005–06 school year. *MMWR Morb Mortal Wkly Rep.* 2006;55:1037–1040.
4. Ogden CL, Fryar CD, Carroll MD, et al. Mean body weight, height, and body mass index, United States 1960–2002. *Adv Data.* 2004;347:1–17.
5. Eiben OG. Physique of female athletes—anthropological and proportional analysis. In: Borms J, Hebbelink M, Venerando A, eds. *The Female Athlete.* Vol. 15. Rome: Karger; 1981:74–89.
6. Ross WD, Leahy RM, Drinkwater DT, et al. Proportionality and body composition in male and female Olympic athletes: a kinanthropometric overview. In: Borms J, Hebbelink M, Venerando A, eds. *The Female Athlete.* Vol. 15. Rome: Karger; 1981:74–89.
7. Eiben OG. Recent data on variability in physique: some aspects of proportionality. In: Ostyn M, Beunen G, Simons J, eds. *Kinanthropometry II.* Vol. 9. Baltimore: University Park Press; 1978:69–77.
8. Malina RM, Zavaleta AN. Androgeny of physique in female track and field athletes. *Ann Hum Biol.* 1976;3:441–446.

9. Bale P. Body composition and somatotype characteristics of sportswomen. In: Borms J, Hebbelink M, Venerando A, eds. *The Female Athlete*. Vol. 15. Rome: Karger; 1981: 150–156.

10. Komi PV. Fundamental performance characteristics in female and males. In: Borms J, Hebbelink M, Venerando A, eds. *Women and Sport*. Vol. 14. Rome: Karger; 1981: 102–108.

11. Slaughter MH, Lohman TG, Boileau RA, et al. Physique of college women athletes in five sports. In: Borms J, Hebbelink M, Venerando A, eds. *The Female Athlete*. Vol. 15. Rome: Karger; 1981:186–191.

12. Wojtys EM, Huston LJ, Lindenfeld TN, et al. Association between the menstrual cycle and anterior cruciate ligament injuries in female athletes. *Am J Sports Med*. 1998;26: 614–619.

13. Hewett TE, Zazulak BT, Myer GD. Effects of the menstrual cycle on anterior cruciate ligament injury risk: a systematic review. *Am J Sports Med*. 2007;35:659–668.

14. Beynnon BD, Bernstein IM, Belisle A, et al. The effect of estradiol and progesterone on knee and ankle joint laxity. *Am J Sports Med*. 2005;33:1298–1304.

15. Wilkerson RD, Mason MA. Differences in men's and women's mean ankle ligamentous laxity. *Iowa Orthop J*. 2000;20:46–48.

16. Shultz SJ, Gansneder BM, Sander TC, et al. Absolute serum hormone levels predict the magnitude of change in anterior knee laxity across the menstrual cycle. *J Orthop Res*. 2006;24:124–131.

17. Shultz SJ, Kirk SE, Johnson ML, et al. Relationship between sex hormones and anterior knee laxity across the menstrual cycle. *Med Sci Sports Exerc*. 2004;36: 1165–1174.

18. Shultz SJ, Sander TC, Kirk SE, et al. Sex differences in knee joint laxity change across the female menstrual cycle. *J Sports Med Phys Fitness*. 2005;45:594–603.

19. Hewett TE. Neuromuscular and hormonal factors associated with knee injuries in female athletes. Strategies for intervention. *Sports Med*. 2000;29:313–327.

20. Janowsky JS, Chavez B, Zamboni BD, et al. The cognitive neuropsychology of sex hormones in men and women. *Dev Neuropsychol*. 1998;14:421–440.

21. Kimura D. Sex differences in the brain. *Sci Am*. 267;1992: 119–125.

22. Kimura D, Hampson E. Chapter 9: Neural and hormonal mechanisms mediating sex differences in cognition. *Biological Approaches to the Study of Human Intelligence*. Norwood, NJ: Ablex; 1993:375–397.

23. Williams CL. Estrogen effects on cognition across the life span. *Horm Behav*. 1998;34:80–84.

24. Reinisch JM, Ziemba-Davis M, Sanders SA. Hormonal contributions to sexually dimorphic behavioral development in humans. *Psychoneuroendocrinology*. 1991;16: 213–278.

25. Aloisi AM. Gonadal hormones and sex differences in pain reactivity. *Clin J Pain*. 2003;19:168–174.

26. Aloisi AM, Bachiocco V, Costantino A, et al. Cross-sex hormone administration changes pain in transsexual women and men. *Pain*. Mar 20, 2007;1:560–567.

27. Aloisi AM, Bonifazi M. Sex hormones, central nervous system and pain. *Horm Behav*. 2006;50:1–7.

28. DiPietro L, Stachenfeld NS. The myth of the female athlete triad. *Br J Sports Med*. 2006;40:490–493.

29. Beals KA, Meyer NL. Female athlete triad update. *Clin Sports Med*. 2007;26:69–89.

30. Sherman RT, Thompson RA. Practical use of the International Olympic Committee Medical Commission Position Stand on the Female Athlete Triad: a case example. *Int J Eat Disord*. 2006;39:193–201.

31. Kramer MS, McDonald SW. Aerobic exercise for women during pregnancy. *Cochrane Database Syst Rev*. 2006;3: CD000180.

32. Dempsey JC, Butler CL, Williams MA. No need for a pregnant pause: physical activity may reduce the occurrence of gestational diabetes mellitus and preeclampsia. *Exerc Sport Sci Rev*. 2005;33:141–149.

33. Giroux I, Inglis SD, Lander S, et al. Dietary intake, weight gain, and birth outcomes of physically active pregnant women: a pilot study. *Appl Physiol Nutr Metab*. 2006;31: 483–489.

34. Mottola MF, Davenport MH, Brun CR, et al. V_{O2} peak prediction and exercise prescription for pregnant women. *Med Sci Sports Exerc*. 2006;38:1389–1395.

35. Davies GA, Wolfe LA, Mottola MF, et al. Joint SOGC/CSEP clinical practice guideline: exercise in pregnancy and the postpartum period. *Can J Appl Physiol*. 2003;28:330–341.

36. Urabe Y, Kobayashi R, Sumida S, et al. Electromyographic analysis of the knee during jump landing in male and female athletes. *Knee*. 2005;12:129–134.

37. Agel J, Arendt EA, Bershadsky B. Anterior cruciate ligament injury in national collegiate athletic association basketball and soccer: a 13-year review. *Am J Sports Med*. 2005;33:524–530.

38. Powell JW, Barber-Foss KD. Sex-related injury patterns among selected high school sports. *Am J Sports Med*. 2000;28:385–391.

39. Gwinn DE, Wilckens JH, McDevitt ER, et al. The relative incidence of anterior cruciate ligament injury in men and women at the United States Naval Academy. *Am J Sports Med*. 2000;28:98–102.

40. Messina DF, Farney WC, DeLee JC. The incidence of injury in Texas high school basketball. A prospective study among male and female athletes. *Am J Sports Med*. 1999;27:294–299.

41. Ireland ML. The female ACL: why is it more prone to injury? *Orthop Clin North Am*. 2002;33:637–651.

42. Rozzi SL, Lephart SM, Gear WS, et al. Knee joint laxity and neuromuscular characteristics of male and female soccer and basketball players. *Am J Sports Med*. 1999;27:312–319.

43. Leetun DT, Ireland ML, Willson JD, et al. Core stability measures as risk factors for lower extremity injury in athletes. *Med Sci Sports Exerc*. 2004;36:926–934.

44. Willson JD, Ireland ML, Davis I. Core strength and lower extremity alignment during single leg squats. *Med Sci Sports Exerc*. 2006;38:945–952.

45. Harty CM, Kawaguchi J, Chmielewski TL, et al. Relationship between muscular strength and lower extremity posture of female athletes during drop vertical jumps. *Med Sci Sports Exerc*. 2007;39(suppl):S23.

46. Ford KR, Myer GD, Toms HE, et al. Gender differences in the kinematics of unanticipated cutting in young athletes. *Med Sci Sports Exerc*. 2005;37:124–129.

47. Fletcher RM, Chmielewski TL, Kawaguchi J, et al. The relationship between hip mechanics and knee landing during single leg landing in female athletes. *Med Sci Sports Exerc.* 2007;39(suppl):S22.

48. Speer SM, Kawaguchi J, Chmielewski TL, et al. Can muscular strength within the kinetic chain predict athletes' improvement in performance with landing training? *Med Sci Sports Exerc.* 2007;39(suppl):S23.

49. Krosshaug T, Nakamae A, Boden BP, et al. Mechanisms of anterior cruciate ligament injury in basketball: video analysis of 39 cases. *Am J Sports Med.* 2007;35:359–367.

50. Grindstaff TL, Hammill RR, Tuzson AE, et al. Neuromuscular control training programs and noncontact anterior cruciate ligament injury rates in female athletes: a numbers-needed-to-treat analysis. *J Athl Train.* 2006;41:450–456.

51. Arendt EA. Dimorphism and patellofemoral disorders. *Orthop Clin North Am.* 2006;37:593–599.

52. Taunton JE, Ryan MB, Clement DB, et al. A retrospective case-control analysis of 2002 running injuries. *Br J Sports Med.* 2002;36:95–101.

53. Wilson JD, Davis I. Mechanics of single leg jumps during exertion in females with and without patellofemoral pain syndrome. *Med Sci Sports Exerc.* 2007;39(suppl):S23.

54. Malone T, Davies G, Walsh WM. Muscular control of the patella. *Clin Sports Med.* 2002;21:349–362.

55. Foley BS, Buschbacher RM. Sacroiliac joint pain: anatomy, biomechanics, diagnosis, and treatment. *Am J Phys Med Rehabil.* 2006;85:997–1006.

56. Rost CC, Jacqueline J, Kaiser A, et al. Pelvic pain during pregnancy: a descriptive study of signs and symptoms of 870 patients in primary care. *Spine.* 2004;29:2567–2572.

57. Dreyfuss P, Dryer S, Griffin J, et al. Positive sacroiliac screening tests in asymptomatic adults. *Spine.* 1994;19:1138–1143.

58. Hancock M, Maher CG, Latimer J, et al. Systematic review of tests to identify the disc, SIJ or facet joint as the source of low back pain. *Eur Spine J.* 2007;16(10):1539–1550.

59. Laslett M, Aprill CN, McDonald B, et al. Diagnosis of sacroiliac joint pain: validity of individual provocation tests and composites of tests. *Man Ther.* 2005;10:207–218.

60. Young S, Aprill C, Laslett M. Correlation of clinical examination characteristics with three sources of chronic low back pain. *Spine J.* 2003;3:460–465.

61. Malanga GA, Nadler S. *Musculoskeletal Physical Examination: An Evidence-Based Approach.* Philadelphia: Mosby; 2006.

62. Sapsford R. Rehabilitation of pelvic floor muscles utilizing trunk stabilization. *Man Ther.* 2004;9:3–12.

63. Slipman CW, Lipetz JS, Plastaras CT, et al. Fluoroscopically guided therapeutic sacroiliac joint injections for sacroiliac joint syndrome. *Am J Phys Med Rehabil.* 2001;80:425–432.

Musculoskeletal Issues in the Elderly

Musculoskeletal disorders are a frequent cause of pain in the elderly. While such problems are not unique to this population, they are certainly more prevalent and may lead to a higher degree of disability than in a younger population. Chronic pain is growing as a major source of morbidity among the elderly, with musculoskeletal pain in general, and chronic back pain in particular, being prominent complaints. Treatment in this group of patients has its own set of challenges due to the natural aging process (Table 22-1) and the higher prevalence of comorbidities.[1-4] This chapter addresses some of the special musculoskeletal issues that arise more often in the elderly.

THORACIC AND LUMBAR BACK PAIN

Chronic low back pain is very common in the elderly. The differential diagnosis of low back pain in older patients is broad, and includes nonmusculoskeletal problems such as infection, cancer, and abdominal aortic aneurism as well as the sprains and strains seen in younger subjects. Older patients, particularly women, are at risk for vertebral compression fractures due to osteoporosis. They are less likely to suffer from herniated discs and more likely to suffer from spinal stenosis and degenerative changes.

Back pain is often caused by mechanical disorders. Degenerative joint disease (DJD) commonly affects the facet joints. If significant facet arthropathy develops, extension or rotation of the spine may cause pain (although these maneuvers are not particularly useful in diagnosing a problem with these joints). Treatment consists of instruction in proper back mechanics (reducing lordosis), weight loss, strengthening of back muscles, and nonsteroidal anti-inflammatory drugs (NSAIDs). The hip flexors are often tight in these

persons, so stretching of these muscles may be beneficial as well. Stomach sleeping is generally to be discouraged. Sometimes facet joint injections may be necessary; they can be of both diagnostic and therapeutic value.

DJD may also lead to degenerative spondylolisthesis (Fig. 22-1). In this case, facet degeneration allows one vertebra to slip on another. Persons with this condition may benefit from an abdominal flexion strengthening program and possibly an anti-extension back brace. The treatments described above for facet pain are also useful for this condition, as they are related.

Osteoporosis may lead to compression fractures in the thoracic or lumbar spine (Fig. 22-2). If no neurologic deficit occurs, the acute compression fracture is treated with a short period of rest, analgesics, and return to activity as soon as tolerated. Long-term functional loss and pain occur because of the development of a kyphotic posture from repeated fractures, so prolonged immobilization, especially in flexion, is avoided. Very painful fractures can in some cases be treated with vertebroplasty or kyphoplasty, which involve stabilization of the fracture with bone cement. Flexion exercises are avoided, both to allow healing of the fracture and to prevent future fractures. Good back extensor strength has been shown to reduce the incidence of fractures.[5]

Lumbar spinal stenosis (LSS) is a narrowing of the spinal canal. It can be congenital in some cases, but usually occurs or worsens with age. For unknown reasons it is not symptomatic in all persons. If the narrowing is significant enough, symptoms can include radicular pain (sometimes multilevel), numbness, tingling, and weakness. This is in the nature of a "neurogenic" claudication (pseudoclaudication), which must be differentiated from "vasculogenic" or true claudication (Table 22-2). In most cases symptoms remain stable and do not progress.[6] Conservative treatment may

TABLE 22-1	Physiologic Effects of Aging on the Musculoskeletal System[1-4]

1. Decrease in muscle mass, including the number of myofibrils and the concentration of mitochondrial enzymes
2. Decrease in the number of functional motor units
3. Increase in body fat proportion (with a concomitant increase in retention of fat-soluble medications)
4. Increase in type I muscle fiber proportion
5. Decrease in strength but with maintenance of relative endurance
6. Decrease in bone mineral density
7. Decrease in water content of cartilage
8. Increase in prevalence of degenerative joint disease

include medications, physical therapy (flexion exercises), and epidural steroid injections.[7] Severe disease may need to be treated with surgical decompression.[8]

CERVICAL PAIN

The cervical spine is prone to injury due to the multiple articulating structures and great cumulative motion of the neck. In the elderly this is compounded by the ubiquitous presence of degenerative changes. The spinal cord in this area is more prone to injury, both because of the relative lack of stabilizing structures and also because the cord itself is wider around the midcervical area.

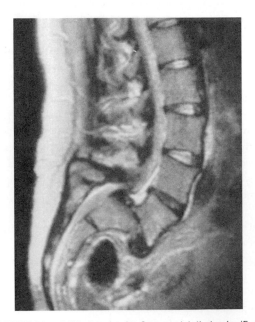

FIGURE 22-1 MRI showing L5-S1 spondylolisthesis. (From Anderson MK, Hall SJ, Martin M. *Sports Injury Management*. 2nd ed. Baltimore: Lippincott Williams & Wilkins; 2000.)

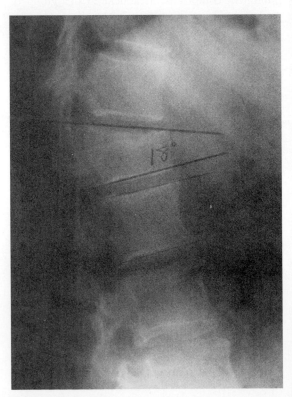

FIGURE 22-2 Thoracic vertebral compression fracture. Wedge compression fracture. (From Anderson MK, Hall SJ, Martin M. *Sports Injury Management*. 2nd ed. Baltimore: Lippincott Williams & Wilkins; 2000.)

TABLE 22-2	**Hallmarks of Neurogenic versus Vasculogenic Claudication**
Neurogenic	**Vasculogenic**
Nerve compression in the spine	Arterial insufficiency in the legs
Worse walking downhill (back placed in extension)	Equal walking up or downhill
Relieved by back flexion	Relieved by rest

As with the rest of the spine, many afflictions of the cervical spine are due to mechanical causes. Degenerative arthritis can affect the facet joints, causing neck pain. These joints can also be injured in trauma, such as a whiplash injury. Management initially consists of conservative measures such as modalities, medications, biomechanics and strength training, and gentle range-of-motion exercises. Cervical collars can give good relief in the acute stages, but are discouraged for long-term use. Traction can also provide pain relief in some cases. Injections can be both diagnostic and therapeutic. In cases where symptoms recur and are significant enough, a radiofrequency ablation procedure may be considered.[9]

Cervical stenosis can occur in the lateral recess, causing a radiculopathy, or centrally, causing a myelopathy. While stenosis can be congenital or acquired, in most cases it is related to arthritic change and bone/disc encroachment. The onset is often insidious. If the stenosis causes a radiculopathy, the customary symptoms predominate. In the case of a myelopathy, there can be complaints of numbness, tingling, and weakness, as well as neck pain. The symptoms may be more prominent in the legs than in the arms, but with intrinsic hand muscle wasting. Upper motor neuron signs may be present below the level of the lesion and bladder disturbances can occur. Most cases do not progress and can be managed with gentle exercises, modalities, braces, and medication. In case of progression of the neurologic deficit or if symptoms are significant enough, surgical decompression is warranted.[10]

HIP PAIN

The hip is one of the joints more frequently afflicted with DJD. Unfortunately, there is nothing that can be done to reverse this condition, and treatment options are limited. Range-of-motion exercises, aquatic

therapy, and strengthening may relieve symptoms to some extent. A cane used on the opposite side, while bearing only a small part of the body weight, can reduce joint compressive forces by a large amount and may help relieve symptoms. If symptoms are significant enough, a joint replacement surgery should be considered.

Trochanteric bursitis is a relatively common problem in the elderly. It can be associated with iliotibial tract problems and hip abductor inflexibility, so stretching of these structures as well as improving the leg biomechanics in general can be beneficial. Often one or more corticosteroid injections, when used in conjunction with an exercise program, can resolve symptoms. Padding or a memory foam mattress can also relieve symptoms caused by direct pressure when side-sleeping.

KNEE PAIN

The most common knee problems in the elderly are degenerative meniscal tears and DJD. Degenerative changes accelerate with age and are more pronounced in women.[11] Squatting, lotus position, and side-knee bending (sitting on the floor with the knees bent and the feet splayed out at the sides) appear to increase the risk for knee degeneration.[12] Sporting injuries are also a risk factor.[13]

Treatment of degenerative meniscal tears is often conservative and includes a knee sleeve for comfort, medications, and a strengthening exercise program. In refractory cases, injection, arthroscopic debridement, or meniscectomy may be considered.

Knee DJD may also respond to the above treatments. In the case of more significant medial compartment arthritis, an unloader (valgus) knee brace is recommended for pain reduction in patients. This type of brace shifts more of the body weight to the less affected lateral component.[14] In refractory cases, injections or joint arthroplasty can be considered.

ANKLE PAIN

Ankle sprains are common in all age groups. Previous injuries or limited joint flexibility may contribute to the risk of ankle sprains. Therapy for ankle sprains focuses on controlling pain and swelling. PRICE (protection, rest, ice, compression, and elevation) is a well-established protocol for the treatment of ankle injury. Ice and NSAIDs improve healing and speed recovery. Functional rehabilitation (e.g., motion restoration and strengthening exercises) is preferred over immobilization.[15]

The elderly often have decreased joint mobility and so immobilization is particularly to be avoided in this age group. Lack of proprioception may predispose to recurrent ankle injury. Because the prevalence of neuropathy rises with age, poor proprioception may be a particular concern in the elderly.

FOOT PAIN

Most foot problems are probably caused or exacerbated by a lifetime of wearing improper footwear. Women are usually more affected than men. In addition, the elderly are predisposed to a number of other foot problems. First, they can have problems with the fat pads on the plantar surface. With aging, these fat pads become atrophic (Fig. 22-3). This causes increased stress on the foot and may lead to metatarsalgia and increased symptoms from DJD. Symptoms of metatarsalgia may be decreased with foam shoe inserts, custom orthotics, or even custom shoes.

A Morton neuroma is a painful neuroma between the distal metatarsals, usually between the third and fourth metatarsals (Fig. 22-4). It is usually caused by compression of the ball of the foot by shoes that are too narrow, especially if high heels force the foot forward. Manual compression of the foot reproduces the symptoms. It can be treated with improved footwear, NSAIDs, stretching, and injection.

DJD can affect multiple joints in the foot, especially in the great toe. This can cause hallux rigidus, a loss of flexibility of the great toe. This can lead to a painful push-off part of the gait cycle. Stretching, NSAIDs, orthotics, and a rocker bottom shoe can help improve symptoms.

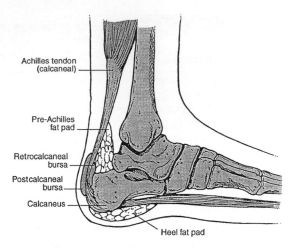

FIGURE 22-3 Fat pad and other structures of the foot. (From Anderson MK, Hall SJ, Martin M. *Sports Injury Management.* 2nd ed. Baltimore: Lippincott Williams & Wilkins; 2000.)

Hallux valgus, with its associated painful bunions is a particular problem in elderly women. It is largely due to a lifetime of wearing inappropriate footwear. Symptoms may be improved with custom footwear and NSAIDs. In more significant cases surgical correction may be necessary.

Acquired pes planus (Fig. 22-5) can be due to a rupture of the tibialis posterior tendon. This muscle tends to support the arch of the foot, and without its help, a painful flat foot can result. This can often be treated successfully if addressed early with a custom orthotic to provide adequate arch support. If an inflexible pes planus has developed, treatment is less successful, but can still include custom orthotics or shoes.

In addition to these musculoskeletal problems, the elderly also have problems with increased incidence of neuropathies and vascular and connective tissue disease, which can lead to a number of deforming foot and toe conditions, such as hammer toe, claw toe, and skin breakdown.

SHOULDER PAIN

Shoulder problems are common in the elderly, and the types of problems are different than in a younger group. More common are degenerative rotator cuff tears, adhesive capsulitis, and of course DJD. Less

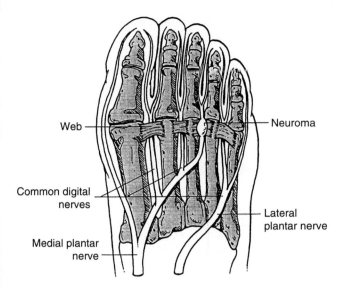

FIGURE 22-4 Morton's neuroma. (From Anderson MK, Hall SJ, Martin M. *Sports Injury Management.* 2nd ed. Baltimore: Lippincott Williams & Wilkins; 2000.)

common are instability and acute rotator cuff tears. Because of the risk of developing contractures and adhesive capsulitis, treatment in the elderly, especially in diabetics, involves less immobilization than is possible in younger patients. It must also be remembered that other problems, such as cervical radiculopathy or referred pain, can present as shoulder symptoms.

The prevalence of rotator cuff disease increases with age, with cuff tears found in over half of those over age 60.[16] When an event occurs and these people become symptomatic, they can often be managed conservatively. The risk of developing adhesive capsulitis is a serious reason to consider nonoperative care, if possible. Such treatment can include NSAIDs, below-shoulder rotator cuff internal and external rotation strengthening, modalities, and corticosteroid injections. In persons who are not particularly active,

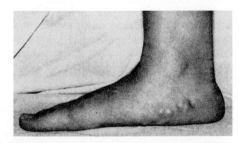

FIGURE 22-5 Pes planus. (From Anderson MK, Hall SJ, Martin M. *Sports Injury Management.* 2nd ed. Baltimore: Lippincott Williams & Wilkins; 2000.)

especially with overhead sporting activities, such treatment is often successful. The rate of successful nonoperative treatment varies from less than 50% to greater than 90%.[17] Earlier surgical intervention may be indicated in the setting of weakness and substantial functional disability. Importantly, older age does not necessarily predict a less successful surgical result. Although older patients may have slightly worse tendon quality and outcomes, surgical outcomes are not necessarily poor, with some studies showing generally favorable results. Significant weakness and decreased preoperative active range of motion appear to be associated with worse surgical outcomes.[17]

Adhesive capsulitis, often known by the descriptive name of frozen shoulder, is much more common in the elderly, especially in diabetics, in persons with thyroid and autoimmune disease, and in women.[18] It can occur spontaneously, but is more commonly triggered by some event such as trauma, immobilization, or surgery. The pathophysiology of the condition is controversial, but the effect is a loss of active and passive range of motion. The condition is also painful. It can result in severe loss of function. Obviously, it is a condition to be avoided, if at all possible. In the elderly it is particularly important to avoid shoulder immobilization. Treatment is with physical therapy, corticosteroid injection, and in some cases operative manipulation. Subscapular blocks have also been described as being effective.[18,19]

Ruptures of the long head of the biceps tendon are also more common as one ages (Fig. 22-6). This is generally a self-limiting problem. It causes a visual deformity, but little functional deficit. In persons who develop weakness, a surgical repositioning may be useful.

FALLS

Falls and the fear of falling are major problems in the elderly. In one study, the mean age of persons experiencing a fall was 67 years. Most subjects were female (80%). The majority of falls (76%) leading to fracture occurred outdoors. Three months after fracture, almost half of the subjects (48%) reported an increased fear of falling and 11% reported falling again.[20] Risk of fracture is associated with slow motor speed and poor strength.[21,22] It is not entirely clear

what kinds of interventions may be useful in preventing falls. However, it seems reasonable to suppose that maintenance of an active lifestyle and exercise, coupled with common sense measures such as adequate lighting and removal of obstacles in the home, would be effective to at least some extent.

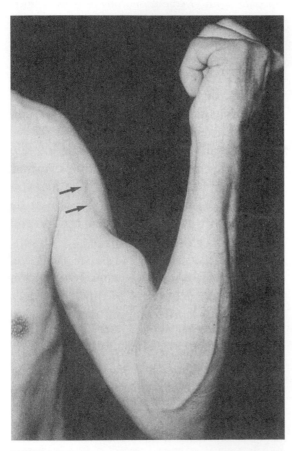

FIGURE 22-6 Biceps tendon rupture. (From Anderson MK, Hall SJ, Martin M. *Sports Injury Management.* 2nd ed. Baltimore: Lippincott Williams & Wilkins; 2000.)

REFERENCES

1. Anniasonn A, Hedberg M, Henning G, et al. Muscle morphology, enzymatic activity and muscle strength in elderly men: a follow up study. *Muscle Nerve.* 1986;9:585–591.
2. Lexell J. Aging and human muscle: observations from Sweden. *Can J Appl Physiol.* 1983;18:2–18.
3. Brown M. Selected physical performance changes with aging. *Top Geriatr Rehabil.* 1987;2:68–76.
4. Campbell M, McComas A, Petito F. Physiological changes in aging muscle. *J Neurol Neurosurg Psychiatry.* 1973;36: 174–182.
5. Sinaki M, Itoi E, Wahner HW, et al. Stronger back muscles reduce the incidence of vertebral fractures: a prospective 10- year follow up of postmenopausal women. *Bone.* 2002;30:836–841.
6. Amundsen T, Weber H, Nordal HJ, et al. Lumbar spinal stenosis: conservative or surgical management? A prospective 10-year study. *Spine.* 2000;25:1424–1435.
7. Botwin KP, Gruber RD, Bouchlas CG, et al. Fluoroscopically guided lumbar transforaminal epidural steroid injections in degenerative lumbar stenosis: an outcome study. *Am J Phys Med Rehabil.* 2002;81:898–905.
8. Englund J. Lumbar spinal stenosis. *Curr Sports Med Rep.* 2007;6:50–55.
9. Slipman CW, Lipetz JS, Plastaras CT, et al. Therapeutic zygapophyseal joint injections for headaches emanating from the C2-3 joint. *Am J Phys Med Rehabil.* 2001;80: 182–188.
10. Mazanec D, Reddy A. Medical management of cervical spondylosis. *Neurosurgery.* 2007;60:S43–S50.
11. Ding C, Cicuttini F, Blizzard L, et al. A longitudinal study on the effect of sex and age on rate of knee cartilage volume in adults. *Rheumatology.* 2007;46:273–279.
12. Boonsin T, Virasakdi C, Geater AF. Habitual floor activities increase risk of knee osteoarthritis. *Clin Orthop Rel Res.* 2006;454:147–154.
13. Thelin N, Holmberg S, Thelin A. Knee injuries account for the sports-related increased risk of knee osteoarthritis. *Scand J Med Sci Sports.* 2006;16:329–333.
14. Gravlee JR, Van Durme DJ. Braces and splints for musculoskeletal conditions. *Am Fam Physician.* 2007;75:342–348.
15. Ivins D. Acute ankle sprain: an update. *Am Fam Physician.* 2006;74:1714–1720.
16. Sher JS, Uribe JW, Posada A, et al. Abnormal findings on magnetic resonance imaging images of asymptomatic shoulders. *J Bone Joint Surg Am.* 1995;77:10–15.
17. Oh LS, Wolf BR, Hall MP, et al. Indications for rotator cuff repair: a systematic review. *Clin Orthop Rel Res.* 2006;455:52–63.

18. Sheridan MA, Hannafin JA. Upper extremity: emphasis on frozen shoulder. *Orthop Clin North Am.* 2006;37: 531–539.
19. Jankovic D, van Zundert A. The frozen shoulder syndrome: description of a new technique and five case reports using the subscapular nerve block and subscapularis trigger point infiltration. *Acta Anaesth Belg.* 2006;57:137–143.
20. Rucker D, Rowe BH, Johnson JA, et al. Educational intervention to reduce falls and fear of falling in patients after fragility fracture: results of a controlled pilot study. *Prev Med.* 2006;42:316–319.
21. Shigematsu R, Rantanen T, Saari P. Motor speed and lower extremity strength as predictors of fall-related bone fractures in elderly individuals. *Aging Clin Exp Res.* 2006;18:320–324.
22. Chan BKS, Marshall LM, Winters KM, et al. Incident fall risk and physical activity and physical performance among older men: the osteoporotic fractures in men study. *Am J Epidemiol.* 2006;165:696–703.

Health Benefits of Exercise

P hysical activity is defined as any bodily movement produced by contraction of skeletal muscle that results in an increase in the expenditure of energy (calories). "Exercise is a subcategory of physical activity in which planned, structured, and repetitive bodily movements are performed to improve or maintain one or more components of physical fitness."[1] Exercise provides a multitude of health benefits for those who participate on a frequent and regular basis. These health benefits include reduced risk of developing cardiovascular diseases (hypertension and coronary artery disease), type 2 diabetes, ischemic stroke, breast and colon cancer, osteoporosis, depression, and dementia, as well as reduced fall-related injuries.[2] There has been a tremendous amount of published research that defines the type, intensity, frequency, and duration of activity needed to achieve enhanced physical fitness, health, and to improve quality of life.

EXERCISE DOSING

The minimum effective dose (intensity, frequency, and duration) that can bring about a significant improvement in overall health is engaging in physical activity that expends 1,000 kcal (450 to 750 metabolic equivalent [MET] min) per week.[2,3] Despite our increased understanding of the biological mechanisms by which exercise benefits the body, clinicians and public health officials are challenged with the increasingly sedentary lifestyle of industrialized societies. In the United States, only about 45% to 50% of the American population participates in a regular exercise program that meets the Centers for Disease Control and Prevention (CDC) and the American College of Sports Medicine (ACSM) physical activity

recommendations.[4] This may be due in part to the cultural biases toward sedentary activities such as video and computer games and higher-paying desk jobs versus lower-paying physical labor.

Recently, the ACSM and the CDC updated their physical activity recommendations in order to "provide a more comprehensive and explicit public health recommendation for adults (less than 65 years old)" that was first published in 1995.[3,5] The new recommendations are more explicit with regard to type of exercise and dose that will afford the individual the most benefit. It is recommended that an individual engage in at least 30 to 60 minutes of continuous or intermittent (10-minute bouts accumulated throughout the day) of moderate aerobic activity 5 days per week, or 20 minutes of vigorous aerobic activity 3 days per week. Table 23-1[3,6] lists examples of aerobic activities that can be incorporated into everyday living to achieve these benefits. Along with aerobic exercise, muscle strengthening activities are also recommended. It is recommended that 8 to 10 exercises be performed on two or more nonconsecutive days each week using the major muscle groups. To increase strength, 8 to 12 repetitions of each exercise that results in volitional muscle fatigue are required.[3] A good exercise program should also include muscle flexibility or stretching exercises to maintain range of motion of the major joints.

Most individuals will want to participate in a combination of vigorous and moderate aerobic activities to meet the recommended requirements. So what combination of exercises will meet the intent of the above recommendations? What activity dose is necessary to achieve health benefits? (The dose is equivalent to the energy expended during a physical activity.) It is suggested that using the MET method is an easy way of determining energy expenditure during physical activity. One MET is equivalent to the amount of

TABLE 23-1	MET Equivalent of Common Physical Activities Classified as Light, Moderate, or Vigorous Intensity

Light (< 3.0 MET)	Moderate (3.0–6.0 MET)	Vigorous (> 6.0 MET)
Walking	**Walking**	**Walking, Jogging, & Running**
Walking slowly around home, store, or office = 2.0[a]	Walking 3.0 mph = 3.3[a] Walking at very brisk pace (4 mph) = 5.0[a]	Walking at very brisk pace (4.5 mph) = 6.3[a] Walking/hiking at moderate pace and grade with no or light pack (< 10 lb) = 7.0 Hiking at steep grades and pack 10–42 lb = 7.5–9.0 Jogging at 5 mph = 8.0[a] Jogging at 6 mph = 10.0[a] Running at 7 mph = 11.5[a]
Household & Occupation	**Household & Occupation**	**Household & Occupation**
Sitting—using computer, work at desk, using light hand tools = 1.5 Standing—performing light work such as making bed, washing dishes, ironing, preparing food or store clerk = 2.0–2.5	Cleaning, heavy: washing windows, car, clean garage = 3.0 Sweeping floors or carpet, vacuuming, mopping = 3.0–3.5 Carpentry, general = 3.6 Carrying & stacking wood = 5.5 Mowing lawn walking; power mower = 5.5	Shoveling sand, coal, etc. = 7.0 Carrying heavy loads such as bricks = 7.5 Heavy farming such as bailing hay = 8.0 Shoveling, digging ditches = 8.5
Leisure Time & Sports	**Leisure Time & Sports**	**Leisure Time & Sports**
Arts & crafts, playing cards = 1.5 Billiards = 2.5 Boating, power = 2.5 Croquet = 2.5 Darts = 2.5 Fishing, sitting = 2.5 Playing most musical instruments = 2.0–2.5	Badminton, recreational = 4.5 Basketball, shooting around = 4.5 Bicycling on flat: light effort (10–12 mph) = 6.0 Dancing, ballroom, slow = 3.0; ballroom, fast = 4.5 Fishing from riverbank & walking = 4.0 Golf, walking, pulling clubs = 4.3 Sailing boat, windsurfing = 3.0 Swimming leisurely = 6.0[b] Table tennis = 4.0 Tennis doubles = 5.0 Volleyball, noncompetitive = 3.0–4.0	Basketball game = 8.0 Bicycling on flat: moderate effort (12–14 mph) = 8.0; fast (14–16 mph) = 10 Skiing cross country, slow (2.5 mph = 7.0); fast (5.0–7.9 mph) = 9.0 Soccer, casual = 7.0; competitive = 10.0 Swimming, moderate/hard = 8–11[b] Tennis singles = 8.0 Volleyball, competitive at gym or beach = 8.0

[a]On flat, hard surface.
[b]MET values can vary substantially from person to person during swimming as a result of different strokes and skill levels.
(Reprinted from Haskell [3])

energy expended when an individual sits quietly (1 kcal/kg/hr). Table 23-1 lists the MET equivalents of common physical activities. If the minimum dose of physical activity needed to achieve a significant health benefit is 450 to 750 MET·min per week, then an individual who bicycles at 10 to 12 mph for 30 minutes 2 times in a week and plays singles tennis for 30 minutes 1 day in a week will have expended 6 MET × 30 min × 2 days plus 8 MET × 30 min × 1 day, or 600 MET·min, thus meeting the recommendations proposed above.

There are limitations to using MET values to determine total energy expenditure. There is a wide variability among individuals that influences the amount of energy a given person expends. This depends on a variety of factors including body composition,

TABLE 23-2	Example of a Recommended Exercise Program		
	Flexibility	**Cardiopulmonary**	**Strengthening**
Sunday		Walk dog for 30 min	Lift weights
Monday	Stretching	Jogging	
Tuesday		Walk dog for 30 min	Lift weights
Wednesday	Pilates or Tai Chi		
Thursday		Walk dog for 30 min	Lift weights
Friday	Yoga	Walk dog for 30 min	
Saturday	Stretching	Tennis with friend	

physical fitness, and skill level. These guidelines and MET values should be applied to generally healthy adults, age 18 to 65 years. Older adults (age > 65), adults with chronic conditions, and adults with functional limitations should use a relative scale of activity intensity as measured by the Borg Scale of Perceived Effort.[7,8] Table 23-2 gives an example of a simple well-rounded exercise program that will provide the health benefits discussed in this chapter.

EXERCISE BENEFITS FOR SPECIFIC MEDICAL CONDITIONS

Cardiovascular and Cerebrovascular Health

Coronary artery disease (CAD) is the leading cause of death in the United States. In 2004, it claimed the lives of over 650,000 people.[9] Physical inactivity is among the risk factors in the development of CAD. Physically active individuals are less likely to develop CAD than their age-related sedentary peers.[10–12] In the Harvard alumni study there was a 20% risk reduction in the men who participated in moderate level of activity or expended at least 1,003 kcal (450–750 MET·min) of energy per week in physical activity.[11] Two studies found that the pace of walking (>3 mph) was more strongly associated with CAD risk reduction when compared with total walking time.[12,13] In contrast, Lee et al.[10] found that walking at least 1 hour per week was sufficient to lower the risk of CAD independent of walking pace. In one large cohort study, weight training was also associated with decreased risk of CAD,[12] which supports the recommendation to incorporate muscle strengthening activities into one's exercise program.

In peripheral vascular occlusive disease (PVOD), walking for greater than 30 minutes, at least 3 times per week, has been shown to improve symptoms of claudication, walking time, and to increase walking distance. Furthermore, improvements in walking distance are associated with improved ability to perform activities of daily living.[14]

Hypertension (HTN) is a common risk factor for CAD and stroke. It affects about 72 million Americans age 20 years and older.[15] With increasing age, the risk of developing HTN increases. There is evidence that a higher level of activity in normotensive white males reduces the incidence of developing HTN later in life.[16] Moderate-intensity exercise is beneficial in reducing systolic and diastolic blood pressures. A meta-analysis of 29 studies revealed a significant reduction in blood pressure when study participants engaged in moderate to vigorous exercise 3 or more times per week.[17] Overall, systolic blood pressure can be reduced by 3.8 to 4.7 mm Hg and diastolic pressures can be reduced by 2.6 to 3.1 mm Hg.[17,18] Although this change may seem small, the public health impact can be very large, with a significant reduction in the incidence of HTN, CAD, and stroke.[17] This reduction will also lead to reduced medicine utilization, side effects, and cost.

Increased blood levels of triglycerides (TG) and low-density lipoproteins (LDL), and low levels of high-density lipoprotein (HDL), increase the risk of CAD, atherosclerosis, HTN, congestive heart failure, and stroke. Aerobic endurance activities have been shown to increase HDL levels by as much as 7% after 9 months of vigorous jogging (10–11 min/mile and a MET of 9), 3 to 5 times per week, for up to 10 to 14 miles per week in men.[19] In studies focusing on women, physically fit or physically active women have higher levels of HDL than their sedentary counterparts; however; studies have failed to establish what dose of activity is needed to increase HDL in women. It is suggested that women participate in activities that expend at least 1,000 to 1,200 kcal/week.[19] For example, a 70-kg woman would need to walk briskly at 4 mph (13 min/mile), for 35 minutes, 5 days per week.

A recent meta-analysis showed a 5% reduction in LDL but no significant change in HDL, total cholesterol, and triglyceride levels in type II diabetics who participated in an aerobic program that lasted at least 8 weeks. This is clinically significant in the risk reduction of CAD; it has been shown that every 1% reduction in LDL reduces coronary risk by about 1.7%. Thus, these observed changes in LDL would be equivalent to an 8.5% reduction in coronary risk.[20] In addition to aerobic activities, resistance exercises have been shown to decrease triglyceride levels with no effect on total cholesterol or HDL levels.[21]

Stroke shares the same risk factors as CAD. By controlling risk factors through medications and lifestyle choices, risk reduction is significant. Those individuals who are physically active throughout adulthood are less likely to have a stroke later in life. In the chronic stroke survivor, exercise can also improve functional capacity and functional recovery. A recent meta-analysis of aerobic training in mild to moderately disabled stroke survivors showed a strong positive effect, with improved peak VO_2, peak workload, walking velocity, and walking endurance.[22] Progressive resistance training programs have also shown significant improvements in muscle strength and improvement in walking ability.[23] Community exercise programs have been shown to improve balance, functional capacity, and mobility, even in chronic (>6 month) stroke survivors.[24]

Pulmonary Health

Pulmonary function declines with age. The rate of this decline is dependent on several factors including genetics, environmental exposures (pollution and toxins), and lifestyle choices (smoking and physical activity). In a longitudinal study of 189 men followed for 25 years, men who regularly engaged in vigorous exercise lost significantly less forced expiratory volume (FEV) than their sedentary counterparts. A slower rate of decline was also observed among those who continued to smoke but who engaged in vigorous activity.[25] A more recent study confirmed that active smokers with moderate and high physical activity levels had a

reduced decline of FEV_1 and forced vital capacity (FVC) compared with those who engaged in low physical activity levels. The active groups also had a reduced risk of developing chronic obstructive pulmonary disease (COPD) as compared with the low physical activity group.[26]

Diabetes Mellitus

Diabetes is the most common serious metabolic disease in the world; it affects 120 million people worldwide.[27] Along with diet and hypoglycemic medications, exercise has been established to have metabolic and cardiovascular benefits in patients with both type I and type II diabetes mellitus. In patients with type I diabetes, exercise reduces insulin requirements by increasing the utilization of energy stores. In patients with type II diabetes, exercise increases the sensitivity of skeletal and adipose tissue to insulin. Exercise increases the number and activity of glucose transporter proteins in adipocytes and myocytes, resulting in more effective glucose transportation into the cell.[28] Additionally, hepatic production of glucose is reduced by exercise.[29] Therefore, regular exercise can reduce oral hypoglycemic requirements in patients with type II diabetes.

The effectiveness of physical exercise in the primary and secondary prevention of diabetes has long been recognized. A prospective, controlled study of patients with impaired glucose tolerance demonstrated that increasing physical activity, combined with weight loss and dietary modification, resulted in a 58% reduction in the development of type II diabetes.[30] In a large prospective study, each increase of 500 kcal in energy expenditure per week was associated with a 6% decrease in incidence of type 2 diabetes.[31] Another prospective cohort study showed that walking at least 2 hours per week was associated with a reduction in the incidence of premature death of 39% to 54% from any cause and of 34% to 53% from cardiovascular disease among patients with diabetes.[32]

Exercise interventions can also be used in the management of diabetes. Resistance training may have even greater benefits for glycemic control than aerobic training. A meta-analysis of 14 controlled trials (11 randomized) revealed that exercise interventions resulted in a small but clinically and statistically significant reduction (0.66%) in glycosylated hemoglobin compared with no exercise intervention.[33] This compares well with reported reductions achieved through medications. Metformin can lower glycosylated hemoglobin levels by 0.9% compared to placebo, and sulphonylureas have been shown to have a similar effect.[34] Reducing the glycosylated hemoglobin by this amount can lead to significant reductions in morbidity and mortality. Each 1% reduction in glycosylated hemoglobin has been associated with risk reductions of 21% for any diabetic related end-point, 21% for diabetes-related deaths, 14% for myocardial infarction, and 37% for microvascular complications.[35]

Osteoporosis

Osteoporosis is defined as decreased bone mass per unit of bone volume. It occurs as a complication of various conditions such as prolonged immobilization, hyperthyroidism, COPD, Cushing disease, certain malignancies, and so forth. Postmenopausal osteoporosis remains the most common manifestation. Ten million people are directly affected, and an additional 34 million are at risk for developing this disease in the United States. Of the 10 million Americans estimated to have osteoporosis, 8 million are women and 2 million are men.[36]

The best way to address osteoporosis is prevention. Physical activity can regulate bone maintenance and stimulate bone formation. Weight-bearing exercise, especially resistance exercise, appears to have the greatest effects on bone mineral density, thus having the greatest osteogenic effect on a specific bone site.[37] Weight-bearing exercises can include aerobics, circuit training, jogging, jumping, and sports (volleyball, basketball, football, etc.) that generate impact forces on the skeleton.

Bone mass increases during childhood and puberty, consolidates during young adulthood, and declines with age.[38] There is evidence to suggest that the years of childhood and adolescence represent an opportune period during which bone adapts particularly efficiently to loading activities.[39]

In perimenopausal and postmenopausal women, regular physical activity has been shown to maintain and increase bone mineral density and to reduce the risk of falls and bone fractures. The results of a prospective cohort study of more than 60,000 postmenopausal women (aged 40–77 years) showed that women who engaged in brisk walking (≥3 mph) 5 hours per week, as well as other leisure-time activities were 55% less likely to suffer a hip fracture than sedentary women.[40] It was also noted in this study that walking at a leisurely pace 1 hour per week led to a risk reduction of 6%.

Exercise has also been shown to be effective in those who have already developed osteoporosis. Although there is no evidence that exercise prevents fractures, randomized clinical trials have shown that regular exercise can reduce the risk of falls by approximately 25%.[41] Weight-bearing exercises that can increase bone strength and improve balance are beneficial for those with osteoporosis. It is recommended that persons with severe osteoporosis perform daily nonstraining exercise such as walking or water exercises for at least 30 minutes. Low-resistance exercises can be done safely and can be advanced as tolerated to increase strength. Spinal extension exercises and isometric abdominal exercises are safe and effective in severe osteoporosis and should be used to prevent spinal compression fractures, to improve posture, and to improve balance.[37]

Cancer

A progressive increase of cancer, with an estimated 15 million new cases and 1 million deaths per year, is expected by the year 2020.[42] There is a significant body of evidence that moderate to vigorous physical activity can reduce the risk of colon and breast cancer.[43,44] Although no activity dose has been established to prevent colon cancer, a large cohort study of African-American women showed that there was a significant reduction in the incidence of polyps (a precursor to cancer) of ~20% with 20 to 39 MET-hours/wk of physical activity (walking at a very brisk pace for 1 hour, 4–7 times per week) and of 30% with ≥40 MET-hours/wk (jogging or running for 1 hour, 4 times per week).[45]

Cancer- and treatment-related side-effects such as fatigue, muscle weakness, declines in functional status, psychological distress, and decreased body mass have been well documented. In recent years, there has been a growing interest in the use of exercise as an intervention for cancer patients. Patients on high-dose chemotherapy who participated in a cycling program at 50% maximum heart rate have been shown to have a reduction in the decline in physical performance and psychological distress relative to a control group.[46]

Researchers have found that walking on a regular basis helps breast cancer patients. Those who regularly walked 3 to 5 hours a week (or did comparable exercise) were 50% less likely to have a recurrence of their cancer than women who exercised less than an hour per week.[47] Although the reason behind the benefits of exercise in breast cancer patients is not clearly understood, researchers have developed some possible theories. Exercise activity has been shown to reduce blood levels of estrogen as well as one type of insulin-like growth factor (IGF), both of which have been shown to promote cancer cell growth.[48]

Prescriptions for physical activity must be individualized for the cancer patient since the site of cancer may impact the ability to participate in an exercise program. Appropriate precautions should be incorporated into the exercise program. Various limiting factors may require decreasing or discontinuing an exercise program to minimize pain and other complications (Table 23-3).[49]

Fibromyalgia, Osteoarthritis, and Rheumatoid Arthritis

Fibromyalgia is a chronic syndrome of diffuse muscle pain with multiple tender points throughout the upper and lower extremities. There are associated symptoms of fatigue, poor sleep pattern, depression, muscle stiffness, and joint pain. Exercise is advocated

as part of an overall treatment plan in fibromyalgia patients. This is often met with great resistance due to the fact that regular daily activities initially seem to exacerbate symptoms. However, a meta-analysis of several randomized trials showed there to be an improvement in tender point pain pressure threshold, global well-being, and physical fitness after a structured moderately intense aerobic exercise program was implemented.[50] Many studies in fibromyalgia patients have large attrition rates that make it difficult to draw conclusions with regard to type of exercise, frequency, and duration that would give maximum benefit. Most clinicians would likely agree that a structured program that starts at a low intensity and gradually increases over time to a moderate intensity level may have better compliance than starting directly with a moderate intensity level program. Water-based exercise is a reasonable option, and may provide better improvements in mood and sleep duration than land-based exercise.[51]

Strengthening programs have also been shown to be of benefit in fibromyalgia patients. Not only does strength improve, but there is also a trend toward

TABLE 23-3	Exercise Precautions for Cancer Patients	
Medical Problem	**Lab Values**	**Recommendations**
Thrombocytopenia	30,000–50,000/m^3	Low-intensity activities, active range of motion (ROM), light weights ($\leq$2 lb), no heavy resistance
	20,000–30,000/ m^3	Self-care activities, functional ambulation, gentle ROM
	<20,000/m^3	Essential activities of daily living (ADL) & ambulation, no exercise
Anemia	Hematocrit <25%, Hemoglobin <8 g/dL	Avoid aerobic and progressive resistance programs; light ROM and isometric exercises are permitted
	Hematocrit 25–35%, Hemoglobin 8–10 g/dL	Essential ADL, assistance as needed for safety; light aerobics; light weights ($\leq$2 lb)
	Hematocrit >35%, Hemoglobin >10 g/dL	Light to moderate aerobics as tolerated, resistance exercises
Bone metastasis	>50% cortex involved	Non- or foot flat weight-bearing, use crutches, gentle ROM, no twisting
	>25–50% cortex involved	Partial weight-bearing, light aerobic low-impact activities, no stretching, no progressive resistance
	0–25% cortex involvement	Exercise as tolerated
Pulmonary dysfunction	<50% of predicted FEV$_1$	No aerobic exercise
	50–75% of predicted FEV$_1$	Light aerobic exercise
	>75% of predicted FEV$_1$	No restrictions
Cardiac dysfunction	Arrhythmias	No aerobics, consult a cardiologist

ADL, activities of daily living
Adapted from Gerber LH, Vargo MM, Smith RG. Rehabilitation of the cancer patient. In: DeVita JT Jr., Hellman S, Rosenberg SA, eds. *Cancer: Principles & Practice of Oncology.* 6th ed. Philiadelphia: Lippincott Williams & Wilkins; 2005:2725–2729.

increased endurance and a significant increase in perceived functionality.[52] In a 21-week strength training study, subjects with fibromyalgia developed increased strength, improved mood, and decreased neck pain, and reported increased functional capacity.

Osteoarthritis (OA) is the leading cause of disability in the United States. It is estimated that 46 million Americans have been diagnosed with osteoarthritis, and that by 2030 there will be 67 million Americans that share this diagnosis.[53] It has been difficult to identify the pathogenesis of OA because of the complex interactions between biomechanical and biochemical factors on the cartilage and bone interface. Good muscle strength and balance, full joint range of motion, and proper body weight help to maintain even pressure loads across a joint and to maintain healthy cartilage physiology. Age, obesity, genetics, trauma, and muscle weakness are some of the risk factors in the development of OA. Persons with OA tend to be less active as well as overweight or obese.[54]

Recent studies have shown that moderate activity can increase functional capacity and decrease pain in OA sufferers. Pain relief from exercise is as effective as nonsteroidal anti-inflammatory drugs (NSAIDs) and has a better safety profile.[55] Exercise can also help with weight loss, either alone or in combination with diet. A 6% weight loss can result in a 30% reduction in pain.[56] Aerobic exercise, land based or water based, is just as effective in controlling pain as muscle strengthening exercises.[57]

Rheumatoid arthritis (RA), an autoimmune condition, is a chronic inflammatory polyarthritis. It is a progressively degenerative disorder that affects joints and connective tissue. It causes significant destruction and deformities to small and large joints, limiting range of motion and inducing muscle weakness. Chronic fatigue, pain, and depression are associated with this disorder and typically lead to functional decline. Low-impact aerobic exercise programs have been shown to positively impact fatigue, pain, and depression without hastening disease progression.[58,59] All forms of medium- and low-impact aerobic exercise improve aerobic capacity, muscle strength, and joint mobility.[60] Exercise of moderate to high intensity has been shown to be a safe and effective way to slow the rate of functional decline, to improve aerobic capacity, and to minimize depression and fatigue without causing a rapid progression of the disease. However, long-term (>2 years), high-intensity weight-bearing exercises appear to accelerate radiographic joint damage progression in patients with preexisting extensive damage.[61] One study comparing aquatic exercises to land-based exercises revealed no difference between groups in the 10-meter walk times, functional scores, pain scores, and quality-of-life measures. Those who participated in the aquatic group were more likely to report feeling much better than those treated with land-based exercises.[62] In general, high-impact exercises such as jumping, running, and basketball should be avoided in patients with significant RA. Medium- and low-impact exercises, such as swimming or aquatics, bicycling, and walking, are more appropriate unless there is significant inflammation.[63] When acute inflammation is present, only gentle active or active assistive ROM (within the available range of motion) and isometric exercises should be performed until the inflammation subsides.[64]

Mental Health

Physical activity has been studied as a form of prevention and treatment for dementia. In one study, leisure time activities such as playing board games, crossword puzzles, playing a musical instrument, and dancing, but not exercise, reduced the risk of dementia.[65] However, in two longitudinal studies involving large cohorts, exercise has also been shown to decrease risk of dementia.[66,67] In those who already have dementia or cognitive impairments, regular physical exercise, such as walking or using an exercise bicycle, has been shown to improve nutritional status and cognitive function and to decrease the risk for falls and behavioral problems.[68] Resistive exercises have equally beneficial effects on cognitive functioning as aerobic activity. The beneficial effects do not appear to depend on the exercise intensity (moderate versus high) being performed; however, moderate-intensity exercises might be more appropriate for the elderly because there appears to be a more significant improvement in their mood profile at this intensity level.[69]

Physical activity is associated with improved psychological well-being, physical health, life satisfaction, and cognitive functioning. Clinical and epidemiologic studies have also shown an association between physical activity and decreased prevalence of anxiety and depression.[70,71] The causal relationship is unclear. Does physical inactivity increase risk of depression and anxiety or does depression and anxiety lead to physical inactivity? In most of the studies previously mentioned in this chapter, improvements in mood have been reported as a secondary measure.[2,51,57-59]

In a review article by Phillips et al.[72] and recent randomized control studies in which physical activity was used as a treatment for depression, promising data support that any type of physical activity can be as effective as pharmacotherapy with few to no side effects.[72–74] Future research is needed to compare aerobic, weight-training, and combined exercise interventions with adequate follow-up to determine the most effective exercise regimen and the dose response in varied populations.

Obesity

Since the mid-1970s, the prevalence of overweight and obesity has increased twofold for both adults and children.[75] The health consequences have been well documented. They include hypertension, coronary artery disease, pulmonary disease, sleep apnea, hyperlipidemia, type 2 diabetes, OA, stroke, and some cancers. Weight loss is essential to decreasing the morbidity and mortality associated with obesity. Caloric intake as well as an increase in energy expenditure at rest and with activity are cornerstones for the prevention and treatment of overweight and obesity. Diet alone has been shown to be largely ineffective in maintaining successful weight loss. Those who have successfully managed to keep the weight off are individuals who, on average, exercise about 1 hour per day.[76] Studies indicate that increases in physical activity may protect against metabolic disease (hyperlipidemia, diabetes) even in the absence of improved aerobic fitness and reduced body fatness.[77,78] However, the greatest benefits are seen in those persons who lose fat mass. Therefore, the combination of increasing levels of physical activity and reduction in fat mass is likely to be the most successful approach for preventing cardiovascular and metabolic disease.

SUMMARY

The health benefits of exercise are expansive in terms of prevention and treatment of the world's most common ailments. Exercise can slow the aging process by minimizing the natural functional declines that are seen in older age. Exercise is recognized as an important intervention in a world that is getting older, heavier, and more sedentary. Currently, it has not been established what type of exercise or dose provides the maximum benefit; however, any aerobic activity combined with resistance training is as important as

proper eating and sleeping to sustain a healthy life. An exercise program should be tailored to an individual's preferences and abilities. This will also improve adherence to a lifetime of exercise. Variety can also help with boredom and decrease drop-out. Health care professionals should continually promote physical activity as part of their preventive medicine and treatment plans.

REFERENCES

1. Howley ET. Type of activity: resistance, aerobic and leisure versus occupational physical activity. *Med Sci Sports Exerc.* 2001;33:S364–S369.
2. Kesaniemi YA, Danforth E Jr., Jensen MD, et al. Dose-response issues concerning physical activity and health: an evidence-based symposium. *Med Sci Sports Exerc.* 2001;33: S531–S538.
3. Haskell WL, Lee IM, Pate RR, et al. Physical activity and public health: updated recommendation for adults from the American College of Sports Medicine and the American Heart Association. *Med Sci Sports Exerc.* 2007;39:1423–1434.
4. Centers for Disease Control and Prevention. *U.S. Physical Activity Statistics 2005.* Available at http://apps.nccd.cdc.gov/ PASurveillance/StateSumV.asp. Accessed April 15, 2007.
5. Pate RR, Pratt M, Blair SN, et al. Physical activity and public health. A recommendation from the Centers for Disease Control and Prevention and the American College of Sports Medicine. *JAMA.* 1995;273:402–407.
6. Ainsworth B, Haskell WL, White MC, et al. Compendium of physical activities: an update of activity codes and MET intensities. *Med Sci Sports Exerc.* 2000;32:S498–S516.
7. Nelson ME, Rejeski WJ, Blair SN, et al. Physical activity and public health in older adults: recommendation from the American College of Sports Medicine and the American Heart Association. *Med Sci Sports Exerc.* 2007;39: 1435–1445.
8. Lee IM, Sesso HD, Oguma Y, et al. Relative intensity of physical activity and risk of coronary heart disease. *Circulation.* 2003;107:1110–1116.
9. Minino AM, Heron MP, Murphy SL, et al. Deaths: final data for 2004. *National Vital Statistics Reports.* Available at http://www.cdc.gov/nchs/data/nvsr/nvsr55/nvsr55_19.pdf. Accessed October 27, 2007.
10. Lee IM, Rexrode KM, Cook NR, et al. Physical activity and coronary heart disease in woman. Is "no pain, no gain" passé? *JAMA.* 2001;285:1447–1454.
11. Sesso HD, Paffenbarger RS Jr., Lee IM. Physical activity and coronary heart disease in men. The Harvard alumni health study. *Circulation.* 2000;102:975–980.
12. Tanasescu M, Leitzmann MF, Rimm EB, et al. Exercise type and intensity in relation to coronary heart disease in men. *JAMA.* 288:2002;1994–2000.
13. Manson JE, Hu FB, Rich-Edwards JW, et al. A prospective study of walking as compared with vigorous exercise in the prevention of coronary heart disease in women. *N Engl J Med.* 1999;341:650–658.

14. Gardner AW, Poehlman ET. Exercise rehabilitation programs for the treatment of claudication pain: a meta-analysis. *JAMA*. 1995;274:975–980.

15. American Heart Association. High blood pressure statistics. Available at http://www.americanheart.org/presenter.jhtml?identifier=4621. Accessed October 28, 2007.

16. Pescatello LS, Franklin BA, Fagard R, et al. American College of Sports Medicine Position Stand. Exercise and hypertension. *Med Sci Sports Exerc*. 2004;36:533–553.

17. Halbert JA, Silagy CA, Finucane P, et al. The effectiveness of exercise training in lowering blood pressure: a meta-analysis of randomized controlled trials of 4 weeks or longer. *J Hum Hypertens*. 1997;11:641–649.

18. Whelton SP, Chin A, Xin X, et al. Effect of aerobic exercise on blood pressure. A meta-analysis of randomized, controlled trials. *Ann Intern Med*. 2002;136:493–503.

19. Kokkinos PF, Fernhall B. Physical activity and high density lipoprotein cholesterol levels. *Sport Med*. 1999;28:307–314.

20. Kelley GA, Kelley KS. Effects of aerobic exercise on lipids and lipoproteins in adults with type 2 diabetes: a meta-analysis of randomized-controlled trials. *Public Health*. 2007;121:643–655.

21. Thomas DE, Elliott EJ, Naughton GA. Exercise for type 2 diabetes mellitus. *Cochrane Database Syst Rev*. 2006;3: CD002968. DOI: 10.1002/14651858.CD002968.pub2.

22. Pang MY, Eng JJ, Dawson AS, et al. The use of aerobic exercise training in improving aerobic capacity in individuals with stroke: a meta-analysis. *Clin Rehabil*. 2006;20: 97–111.

23. Morris SL, Dodd KJ, Morris ME. Outcomes of progressive resistance strength training following stroke: a systematic review. *Clin Rehabil*. 2004;18:27–39.

24. Eng JJ, Chu KS, Kim CM, et al. A community-based group exercise program for persons with chronic stroke. *Med Sci Sports Exerc*. 2003;35:1271–1278.

25. Pelkonen M, Notkola IL, Lakka T, et al. Delaying decline in pulmonary function with physical activity: a 25-year follow-up. *Am J Respir Crit Care Med*. 2003;168:494–499.

26. Garcia-Aymerich J, Lange P, Bunet M, et al. Regular physical activity modifies smoking-related lung function decline and reduces risk of chronic obstructive pulmonary disease: a population-based cohort study. *Am J Respir Crit Care Med*. 2007;175:458–463.

27. American Association of Diabetes Educators. Diabetes—Facts and Statistics. Available at http://www.aadenet.org/DiabetesEducation/GovStats.shtml. Accessed February 16, 2007.

28. Tabata Y, Suzuki T, Fokunaga T, et al. Resistance training affects the GLUT 4 content in skeletal muscle of humans after 19 days of head down bed rest. *J Appl Physiol*. 1999;86: 909–914.

29. DeFronzo RA, Sherwin RS, Kraemer N. Effect of physical training on insulin action in obesity. *Diabetes*. 1987;36: 1379–1385.

30. Tuomilehto J, Lindstrom J, Eriksson JG, et al. Prevention of type 2 diabetes mellitus by changes in lifestyle among subjects with impaired glucose tolerance. *N Engl J Med*. 2001;344:1343–1350.

31. Helmrich SP, Ragland DR, Leung RW, et al. Physical activity and reduced occurrence of non-insulin-dependent diabetes mellitus. *N Engl J Med*. 1991;325:147–152.

32. Gregg EW, Gerzoff RB, Caspersen CJ, et al. Relationship of walking to mortality among U.S. adults with diabetes. *Arch Intern Med*. 2003;163:1440–1447.

33. Boule NG, Haddad E, Kenny GP, et al. Effects of exercise on glycemic control and body mass in type 2 diabetes mellitus: a meta-analysis of controlled clinical trials. *JAMA*. 2001;286:1218–1227.

34. Johansen K. Efficacy of metformin in the treatment of NIDDM. Meta-analysis. *Diabetes Care*. 1999;22:33–37.

35. Stratton IM, Adler AI, Neil HA, et al. Association of glycaemia with macrovascular and microvascular complications of type 2 diabetes (UKPDS 35): prospective observational study. *BMJ*. 2001;321:405–412.

36. National Osteoporosis Foundation. Fast Facts. Available at http://www.nof.org/osteoporosis/diseasefacts.htm. Accessed October 30, 2007.

37. Sinaki M. Prevention and treatment of osteoporosis. In: Braddom RL, ed. *Physical Medicine and Rehabilitation*. 3rd ed. Philadelphia: Saunders Elsevier; 2007:929–949.

38. Matkovic V, Jelic T, Wardlaw GM. Timing of peak bone mass in Caucasian females and its implication for the prevention of osteoporosis. Inference from a cross-sectional model. *J Clin Invest*. 1994;93:799–808.

39. Khan K, McKay HA, Haapasalo H, et al. Does childhood and adolescence provide a unique opportunity for exercise to strengthen the skeleton? *J Sci Med Sports*. 2000;3:150–164.

40. Feskanich D, Willett W, Colditz G. Walking and leisure-time activity and risk of hip fracture in postmenopausal women. *JAMA*. 2002;288:2300–2306.

41. NIH consensus development conference statement: osteoporosis prevention, diagnosis, and therapy. March 27–29, 2000. Available at http://consensus.nih.gov/2000/2000 Osteoporosis111html.htm. Accessed October 30, 2007.

42. Parkin DM, Bray F, Ferlay J, et al. Estimating the world cancer burden: Globocan 2000. *Int J Cancer*. 2001;94: 153–156.

43. Slattery M. Physical activity and colorectal cancer. *Sports Med*. 2004;34:239–252.

44. Brody JG, Rudel RA, Michels KB, et al. Environmental pollutants, diet, physical activity, body size, and breast cancer: where do we stand in research to identify opportunities for prevention? *Cancer*. 2007;109(suppl):2627–2634.

45. Rosenberg L, Boggs D, Wise LA, et al. A follow up study of physical activity and incidence of colorectal polyps in African-American women. *Cancer Epidemiol Biomarkers Prev*. 2006;15:1438–1442.

46. Dimeo FC, Stieglitz RD, Novelli-Fischer U, et al. Effects of physical activity on fatigue and psychologic status of cancer patients during chemotherapy. *Cancer*. 1999;85:2273–2277.

47. Holmes MD, Chen WY, Feskanich D, et al. Physical activity and survival after breast cancer diagnosis. *JAMA*. 2005;293: 2479–2486.

48. Barnard RJ, Gonzalez JH, Liva ME, et al. Effects of a low-fat, high-fiber diet and exercise program on breast cancer risk factors *in vivo* and tumor cell growth apoptosis *in vitro*. *Nutr Cancer*. 2006;55:28–34.

49. Gerber LH, Vargo MM, Smith RG. Rehabilitation of the cancer patient. In: DeVita JT Jr., Hellman S, Rosenberg SA, eds. *Cancer: Principles & Practice of Oncology*. 6th ed. Philidelphia: Lippincott Williams & Wilkins; 2005: 2725–2729.

50. Busch A, Schachter CL, Peloso PM, et al. Exercise for treating fibromyalgia syndrome. *Cochrane Database Syst Rev.* 2002;3:CD003786.

51. Gowans SE, deHueck A. Pool exercise for individuals with fibromyalgia. *Curr Opin Rheumatol.* 19:2007;168–173.

52. Kingsley JD, Panton LB, Toole T, et al. The effects of a 12- week strength-training program on strength and functionality in women with fibromyalgia. *Arch Phys Med Rehabil.* 2005;86:1713–1721.

53. Centers for Disease Control and Prevention. *Chronic Disease Prevention. Targeting Arthritis. Reducing Disability for Nearly 19 Million Americans. At a Glance 2007.* Available at http://www.cdc.gov/nccdphp/publications/AAG/arthritis.htm. Accessed November 2, 2007.

54. Hootman JM, Macera CA, Ham SA, et al. Physical activity levels among the general U.S. adult population and in adults with and without arthritis. *Arthritis Rheum.* 2003;49:129–135.

55. Baker K, McAlindon T. Exercise for knee osteoarthritis. *Curr Opin Rheumatol.* 2000;12:456–463.

56. Messier SP, Loeser RF, Miller GD, et al. Exercise and dietary weight loss in overweight and obese older adults with knee osteoarthritis. The arthritis diet and activity promotion trial. *Arthritis Rheum.* 2004;50:1501–1510.

57. Ettinger WH Jr., Burns R, Messier SP, et al. A randomized trial comparing aerobic exercise and resistance exercise with health education program in older adults with knee osteoarthritis. The fitness arthritis and seniors trial (FAST). *JAMA.* 1997;277:25–31.

58. Neuberger GB, Aaronson LS, Gajewski B, et al. Predictors of exercise and effect on symptoms, function, aerobic fitness and disease outcomes of rheumatoid arthritis. *Arthritis Rheum.* 2007;57:943–952.

59. Lee EO, Kim JI, Davis AHT, et al. Effects of regular exercise on pain, fatigue, and disability in patients with rheumatoid arthritis. *Fam Community Health.* 2006;29:320–327.

60. Van de Ende CHM, Vliet Vlieland TPM, Munneke M, et al. Dynamic exercise therapy for treating rheumatoid arthritis. *Cochrane Database Syst Rev.* 1998;CD000322. DOI:10.1002/4651858.

61. Munneke M, de Jong Z, Zwinderman AH, et al. Effect of high-intensity weight-bearing exercise program on radiologic damage progression of large joints in subgroups of patients with rheumatoid arthritis. *Arthritis Rheum.* 2005;53:410–417.

62. Eversden L, Maggs F, Nightingale P, et al. A pragmatic randomized controlled trial of hydrotherapy and land exercises on overall well being and quality of life in rheumatoid arthritis. *BMC Musculoskel Disord.* 2007;8:23.

63. Finckh A, Iversen M, Liang MH. The exercise prescription in rheumatoid arthritis: *primum non nocere. Arthritis Rheum.* 2003;49:2393–2395.

64. Galloway MT, Jokl P. The role of exercise in the treatment of inflammatory arthritis. *Bull Rheum Dis.* 1993;42:1–4.

65. Verghese J, Lipton RB, Katz MJ, et al. Leisure activities and the risk of dementia in the elderly. *N Engl J Med.* 2003;348:2508–2516.

66. Laurin D, Verreault R, Lindsay J, et al. Physical activity and risk of cognitive impairment and dementia in elderly persons. *Arch Neurol.* 2001;58(3):498–504.

67. Larson EB, Wang L, Bowen JD, et al. Exercise is associated with reduced risk of dementia among persons 65 years of age and older. *Ann Intern Med.* 2006;144:73–81.

68. Rolland Y, Rival L, Pillard F, et al. Feasibility of regular exercise for patients with moderate to severe Alzheimer disease. *J Nutr Health Aging.* 2000;4:109–113.

69. Cassilhass RC, Viana VAR, Grassman V, et al. The impact of resistance exercise on cognitive function of the elderly. *Med Sci Sports Exerc.* 2007;39:1401–1407.

70. Goodwin RD. Association between physical activity and mental disorders among adults in the United States. *Prev Med.* 2003;36:698–703.

71. Adams TB, Moore MT, Dye J. The relationship between physical activity and mental health in a national sample of college females. *Women Health.* 2007;45:69–85.

72. Phillips WT, Kiernan M, King AC. Physical activity as a nonpharmacological treatment for depression: a review. *Compl Health Prac Rev.* 2003;8:139–152.

73. Singh NA, Clements KM, Fiatarone MA. A randomized controlled trial of progressive resistance training in depressed elders. *J Gerontol Ser A Biol Sci Med Sci.* 1997;52:M27–M32.

74. Atlantis E, Chow CM, Kirby A, et al. An effective exercise-based intervention for improving mental health and quality of life measures: a randomized controlled trial. *Prev Med.* 2004;39:424–434.

75. Centers for Disease Control and Prevention. *Obesity and Overweight.* Available at http://www.cdc.gov/nccdphp/dnpa/obesity/index.htm. Accessed November 6, 2007.

76. National Weight Control Registry. *NWCR Facts.* Available at http://www.nwcr.ws/Research/default.htm. Accessed November 6, 2007.

77. Ekelund U, Franks PW, Sharp S, et al. Increase in physical activity energy expenditure is associated with reduced metabolic risk independent of change in fatness and fitness. *Diabetes Care.* 2007;30:2101–2106.

78. McInnis JK. Exercise and obesity. *Coron Artery Dis.* 2000;11: 111–116.

INDEX

Page numbers followed by *f* refer to figures; *t* refer to tables, respectively.

Clarke sign, 233, 234*f*
Clavicle injuries, 125*t*
Cleat positioning, 110*f*
Clinical excellence, 23
Clipless pedals, 120
Closed kinetic chain (CKC) exercises, 75
Collagen, 18
Compartment syndrome, 19
Compression fracture, 86–87
Computed tomography (CT), 57, 182
Concentration, 13–14
Concussions, 127, 129
Consumer Product Safety Commission, 85
Contusions, 137
Coracoacromial arch, 235*f*
Core stability, 103
Core stabilization program, 186
Coronary artery disease (CAD), 265
Corticosteroids
    for chronic groin pain, 154
    inflammation reduced by, 21
    for plantar fasciitis, 171
Cortisol, 44*f*
Costoclavicular ligaments, 134
Counterforce taping, 171
Cowboy collar, 132
Creatine
    dosage, 46*f*
    force production increased through,
        41–42
Creatine synthesis, 42*f*
Crepitus, 149
Cross-country bike, 121*f*
Cross-country racing, 124, 124*t*, 125*t*
Cross-country skiing, 176
Cross-country skis, 176*f*
Cross-training, 29, 184, 227
Cryotherapy, 185
CTS. *See* Carpal tunnel syndrome
Cue words, 14
Cushing disease, 267
Cycling. *See also* Bicycles; Bicycling;
    Mountain biking; Mountain biking
    injuries
    biomechanics of, 110
    bottom dead center, 111
    fit of frame, 109
    overuse injuries in, 111*t*
    recovery phase, 111
Cysteine, 43*f*

De Quervain tenosynovitis, 91, 113,
    113*f*, 221
"Dead arm," 59
Dead bug, 102
Death by immersion, 179
Decision-making skills, 15
Degenerative joint disease (DJD),
    255, 258
Dehydroepiandrosterone (DHEA), 44*f*, 45

Deltoid
    anatomy of, 54
    bench press for, 227
    gymnastics influence on, 194
    role in shoulder complex, 97
    shoulder press for, 228
    shoulder subluxation and, 236
Dementia, 269
Depression, 269–270
Derivatives, 46*t*
DHEA. *See* Dehydroepiandrosterone
Diabetes mellitus, 266–267
Diffuse cerebral swelling, 131
Dig, 219–220
DIP flexion, 213
Disabled skiing, 176–177, 177*f*
Disc herniation, 86
Discogenic back pain, 231
Dislocations
    of cervical spine, 132–133
    of elbow, 136, 191,
        195–196, 196*f*
    glenohumeral, 56
    of hand, 65, 136, 221
    of hip, 138
    of incus, 127
    of joint, 213
    of knee, 170
    of shoulder, 126
    from snowboarding, 178, 180
    sternoclavicular, 57
Disordered eating, 243
Distal phalanx, 137*f*
Distal radioulnar joint dysfunction
    (DRUJ), 66
Distal radius injuries, 125*t*
Distal tibial plafond fractures, 183
Distal tibiofibular junction, 143*f*
Distal ulnar wrist pain, 198
Diving. *See also* Swimming/diving
    injuries
    history of, 104
    injuries, 104–107
    mechanics of, 105*f*
    phases of, 106*f*
Division 47, 11
Dizziness, 129
DJD. *See* Degenerative joint disease
DO. *See* Doctor of Osteopathy
Doctor of Osteopathy (DO), 3
Dolphin kick, 94
"Doping," 39
Dorsal impaction syndrome, 107
Dorsiflexion, 149
Downhill bike, 121*f*
Downhill racing, 121, 124, 124*t*, 125*t*
Downhill running, 159
Downhill skiing, 175
Downswing, 85
Drag. *See* Form drag; Frictional drag;
    Wave drag

Drawer test
    anterior
        of ACL, 138
        of ankle, 141*f*, 200, 207
        of arm, 99
        of ATF, 140
        of knee, 164
    posterior, of knee, 164
DRUJ. *See* Distal radioulnar joint
    dysfunction
Dual slalom, 124*t*
Dumbbells, 230*f*
Dupuytren's contractures, 37
Dynamic assessment, 23
Dynamic examination, 25, 25*f*

Eating disorders
    female athletes triad and, 246
    young women at risk for, 26
Eccentric strength training, 209*f*, 211
Ecchymosis, 137
Echocardiography, 6, 8
Economics, 7
Edema, 18, 134
EDX. *See* Electrodiagnostics
EKG. *See* Electrocardiogram
Elbow
    anatomy, 60
    flexion test, 64
    joint, 197*f*
    recovery technique, 94*f*
    surgery, 77
Elbow injuries, 60
    in baseball, 59
    collateral ligament, 136
    dislocations, 136, 191,
        195–196, 196*f*
    in football players, 136
    in golf, 89
    from snowboarding, 180–181
    in tennis, 75, 76*f*, 89
    from weight-training, 236
Elderly. *See* Musculoskeletal issues in
    elderly
Electrocardiogram (EKG), 7
Electrodiagnostics (EDX), 86, 232
Electromyographic/nerve conduction
    velocity (EMG/NCV) studies, 64
Electromyography, 223
EMG/NCV. *See* Electromyographic/nerve
    conduction velocity studies
Endocrine system, 244
Ephedrine, 40
Epicondylitis
    in baseball, 63
    in football, 136
    in golf, 89
    stretch for, 38*f*
    in tennis, 75–76
    in weight-training, 236